Good News For People With Bad News

Other titles by the same author:

Co-written with Jon Gamble, *Treat Your Child Yourself: A Parent's Guide To Drug-Free Solutions For Common Complaints* (2007) 2nd edn, ISBN 97809752473 2 7

Available from www.karunapublishing.com.au

GOOD NEWS
for people with
BAD NEWS

Recovery Stories Everyone Must Know About

Nyema Hermiston
RN ND Adv Dip Hom

Karuna Publishing
Australia
2014

Good News For People With Bad News

Published in Australia by
Karuna Publishing
21 Hambridge Road
Yerrinbool NSW 2575
Australia

www.karunapublishing.com.au

GoodNews@karunapublishing.com.au

https://www.facebook.com/GoodNewsforPeoplewithBadNews

National Library of Australia Cataloguing-in-Publication entry
Author: Hermiston, Nyema, author.
Title: Good news for people with bad news : recovery stories everyone must know about / Nyema Hermiston.

ISBN: 9780975247365 (paperback)

Notes: Includes index.

Subjects: Incurables--Treatment--Anecdotes.
Incurable diseases--Treatment--Anecdotes.
Patient self-monitoring--Anecdotes.
Alternative medicine--Anecdotes.
Healing--Anecdotes. Therapeutics--Anecdotes.

Dewey Number: 615.5

Cover design Michael Cowdroy, from an idea by Rose Gamble

Printed in China

To my late friends and colleagues,
Patricia Janssen and John Maitland

The intuitive mind is a sacred gift and the rational mind is a faithful servant. We have created a society that honours the servant and has forgotten the gift.

We will not solve the problems of the world from the same level of thinking we were at when we created them.

More than anything else this new century demands new thinking. We must change our materially based analyses of the world around us to include broader, more multidimensional perspectives.

– Albert Einstein

Contents

Foreword

Doctor Ian Gawler
OAM, BVSc, MCounsHS

Good News for People with Bad News tells the truth of people's experiences – people who chose less well-known therapies in response to their serious illnesses, and flourished! It is a wonderfully provocative book that opens up many new possibilities for people faced with a health crisis.

In Tibet, there is a traditional saying: "An old patient is more useful than a new doctor". This is not to be unkind to doctors, or to the medicine of our day. Both have so many good things on offer. No, what is being spoken of here is the power of free-thinking and the power of shared experience.

So many people who tell their stories in *Good News for People with Bad News* would happily have taken a standard treatment for their condition – if there had been one available. However, united by their poor prognoses, what they have in common is a capacity to think freely, a willingness to seek other options and the perseverance to keep looking until they did find something that worked.

To search outside orthodox avenues, even to think that recovery is possible when well-trained doctors say it is not, requires courage. Some might call it desperation, others might just describe it as a logical thing to do. Why not dare to dream of recovery? Why not try things that are less commonly known – provided that the risk of harm is minimal, given that very few things in life are free of any risk at all!

The reality is that there are always more possibilities than you first thought and *Good News for People with Bad News* provides many examples of real people who found real solutions. So if you, or someone you love, has a difficult health problem, this book is packed with inspiration and fresh ideas. In fact, this book is overloaded with good ideas! People recount finding solutions through many different therapies and if it is a simple solution you are after, it may be hard to find here.

What comes through clearly is the capacity of the human mind and spirit to investigate, assess new information, make good choices, persevere and triumph. Here lies the real message of this important book: never give up!

My wish is that *Good News for People with Bad News* does help many more people to find the answers they need. My sense is that it will!

Doctor Ian Gawler OAM, BVSc, MCounsHS
www.iangawler.com
Yarra Junction, Australia
July 2014

Doctor Ian Gawler has played a major role in pioneering and popularising meditation and other mind-body techniques in the Western world. Doctor Gawler, himself a long term cancer survivor, co-founded the world's first lifestyle-based cancer and multiple sclerosis self-help groups and convened Australia's first Mind-Body Medicine conference. Ian is a regular blogger and has authored six bestselling books including You Can Conquer Cancer, Meditation – An In-depth Guide *and* The Mind that Changes Everything.

A powerful advocate of a healthy lifestyle, Doctor Gawler has appeared widely in the media and presented at many major conferences. He has a gift for combining his years of experience with ancient wisdom and scientific research into a modern, practical context.

Doctor Gawler was awarded the Order of Australia Medal for his services to the community in 1987. His biography, The Dragon's Blessing, *was written by Guy Allenby in 2008.*

INTRODUCTION

Orthodox medicine has given us much to be grateful for. Last century, public health underwent a revolution of infection control with improved sanitation, hygiene, vaccination programmes and antibiotic therapy that saved countless lives. Those of us who live in a country with a modern public health system benefit from medical care from the day we are born. We all know of a loved one whose life was saved by quality medical treatment. Few would argue the benefits of easy access to healthcare, hospital services, screening to detect disease, infection control and public health education. When we get sick, we expect to go to our doctor, receive treatment and recover.

But what happens when the treatment you receive does not work, or there is no treatment available and you are left facing a debilitating disease or a shortened life? Your doctor has sagely shaken his or her head and told you there is no other treatment available for your condition. You are offered palliative treatment to manage your condition and help you enjoy your life as best you can. You do not think about using any other therapies because your doctor has assured you that every possible treatment has been tried.

How some people have responded to this situation is the focus of this book.

The Stories

Here, over 40 people, including parents, describe how they did not accept their bleak medical outlook. Instead, they became determined to seek out treatments that would help them recover and lead them back to a normal life. The therapies they use vary from dietary regimes and intense nutritional therapy, to little-known medical innovations. The people in this book feel that their stories are worthy of sharing, so that others might benefit from their experience.

Many of the patients report that even though orthodox medicine offered them no help, the alternative treatment they considered using was dismissed as "unscientific", with a general attitude of: "Because there's nothing we can do to help you, no-one else will be able to help you either."

I suspect the recovery stories here will have been regarded as 'anecdotal' and therefore dismissed as unreliable data. But anyone willing to look will see that the treatments *have* been researched. Some have achieved the status of 'scientifically proven' and had successful treatment outcomes for almost one hundred years.

These are not isolated cases of recovery; they represent growing numbers of people who are making their own choices about the type of treatment they use. Yet many of these treatments remain obscure to most people.

In the process of listening to over 50 patient stories, 43 of which appear here, it became apparent that the therapies used are a small selection of a myriad of alternative therapies that are available today for most illnesses, making orthodox treatment just one treatment option among many.

The aim of this book is to shed light on therapies available to treat diseases that are believed to be incurable and therefore untreatable. The people in this book challenge that belief.

Awareness

Presented here are patients who have unexpectedly survived after using an alternative treatment, which has engendered anger from their doctor, along with dismissal, that the recovery was "spontaneous" or "due to the 'placebo' effect" – although the patient obviously did not succumb to the placebo effect from any medical treatment they already received.

There is a lack of awareness of alternative therapies. Even when a therapy is a *medical innovation*, doctors are generally unaware of it, due to an attitude of: "If medical orthodoxy doesn't know about it, it lacks validity and we need to test it first." Because of this misguided approach, the public are being asked to believe that there is only one truth: that of mainstream medical science. By its very claim, this is unscientific.

Science

By definition, science[1] considers all possibilities before reaching a conclusion. Science is an unbiased systematic investigation into a field of study that is organised into a body of knowledge – knowledge *gained by the people using and observing that system*. When the unexpected happens and a patient recovers from an alternative treatment, where is the openness and curiosity one would expect from the scientific community? In many cases, the doctors who criticise a non-orthodox therapy have had no direct experience of that therapy.

When alternative treatment methods are successfully used for patients with 'incurable' conditions, they are ignored or ridiculed out of hand, rather than being viewed as a potentially helpful therapy. Without proper investigation, this indicates that we are living more in a world of 'consensus science', rather than one of true investigative science.

Little appears to have changed throughout history.

In the 19th century, Hungarian physician Ignaz Semmelweis discovered that the puerperal fever[2] mortality rate could be drastically reduced by thorough hand washing in obstetric clinics. Despite evidence that this reduced deaths to below one per cent, Semmelweis's discovery was rejected by the medical

1 "Science is the intellectual and practical activity encompassing the systematic study of the structure and behaviour of the physical and natural world through observation and experiment." (Oxford Dictionary)

2 Puerperal fever results from the female reproductive organs becoming infected in the first ten days following childbirth or miscarriage, which can be fatal if untreated.

community, offended by the implication that they should wash their hands before delivering babies. Years after Semmelweis's death in 1847, hand washing before surgical procedures earned widespread acceptance.

We know that thousands of sailors on British shipping expeditions died of scurvy caused by a lack of vitamin C, but it took 40 years and many more deaths for the British admiralty to be convinced by ship surgeon James Lind's suggestion to provide lemon juice for sailors in his 'Treatise of the Scurvy' in 1753. It wasn't until the 1790s that citrus juice for sailors was finally carried onboard sailing ships.

Russian microbiologist Ilya Mechnikov discovered cellular immunity in 1882, for which he encountered considerable hostility, but eventually won a Nobel prize with Paul Erlich in 1908[3] for the discovery of phagocytosis.[4]

Mechnikov also recognised the importance of gut bacteria. In 1907, he discovered a relationship between health and the make-up of gut bacteria, and suggested that senility could be delayed by manipulating gut bacteria with the lactic acid-producing bacteria found in yogurt. Popular for a time, the idea was eventually disregarded, then re-emerged in the 1990s, almost one hundred years later.[5] Probiotics are gaining increasing recognition for their role in resolving chronic gut problems such as Irritable Bowel Syndrome, inflammatory bowel disease and childhood allergies.[6] They are now a popular over-the-counter supplement, receiving intense medical attention and are a multi-billion dollar industry globally. Gut bacteria are a key element in three of the recovery stories in this book.

History is littered with stories of medical discoveries and beneficial treatments that have been dismissed out of hand at one time, then to be accepted many decades later – and it's still happening.

In 1977, Stanislaw Burzynski, MD PhD, pioneered biologically active peptides called antineoplastons for the treatment of cancer and in 1984 founded the Burzynski Research Institute (BRI) in Houston Texas, USA. Antineoplastons have been responsible for curing terminal cancer, including aggressive brain cancers for which there is no medical cure. Rather than drawing positive attention from the medical world, the BRI has spent many years dealing with court cases against it, having been repeatedly hounded by the FDA.[7] Two compelling documentaries have been made recounting these events.[8]

At the Kurume University in Fukuoka, Japan, Japanese pathologists, oncologists and surgeons have conducted independent studies of antineoplastons.[9] They

3 *Ilya Mechnikov, Biographical* http://www.nobelprize.org/nobel_prizes/medicine/laureates/1908/mechnikov-bio.html

4 Phagocytes are immune cells that engulf bacteria. This process is known as phagocytosis.

5 *Recycling Metchnikoff: Probiotics, the Intestinal Microbiome and the Quest for Long Life* http://www.ncbi.nlm.nih.gov/pmc/articles/PMC3859987/

6 *Journal of Clinical Gastroenterology: Food Allergy and Probiotics in Childhood* September 2010, Volume 44, Issue, pp S22-S25http://journals.lww.com/jcge/Abstract/2010/09001/Food_Allergy_and_Probiotics_in_Childhood.7.aspx

7 FDA – US Food and Drug Administration is an agency of the United States Department of Health and Human Services, responsible for protecting and promoting public health.

8 See 'Resources – Cancer' for references to *Burzynski, The Movie* and *Cancer is a Serious Business.*

9 Tsuda, H et al *Demethylation effect of the antineoplaston AS2-1 on genes in colon cancer cells*, Ushijima M et al, Oncol Rep Jan 2014; 31(1): 19-26. http://www.ncbi.nlm.nih.gov/pmc/articles/PMC3868501/

concluded: "After twenty-seven years of independently testing antineoplastons – including randomized clinical trials, we found that Doctor Burzynski was right. It's obviously not 'anecdotal' anymore."

The future of antineoplaston therapy for cancer patients remains uncertain, while criticism of antineoplastons abounds – and of Doctor Stanislaw Burzynski.

In the process of seeking people to interview for this book, a number of doctors who use alternative therapies were not prepared to "go public", for fear of attracting the "wrong kind" of attention. Integrative medicine, where doctors practise both orthodox and non-orthodox medicine, is a risky business.

Penicillin, the First Wonder Drug

One wonders how the case of the first patient whose life was saved with antibiotics would be viewed today. Researchers at Oxford University began developing penicillin for treatment on humans in 1939, at the outbreak of World War II.

In 1942, 33-year-old Anne Miller lay in a New Haven hospital in Connecticut, with a dangerously high temperature, dying from septicaemia[10] caused by a streptococcal infection following a miscarriage. She was treated with a tiny amount of penicillin – at the time an obscure, experimental drug. Overnight, her temperature dropped and she survived. She went on to live until she was 90 years old.[11] Before Mrs Miller's life-saving treatment, only a few experiments had been conducted with penicillin in mice and people, with mixed results.

News of Mrs Miller's miraculous recovery helped inspire the American pharmaceutical industry to begin full production of penicillin, resulting in a dramatic reduction of deaths from infection during World War II. No doctor or scientist needed evidence of successful infection treatment in large numbers of patients to be compelled to use it. The medical community seized upon this 'anecdotal' evidence – the way great discoveries begin.

So, antibiotic therapy heralded the beginning of life-saving drug treatment for serious bacterial infections internationally. Having achieved effective infection control with antibiotics and vaccinations, there evolved an ideology in orthodox medicine that drug therapy could effectively treat other diseases too. Unfortunately, in the decades that followed, death rates from chronic diseases like cancer, cardiovascular disease and diabetes grew, and for which drug therapy has become standard practice.

Where antibiotics treat the cause of illness (the infection), drug therapy for chronic disease does not. Instead, it manages symptoms, as long as the medication is taken, leading to the practice of polypharmacy,[12] where multiple medications for inflammation, diabetes, reflux, high blood pressure, cholesterol and insomnia may

10 Septicaemia is a bacterial infection of the blood, commonly known as 'blood poisoning'.

11 *Anne Miller, 90, First Patient Who Was Saved by Penicillin* http://academics.wellesley.edu/Chemistry/Chem101/antibiotics/obit-a-miller.html

12 Polypharmacy is the use of multiple medications in one patient, generally in people over 65 years.

all be taken together long term, with no resolution of any of the symptoms. This practice is compounded by pressure on doctors to either prescribe the corresponding medication, or be seen as negligent, leaving many people on a growing list of drugs for the rest of their lives. To my knowledge, no scientific studies have been conducted that record the effects – positive or negative – of drug cocktails like this on patients after five, ten or 15 years. One man's story in this book tells how his physician described this process as: "Climbing the [medication] ladder."

Orthodox Medicine

Risks

The clear message from medical orthodoxy is not to trust treatments other than their own, due to their 'unscientific' status. But, let's be equally clear, by comparing the perceived risk of using alternative therapies with the actual risks of orthodox medical treatments. With just a little delving, the following comes to light.

- In the United States, adverse drug reactions (ADRs) are the *fourth leading cause of death*.[13,14] Two million serious ADRs cause 100,000 deaths every year. ADRs in nursing homes amount to 350,00 every year.[15]
- Adverse drug events (ADEs) are also common in the Australian health system. Anticoagulant, anti-inflammatory, and cardiovascular drug accidents, all of which are preventable, collectively make up over one half of all ADEs.[16]
- In Australia, medical errors lead to 18,000 deaths every year and 50,000 people suffer a permanent injury. It has been labelled a 'silent epidemic'.[17] With no systematic data collection for errors, it is impossible to know the true number of medical mistakes that cause serious harm or death.
- A Chief Medical Officer in England has estimated that each year 60,000 to 255,000 National Health Service patients suffer serious disability or death as a result of healthcare interventions.[18]
- At a US Senate hearing in July 2014, Doctor Tejal Gandhi, associate professor of medicine at Harvard Medical School and president of the National Patient Safety Foundation, spoke of preventable medical errors persisting as the number three killer in the US, claiming the lives of some 400,000 people annually, which amounts to over 1,000 per day.[19]

13 Institute of Medicine, National Academy Press, 2000 Lazarou J et al JAMA 1998;279[15]1200-1205 http://www.fda.gov/Drugs/DevelopmentApprovalProcess/DevelopmentResources/DrugInteractionsLabeling/ucm114848.htm

14 *A Problem Too Important to Ignore*, Gurwitz JH et al Am J Med 2000;109(2):87-94 http://www.rxwise.com/images/RxWise.Consumer.Presentation.5-25-05.pdf

15 *How Many Die From Medical Mistakes in US Hospitals?* http://www.scientificamerican.com/article/how-many-die-from-medical-mistakes-in-us-hospitals/

16 *Adverse Drug Events and Medical Events in Australia* http://www.ncbi.nlm.nih.gov/pubmed/14660523

17 *Medical Mistakes – A Silent Epidemic in Australian Hospitals* http://www.abc.net.au/worldtoday/content/2013/s3778256.htm

18 *Preventable deaths due to problems in care in English acute hospitals: a retrospective case record review study* http://qualitysafety.bmj.com/content/early/2012/07/06/bmjqs-2012-001159.full

19 *Deaths by Medical Mistakes Hit Records* http://www.healthcareitnews.com/news/deaths-by-medical-mistakes-hit-records

When medical accidents that cause death and disability are commonplace in orthodox health systems around the world, the warning of the "dangers of alternative therapies" is absurd.

Surgery and drug therapy bring with them high risk to patients, so statistics like this may be inevitable in well-meaning healthcare systems around the world. The two key reasons behind rigorous drug trials are to establish efficacy and safety. The more dangerous the treatment, the more important it is to undergo scientific trials.

Efficacy

The same question should be asked of orthodox medicine: "Is the therapy you are prescribing scientifically proven?"

Professor John Ioannidis, a meta-researcher and one of the world's foremost experts on the credibility of medical research, says as much as 90 per cent of the published medical information that doctors rely on is flawed. His paper, *Why Most Published Research Findings Are False,*[20] was published in the Public Library of Science (PLoS) in August 2005 and in *New Doctor* in December 2008.[21] It outlined the results of a detailed analysis of medical research papers and questioned the results of many of them. An article based on this paper, *Lies, Damned Lies and Medical Science,*[22] appeared in *The Atlantic* online magazine in October 2010. This means that an unknown number of medical treatments that are offered as a first line of treatment may not be scientifically proven.

In December 2003, Allen Roses, the worldwide vice-president of genetics at the pharmaceutical company GlaxoSmithKline, stated that fewer than half of the patients prescribed some of the most expensive drugs actually derived any benefit from them.[23]

Medical Pioneers

Some of the therapies described in this book were developed by doctors who used pharmaceutical drugs in inventive ways and have achieved what orthodox medicine has not.

Two examples are:

Antibiotics to Treat Rheumatoid Arthritis (RA)

Working with Albert Sabin (later of polio vaccine fame) at the Rockefeller Institute in the US, just before World War II, Doctor Thomas McPherson-Brown isolated a bacteria-like agent from the joint fluid of a woman with RA and speculated that it might be the trigger for her disease. Later, Brown headed up arthritis research for the Veterans' Administration and eventually became

20 *Why Most Published Research Findings Are False* http://www.plosmedicine.org/article/info%3Adoi%2F10.1371%2Fjournal.pmed.0020124

21 http://search.informit.com.au/documentSummary;dn=552051393460980;res=IELFSC

22 Lies, Damned Lies and Medical Science http://www.theatlantic.com/magazine/archive/2010/11/lies-damned-lies-and-medical-science/308269/

23 *Glaxo Chief: Our Drugs do Not Work on Most Patients* http://www.independent.co.uk/news/science/glaxo-chief-our-drugs-do-not-work-on-most-patients-575942.html

Dean of Medicine at George Washington University Medical School. He treated some 10,000 patients with RA and other connective tissue diseases using tetracycline therapy. Even during a time when excitement about antibiotics was high, his colleagues ridiculed him and he was progressively cut off from sources of research funding. After his death in 1989, a clinical study sponsored by the National Institutes of Health in 1995 showed that *Minocycline*[24] was safe and effective for treating RA: "We observed significant differences favouring *Minocycline* over placebo in the primary outcome measures."[25] Today, patients with RA and other connective tissue diseases struggle to gain access to this antibiotic. However, if you are a teenager with acne, you can stroll into your doctor's office and be prescribed *Minocycline*, with no questions asked.

Naltrexone to Treat Autoimmune Diseases

In 1985, Harvard educated Doctor Bernard Bihari[26] was the Principal Investigator in a study funded by the Foundation for Integrative Research, at SUNY/Health Science Center at Brooklyn, on Low Dose Naltrexone (LDN)[27] for the Treatment of AIDS. The impact of this and his other work in LDN has been substantial in contributing to the successful treatment of a wide range of autoimmune diseases. As the stories reveal, a patient faced with taking highly toxic medication, who is looking for a safer alternative, has to work hard to find a doctor who will agree to prescribe LDN.

Therapies like these have not been accepted or used by the broad medical community and few are familiar with them, even if they have undergone the gold standard of medicine: the double blind trial. How come?

- What is happening when a child with epilepsy receives medication and brain surgery before trying the ketogenic diet[28] that has an almost one hundred year history of efficacy and has been fully described in medical journals?
- What is happening when a costly drug for pancreatic cancer that extends life for just a few weeks or months is heralded as a great advance, yet successful, nutritional treatments for pancreatic cancer (there are three in this book)[29] are disregarded?

Complementary and Alternative Medicine (CAM)

For a person squarely facing a lifetime of disability or death, with no effective medical treatment available to them, it is difficult to see the harm in trying a therapy that carries no serious medical risk. It may be true that alternative

---

24 *Minocycline* is a tetracycline based broad spectrum antibiotic.

25 Tilley BC et al, *Minocycline in Rheumatoid Arthritis: a 48 Week, Double-Blind, Placebo-Controlled Trial,* Ann Int Med, 1995; 122:2, pg 81-89.

26 Doctor Bernard Bihari, MD, was board certified with the American Board of Psychiatry and Neurology and became Instructor in Neurology at Harvard Medical School.

27 *Low Dose Naltrexone In The Treatment Of Acquired Immune Deficiency Syndrome* http://www.lowdosenaltrexone.org/ldn_aids_1988.htm

28 The ketogenic diet is a scientifically tested high-fat, low-carbohydrate, adequate-protein diet that has been used in medicine since the 1920s to treat epilepsy in children. See the stories of Charlie Abrahams and Emily Wall.

29 See the stories of Sarah Ann Cooper, Arlene Van Straten and David Yoffie.

treatments[30] have not been subjected to the same rigorous testing as standard medical treatments (although some have), but neither do they carry the inherent dangers. The treatment will either work, or it will not.

People are turning to complementary and alternative therapies, because they offer another option. When patients reach a dead end with their medical treatment, they have little choice but to take matters into their own hands if they want to defy their diagnosis. Doctors are alarmed at this and feel the need to 'warn the public' about their patients' errors of judgement. Implicit in this approach is the patriarchal view that people are incapable of making an independent judgement about their own healthcare. This unhelpful approach is increasingly being rejected by people who are looking for treatments that address the *cause* of their illness.[31,32] They are left with the physically and emotionally difficult route of doing their own research without their doctor's approval.

People selecting their own form of healthcare is becoming a more recognised option – and there is some science to it. Doctor Halsted Holman, professor at the Stanford University School of Medicine, advocates four principles of personalised and self-managed medicine that he calls: "patient empowerment".[33,34]

1. There is no complete cure for chronic illness unless the cause of the individual's own disease is discovered and successfully managed.
2. For effective treatment of chronic illness, an individual must engage continually in different approaches to his or her health.
3. The individual knows the most about his or her own condition, the effects of certain therapies and must apply that knowledge in shaping a self-management program.
4. To achieve success, the individual and the individual's health professionals must share knowledge and divide authority.

When their patients turn to CAM, some doctors cite their 'concern' about people being duped against their will into using "unproven, unscientific and risky therapies", yet most CAM therapies carry little risk when used by qualified personnel. People are also discerning about how they spend their well-earned money. When a person pays for treatment out of their own pocket, they are unlikely to continue with that treatment if they do not see a benefit.

A Range of Treatment Options

No single treatment system is able to properly deal with every health issue. Some illnesses lean themselves more to certain types of therapy than others,

30 Alternative indicates any treatment which is not orthodox medical treatment, including natural therapies.

31 *The Rise and Rise of Complementary and Alternative Medicine – A Sociological Perspective* https://www.mja.com.au/journal/2004/180/11/rise-and-rise-complementary-and-alternative-medicine-sociological-perspective

32 *Complementary Medicine On the Rise* http://news.bbc.co.uk/2/hi/uk_news/northern_ireland/6380745.stm

33 *Patient Self Management in Chronic Disease* http://jama.jamanetwork.com/article.aspx?articleid=195525

34 Evidence Suggesting That a Self-Management Program Can Improve Health Status While Reducing Hospitalization: A Randomized Trial http://journals.lww.com/lww-medicalcare/Abstract/1999/01000/Evidence_Suggesting_That_a_Chronic_Disease.3.aspx

and individuals respond better to some therapies than others. Some people are hypersensitive and are unable to tolerate pharmaceutical drugs.

Rather than finding 'the' treatment for a single condition, what transpires in these stories is the variety of effective treatments. *Several* different treatments for one condition can be available. For example, three people diagnosed with lymphoma here were successfully treated with three different therapies – Gerson therapy, antineoplaston therapy and Low Dose Naltrexone.

Although there is a large number of CAM therapies for serious illness to select from, there are no government-sanctioned sources of this information, although the World Health Organisation recognises CAM as viable therapies to improve health status worldwide.[35] This leaves many patients, having received a shattering diagnosis, left to discover suitable therapies for themselves and forge their own treatment path.

Just some of the available therapies are:

Medical:

- Alpha Lipoic Acid for liver disease.
- Antibiotic therapy for rheumatoid arthritis, juvenile rheumatoid arthritis, scleroderma and other connective tissue diseases.
- Antineoplaston therapy for cancers, including aggressive brain tumours.
- SCENAR Therapy (Self Controlled Energy Neuro Adaptive Regulator) for musculo-skeletal pain and immune function.
- Faecal transplants for inflammatory bowel disease.
- Helminth Therapy for autoimmune diseases and allergies.
- Ketogenic diet for epilepsy, autism and other neurological diseases.
- Low Dose Naltrexone for autoimmune and other diseases.
- Orthomolecular medicine for a wide range of illnesses, including heart disease, diabetes and mental/emotional disorders such as autism and schizophrenia.

Natural Therapies:

- Acupuncture
- Ayurvedic medicine
- Buteyko therapy
- Chiropractic
- Dietary therapy, individualised

---

35 WHO Traditional Medicine Strategy 2002-2005 http://apps.who.int/iris/bitstream/10665/67163/1/WHO_EDM_TRM_2002.1.pdf

- Herbal Medicine
- Homeopathy
- Kinesiology
- Nutrition
- Osteopathy
- Traditional Chinese Medicine

Mental, Emotional, Spiritual:

- Meditation and prayer
- Tai Chi
- Yoga

Nutrition

Perhaps the most fundamental element of any treatment plan for any disease is diet and nutrition, which play a vital role in many of the recovery stories. When patients have their nutritional status fully examined, it can reveal the potential cause of their illness. For example, in the stories, vitamin D deficiency emerges in the cases of multiple sclerosis, Crohn's disease and prostate cancer.

In the 1970s, Linus Pauling, the only person ever to be awarded two unshared Nobel prizes (Chemistry in 1954, Peace in 1962), published a substantial work on the benefits of vitamin C as a therapeutic intervention in a wide range of chronic illnesses, including cancer. His work on the impact of high-dose vitamin C for chronic diseases remains largely ignored by medical orthodoxy. He coined the term 'orthomolecular' medicine[36] as treatment for chronic disease and some mental illnesses. Even so, nutrients are not taken seriously by the medical community as potent weapons against chronic disease, so vast bodies of work such as that of Pauling's are overlooked, or diminished by statements like: "We can thank Linus Pauling, who became obsessed with it [vitamin C] as a wondrous cure-all."[37]

Positive media reports on nutrients are rare. A few, such as zinc for viral infections, glucosamine for joint pain and fish oils for arthritis and mental function, have passed muster. On 30th May 2014, the Orthomolecular Medicine News Service (OMNS)[38] announced that two papers from the *Journal of Orthomolecular Nutrition*[39] had been indexed by PubMed,[40] but

36 Orthomolecular medicine describes the practice of preventing and treating disease by providing the body with optimal amounts of substances which are natural to the body. http://orthomolecular.org/library/jom/index.shtml

37 *Pills of Wisdom?* New Scientist, 30th August, 2014.

38 Orthomolecular Medicine News Service http://orthomolecular.org/resources/omns/

39 *Journal of Orthomolecular Medicine* http://www.orthomed.org/jom/jom.html

40 PubMed is a free search engine that accesses MEDLINE. It is maintained by the United States Library of Medicine (NLM) at the National Institutes of Health.

not by MEDLINE.[41] The two papers were on the topic of intravenous vitamin C in cancer therapy.[42,43] OMNS has been publishing research from hundreds of clinical nutrition papers like these for the past 47 years,[44,45] yet they remain excluded by the US National Library of Medicine, the world's largest taxpayer-funded medical library. When it comes to scientifically-based treatments, nutrition just doesn't count.

In the stories of autism and childhood epilepsy, parents did their own research and gave their children special diets and supplements. After years of intensive treatment, these children recovered from the illnesses their parents had been told were incurable. One young child was successfully cured of severe epilepsy after using the ketogenic diet.

Some parents are not prepared to wait ten or 20 years for scientific validation of a harmless dietary therapy. They can and do successfully use dietary regimes guided by nutritionists, naturopaths and integrative doctors to treat their children for autism, epilepsy and other 'untreatable' conditions. As free online access to academic journals worldwide becomes more commonplace, people can educate themselves about their treatment.

Challenging CAM

As more people all over the world move towards using CAM, others are trying to discredit CAM therapies. In Australia, the organisation 'Friends of Science in Medicine' is actively lobbying universities nationwide to remove all tertiary courses on CAM until "adequate scientific investigation is done". Internationally, health authorities are restricting the use of nutritional supplements by non-medical personnel[46,47] on the grounds that their efficacy has not been established.

This approach is not in line with the trend of public opinion. Increasing numbers of the public are choosing to pay for their own healthcare using CAM therapies.[48] In 2000, Australians spent AU$2.3 billion on complementary medicines – more than four times patients' contributions for all pharmaceutical medications.[49] A nationwide US government survey in 2009 revealed adults spent US$33.9 billion on visits to CAM practitioners and CAM products.[50]

41 MEDLINE (Medical Literature Analysis and Retrieval System Online) is a database for science and biomedical information, which includes bibliographic summaries of articles from academic journals on dentistry, general healthcare, medicine, pharmacy, veterinary medicine plus literature on biology and biochemistry. It is freely available on the internet via PubMed.

42 *Schedule Dependence in Cancer Therapy: Intravenous Vitamin C and the Systemic Saturation Hypothesis*, González MJ et al J Orthomol Med 2012 Jan 1;27(1):9-12. PMID: 24860238 [PubMed]

43 *Mitochondria, Energy and Cancer: The Relationship with Ascorbic Acid*, González MJ et al J Orthomol Med. 2010;25(1):29-38. PMID: 23565030 [PubMed]

44 International Society of Orthomolecular Medicine Archives http://orthomolecular.org/library/jom/index.shtml

45 *A Time Line of Vitamin Medicine* http://orthomolecular.org/resources/omns/v10n08.shtml

46 *Regulation of Vitamins – Politics as Usual* http://orthomolecular.org/resources/omns/v10n02.shtml

47 *War Against Natural Medicine* http://www.abc.net.au/news/2012-02-21/schwager-war-against-natural-medicine/3840682

48 *Impact of CAM on PBS Expenditure* http://www.natsem.canberra.edu.au/storage/ Impact of complementary and alternative medicine (CAM) use on PBS expenditure - Thiebaut Jun08.pdf

49 *CAM in Australia* https://www.inkling.com/read/herbs-natural-supplements-braun-cohen-3rd/chapter-1/complementary-medicine-in

50 *National Center for Complementary and Alternative Medicine – Statistics on CAM Costs* http://nccam.nih.gov/news/camstats/costs

However, the opinions and judgements of the consumers of healthcare are being overruled by orthodox medicine, which, despite practising in a world where medical misadventure is commonplace, is compelled to control the practice of safer, milder and more effective options. Patients are encouraged to remain in the medical tunnel of drugs and surgery, even if they are not benefitting from these treatments. They are cautioned that outside this tunnel is dangerous, unchartered territory.

Ethics

When the best hope offered is no hope, and a patient is discouraged from seeking an alternative treatment of "quackery",[51] the issue becomes an ethical one. While it is unethical to treat patients with sham therapies and offer them hope where there is none, it is equally unethical to discourage patients from using potentially beneficial therapies when the medical options are nil.

A vicious cycle is in play. Researchers struggle to have studies on CAM published, leaving the medical community, and the public alike, unaware of the benefits of these therapies. And when successful treatment outcomes of CAM therapies are not recorded, they remain excluded from medical literature, leaving an inaccurate picture of treatment possibilities for consumers.

When it comes to patient safety, a double standard exists. Despite the tens of thousands of deaths in many countries from medical treatment each year, the public is expected to take pharmaceutical drugs without question, based on their 'scientific status', while also being warned against nutritional and other supplements. Deaths on record from CAM are rare,[52] yet a constant stream of warnings about simple nutrients persist, like: "vitamin A can cause cancer", "herbs are dangerous", "diets are unproven". The risks associated with orthodox medicine are accepted as being inevitable, so it is not newsworthy that thousands of people around the world die every day from the effects of their medical treatment. But if a patient dies as a result of using CAM, it is seen as a travesty and makes international headlines. It seems it's okay to die if you take what your doctor prescribes you, but if you use CAM therapies, it is not.

The Future

Most people want to go to a doctor for their healthcare, but if there is no medical treatment on offer, the internet may be the next stop. There, they can find large communities of people who are sharing their experiences of successful treatments and supporting each other. It is a thriving community-health network that has a lot to offer. A strong theme in these stories is that

51 Quackery – promotion of unproven or fraudulent medical practices.

52 The 2013 annual report of the American Association of Poison Control Centers shows zero deaths from multiple vitamins; zero deaths from vitamin A, niacin, vitamin B6, vitamin D, or vitamin E http://orthomolecular.org/resources/omns/v09n03.shtml

when patients find out what others are doing, it helps them to make informed decisions, gives them control and helps take away their fear.

It may not be ideal from a medical perspective, but until practitioners become as well informed as their patients, this trend of 'medicine via social media' will continue, because the internet is a real game-changer. As testified here, several people found treatments on the internet – not from their doctors – and that discovery saved their lives. Not all medical information will be reliable, but it is a forum for all to share freely; one woman in this book says of the internet: "You might get a lot of nonsense, but there's a whole wealth of information there."

Integrative medicine (IM) is another growing trend. Doctors who practice IM are in high demand, because they offer their patients more treatment options and are willing to work with other health professionals. It is a model that must be far more satisfying for doctors than grimly adhering to treatment protocols that they know will never help their patients recover, yet making routine prescriptions for fear of legal action if they do not. When patients have access to IM doctors, it alleviates their angst of having to choose between standard medical practice and CAM therapies.

I hope more doctors will come to familiarise themselves with CAM therapies, or refer their patients to nutritionists, naturopaths, acupuncturists, etc. If they do not, their patients will increasingly 'practitioner shop' until they find someone who will. When a practitioner has reached his or her limits of treatment possibility for their patient, it is professional and ethical to refer to another practitioner. Giving referrals also shows respect to patients. When referring becomes common practice between doctors and CAM practitioners, patients can only benefit from being exposed to more treatment options. As one of these stories ends: "If people worked together, an awful lot would get done."

It would be more satisfying for practitioners of all persuasions if they were willing to share their knowledge and experience with each other. There is no need for the 'orthodox medicine is best and everything else is unproven' mentality. It would make sense if CAM therapists and doctors worked together to find the best treatment for their patients, instead of arguing their case for types of treatments in journals and the media. Understanding *which patients are recovering, and why*, is key.

Sick people are our greatest teachers. Their illnesses signal what's happening in the community. I can remember how, when the number of allergy sufferers coming into my practice really started increasing, it was a great stimulus to learn more about allergies – and quickly.

Patients are also a great resource-army of seekers and searchers. They have the motivation to learn and share what they have discovered. It was a patient who informed me about chemo-sensitivity tests[53] for cancer,

53 Chemo-sensitivity testing is not available within most healthcare systems, due to the cost of testing.

where a patient's blood is sent to Germany or France to find out to which chemotherapy drug their particular type of cancer is the most sensitive. From a sometimes urgent need, patients are their own best advocates and it seems that it is *they* who are driving the increased awareness of available therapies. They discover data about forgotten medical pioneers, discarded yet valuable research, and therapies of value. Practitioners have a lot to learn from patients.

In publishing this book, it is my hope that these stories give confidence to others to find their own way to health, and to broaden their practitioners' experiences. The future holds great promise for people finding an individualised solution for their illness, to achieve recoveries just like those in this book. If current trends continue, this will increasingly be achieved through integrative doctors, CAM practitioners and online patient forums.

When one considers the vast resources of science and medicine, it is a cruel irony that people with serious illness are often left to make life-changing decisions regarding their healthcare alone.

ABOUT THE INTERVIEWS

The 41 live interviews of the 43 people in this book were conducted between October 2012 and May 2014, by Skype, phone and in person, with people from six countries – Australia, Canada, England, Mexico, New Zealand and USA. Most have allowed their full names to be used, others have chosen to use their first name or a pseudonym.

The prime motive for these people to share the personal experiences of their recoveries, is simply to help other people who are currently in a similar position that they were once in. They have told their stories in the hope that others may find the confidence to select the best possible treatment for themselves.

Without exception, these people displayed a generosity of spirit, for which I thank them on behalf of the many people who will inevitably benefit from their knowledge, understanding and experience.

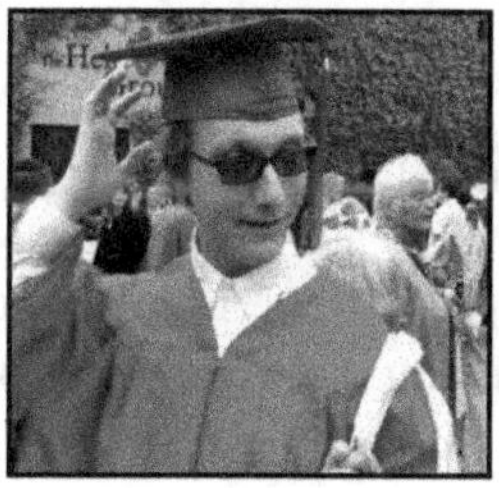

Charlie Abrahams, 21 years

Santa Monica, California, USA

Diagnosed with epilepsy at one year

Interview with Jim Abrahams, Charlie's father

On his first birthday, Charlie started having seizures. At first they were very subtle, but they quickly escalated into much more dramatic seizures, so Nancy and I started taking him to doctors. We felt fortunate because we had access to several of the leading paediatric neurologists in the United States and Charlie had seizures in all of their arms. They were in total agreement about what to do. They all said that as treatment options you can give these kids drugs and you can do brain surgery. They ran through every available drug on Charlie, with all the attending side effects of constipation, sleeplessness or drowsiness. At one point, he was sleeping 18 hours a day – he sort of became a zombie. There was a rash for a while. They used the drugs in combination with each other too and nothing stopped his seizures – nothing ever stopped his seizures. He got sicker and sicker and was having dozens of seizures a day. So then they recommended a brain operation, which was a hideous experience. That didn't stop his seizures either; about a day after he got out of the hospital from the surgery, the seizures returned. We were told by the last doctor we saw that if the surgery didn't work, to expect a life of continued seizures and what they called 'progressive retardation'.

So I started doing research, this is back in 1993 now. Not with any thought of finding a cure for him, or even to improve his health. It wasn't to find any alternate therapy for him. You know, while watching this going on and participating in this devastating diagnosis, it was to try to figure out – how do these kids make it through life? What happens? And how do their families make it through life?

Once I started doing some research – and trust me, I'm not much of a researcher, but if you go to a medical library and you start looking up paediatric epilepsy, you come across the ketogenic diet. It's in all the texts, going back to 1921, when it was invented at the Mayo Clinic in the United States. All the way back from the 1920s through to 1992 at the time, there was anecdotal evidence published by different doctors at different hospitals, saying that the ketogenic diet improved more than half the kids that went on it. A significant percentage, 20-30 per cent, were cured, which is kind of an outstanding thing to come across, especially when your kid's been beat up like that. The last study that I came across had actually been published in 1992, and I was doing my research in 1993. The 1992 study was published in *Epilepsia*, which is the premier epilepsy medical journal, I think worldwide, certainly in the United States. In that study, written by the folks at Johns Hopkins Hospital, they said that they had tried the ketogenic diet on 58 consecutive kids with really bad epilepsy – multiple daily seizures, multiple drugs and all that stuff. Of those 58 kids, 29 percent achieved complete seizure control and another 30 per cent were significantly improved, with fewer seizures and fewer drugs. But none of these world class neurologists that we had taken Charlie to see ever mentioned a syllable about the ketogenic diet to us, and yet their premier journal had this published, just the year before, as well as all the evidence going back to the 1920s.

So I called up the guy from Johns Hopkins who had written the article, the 1992 study, and he said: "Send me Charlie's medical records, bring Charlie and we'll try the diet with him." Nancy, Charlie and I flew across the country from Los Angeles on the West Coast to Baltimore on the East Coast. Johns Hopkins had the benefit of having a dietician on the staff who is very conversant in the ketogenic diet, because she was around during it's heyday – Mrs Kelly, she's kind of an angel. So she put Charlie on the diet. At the time, Charlie was having dozens and sometimes as many as a hundred seizures a day. In two days the seizures were gone. Even though I've told this story hundreds of times, I still get choked up when I tell it.

When Charlie started the diet he was on four medications. Within a month of starting the diet, they took him off all the medicine. He was drug free and seizure free. He was on the diet for five years. He was cured. He's never taken another pill, he eats anything he wants and just lives a normal life.

Before the diet, Charlie had that surgery, for which Nancy and I will forever feel guilty. I think he has been affected by the seizures, the medication and the surgery. They say that the first two years of a child's life are the most important in terms of brain development and his brain got robbed of its second year. He has some autism. He's a happy kid now, but did the surgery take a bite out him? Absolutely.

It was tough doing the diet. Today, one of the primary excuses for not telling families about the diet, the popular phrase used by the medical profession is that it's a drastic lifestyle change. Granted, it is a drastic lifestyle change, and I wouldn't recommend it for you or for me, but if you have a kid who is experiencing multiple seizures every day and who's on multiple drugs, then it's a vastly improved lifestyle change. Everything is 'as compared to what?' Compared to eating just a normal diet, it's not that great, but compared to a lifetime of drugs and seizures, it's a walk on the beach.

The ketogenic diet is basically a high-fat, no-sugar, limited-carbohydrate diet that mimics the effects of fasting. When you burn fat for energy (instead of carbohydrates the way you and I are doing right now) you produce ketone bodies. The thought is that a combination of these ketone bodies in combination with low blood glucose help to suppress seizures. The diet actually switches body and brain metabolism. Meals have to be calculated for each person, based on a specific number of calories each day. The person must eat every meal – no more, or no less, so it's not easy. It's much easier today though than when Charlie was on the diet, because now there are computer programmes that help to calculate the meal plans. Also, the foods that are available are much more attractive and much more palatable than when Charlie was on the diet.

There are a number of myths that the doctors use to dissuade people to try the diet. One is that: yes, it's difficult. But in response to that, I ask the question: "Where in medical school do they teach a course in deciding what is too difficult for any parent of a critically ill child to go through? Where do they teach that course? What is the name of the course that teaches a doctor to evaluate that?" So I don't think that's a particularly fair argument to make. It should be the doctor's job to explain what all the available alternatives are, and then in a process of joint, informed decision making, come up with a solution that's appropriate for that family. I don't think that it's really a doctor's job to decide for me what's too difficult for me to endure.

Another of the myths that doctors use to talk parents out of diet therapy is that there's no science in it. I find this incredibly insidious, because there is science today that talks about both the mechanisms and the efficacy of diet therapy. But if you say to a parent that there's no science to diet therapy, you're sort of saying that there is science to the other stuff that they do – and there isn't. There isn't a study in the world that talks about the interactions of the drugs, and no study that talks about the effect of drugs on children. You're not allowed to experiment with drugs on children, so how can there be science to it? That's a particularly dangerous double standard that they use to talk people out of diet therapy and into the next drug.

The conclusion I can't help but draw – and nobody argues with me about this – is that the ketogenic diet is not financially remunerative to doctors and to hospitals. In the United States, hospitals are businesses just like any other business, and they need to turn a profit. There are epilepsy treatments that are incredibly remunerative, and diet therapy is not, despite the fact that it's been scientifically proven and that more than half the people with epilepsy who've tried diet therapy are improved.

Only a tiny fraction of people who deserve the diet are even told about it. In the United States, there are paediatricians who just don't know about it. But more disturbing is that there are paediatric neurologists – people who specialise in treating neurological disorders in children – who either don't know or don't tell caregivers about this option. I don't think there's any question that drug companies have an enormous influence, not just on a practising physician, but on the way they're taught. They help finance medical schools, so it's not mysterious how this situation has occurred – at least not to me.

I thought when we started the Charlie Foundation that we'd be in business for a year or two, because it was so obvious. Why wouldn't you change your diet rather than cut your brain? It never occurred to me that 18 years later, I'd still be on a soap box trying to tell people this stuff. I thought, well, we'll just blow the whistle here, and there'll be a revolution. Of course, there has been no revolution. The people I work with and myself have downgraded our expectations now to one kid at a time.

We did a symposium in 2008 and now 2012. At the 2012 International Symposium[1] there was great reason for optimism. In the medical portion, there were 450 doctors, scientists and dieticians from 30 different countries in attendance. It was really exciting. For once it wasn't like pushing a boulder uphill. Everybody wouldn't have gone to the trouble being there unless they had some sort of belief that you can get better by changing what you eat.

As the diet is becoming more popular, they're using it with other neurological disorders too. There were speakers talking about the use of the same diet, the ketogenic diet, with Type 2 diabetes, early onset Alzheimer's, malignant brain tumours and with motor neurone disease.[2] They've found significant improvement with all these diseases, with this same ketogenic diet. So it's very hopeful now, that as this diet becomes a therapy for more disorders than just epilepsy, hospitals won't be able to get away with not having a ketogenic diet department with dieticians who specialise in it among their staff.

I think everybody walked out of the symposium having seen great progress and had great optimism about the future. Nonetheless, when you get back home and back to work, it still feels like you're pushing a boulder uphill again.

We have a sister organisation in London called Matthew's Friends[3] created by a mum, Emma Williams, who started the diet, but too late for her son. He improved on the diet, but he was eight years old by the time she got him onto it. He's very impaired, but it did help his seizures go away. When a child has a seizure, they black out instantly and can fall and hit their head. I think he had damage from the seizures, the drugs and the falls. We did the symposium in 2008 and 2012 here, and she did the 2010 one in Scotland.[4] She's going to do another one in 2014 in Liverpool in the UK.

At the symposiums, we have a fundraiser and a family day, which is also very well attended. Meryl Streep has been very helpful with promoting The Charlie Foundation and the diet. She came to the family day at the recent symposium, so we got some publicity, but not nearly enough. It still mysteriously doesn't get much publicity. I don't know the explanation.

1 Third International Symposium – Dietary Therapy for Epilepsy & Other Neurological Disorders, Chicago, September 2012.

2 Motor Neurone Disease (MND) is also known as Lou Gehrig's Disease, or ALS - amyotrophic lateral sclerosis.

3 http://www.matthewsfriends.org

4 International Symposium on Dietary Treatments for Epilepsy & Other Neurological Disorders Edinburgh, Scotland 2010.

In three weeks, I'm going to the Epilepsy Society meeting, where there will be 7000 professional attendees, and there will be one little satellite meeting about diet therapy. They're really depressing to go to. We'll have a booth and some people will come and talk to us, but there will be thousands of people there and no mention of diet therapy among the speakers.

Nonetheless, there is progress. In 1994, there was one hospital in the world with the ketogenic diet programme, and today there are 200, so a lot of kids have improved and gotten better and now adults are also using the diet. There's a list of those hospitals on the Charlie Foundation website.[5]

We do everything we can to get the word out. The large message though is that the medical destiny of us and of our children is up to us. We have to embrace that and not be intimidated by it. I sleep much better knowing that we have a website. There's a section there of 'keto-kids', who have benefitted from the diet.

Charlie is 21 years old now. He's been cured. He hasn't had a seizure in 15 or 16 years. He's been off the diet since he was six or seven years old. He has been playing piano for 13 years, boxes twice a week, and is in his second year of college studying early childhood education. When he was sick, Nancy's first question to a new doctor was not about stopping the seizures, or even improving his health, but always: "Can he be happy?" He's certainly the happiest of our three kids and really proud of himself. He doesn't remember epilepsy and he barely remembers being on the diet. He's not quite sure what all the hoopla's about.

Charlie Abraham's presentation at the International Symposium on Diet Therapies, Phoenix Arizona, April 2008

"I want to thank you all for being here. My name is Charlie Abrahams. I used to have epilepsy. When I arrived at John's Hopkins just before Thanksgiving in 1993, I was 20 months old. I weighed about 16 pounds and was taking Dilantin, Felbatol, Tegretol and Tranxene several times every day.

I still had a bandage on the back of my head from when they operated on my brain. I had been having dozens, sometimes as many as a hundred, seizures a day for a year. Then Doctor Friedman and Diana Tellis and Mrs Kelly changed what I ate. My seizures were gone in two days. I was off all those drugs in a month. I'm not sure what would have become of me if my family hadn't found the ketogenic diet, but I doubt that today I would be an A student in high school with lots of friends. I doubt I would have been playing piano for the last eight years and I doubt that I could hit an eight iron 160 yards. I even think I will soon reach a lifetime goal by being able to kick my older brother's butt.

I do admit that science is my hardest subject. A lot of it I just don't understand.

5 *The Charlie Foundation* www.charliefoundation.org

So, it was fun to see my teacher's reaction when I told her I was going to miss a couple of days of school this week because I was addressing an international symposium on dietary therapies for epilepsy and other neurological disorders.

But I was one of the lucky ones. Since the diet was invented, there have been millions of kids just like me who were as sick as I was, but whose families had either never heard about the diet, or who were talked out of it.

So, when I say thank you for being here, I really mean it. Not just for me, but for all the kids and their families you are helping. Especially, I want to thank Mrs Kelly, the dietician at Johns Hopkins, who told my parents what I was supposed to eat. It was complicated, and knowing them as well as I do today, I'll bet that working with them was a real challenge for Mrs Kelly. But Mrs Kelly patiently hand calculated every bite that went in my mouth for five years. The truly amazing thing is that Mrs Kelly had been doing the same thing for hundreds of children for over 40 years before I got there, and continued for several years after I left.

When you think about it, a big reason we're all here today is because of Mrs Kelly. And now, we can all say thank you. So I would like to present this award to Mrs Kelly, with gratitude and admiration for a lifetime of helping children with epilepsy."

Jim Abrahams is an LA-based film director and producer. Among his many other movies, he directed the Telemovie First Do No Harm[6] *starring Meryl Streep, about a boy with life-threatening epilepsy who eventually recovered using the ketogenic diet. The boy, whose story the movie was based on, is now 37 years old and spoke at the 2012 Charlie Foundation Symposium. Jim Abrahams also created* The Charlie Foundation *website, http://www.charliefoundation.org which has a Vimeo introduction by Meryl Streep on the homepage.*

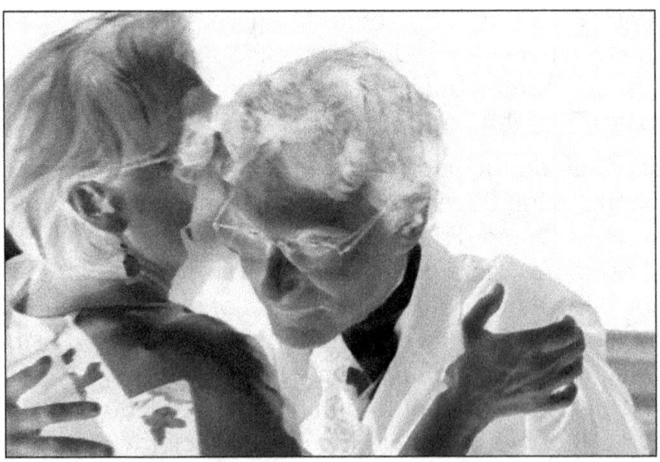

Charlie with Meryl Streep at his presentation at the International Symposium on Diet Therapies. Phoenix, Arizona, April 2008.

6 A DVD of *First Do No Harm* is available from The Charlie Foundation 515 Ocean Ave. #602N Santa Monica, CA 90402.

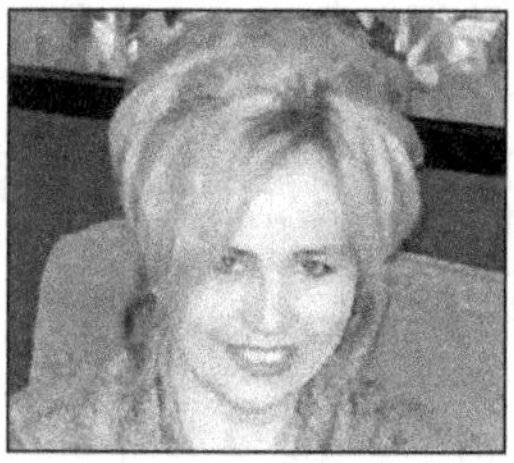

Elaine Bakos, 53 years

British Colombia, Canada

Fibromyalgia, with symptoms since childhood

I have always suffered from aching and pain. From about ten years old, my legs ached all the time. All we heard was, "Oh, it's growing pains." I never had any endurance – like when I tried track, I was told I was lazy. For as long as I can remember, I always had to push myself and needed a lot of sleep. I figured that's just the way I'm built.

When I was 17 years old, chronic fatigue wasn't really diagnosed. It was fatigue that you just couldn't get off the couch, you just survived – that's all. I'll never forget my GP[1] who, when I first started seeing him for my thyroid, said: "Well, we don't want to diagnose you with chronic fatigue, because that's a dead end."

As an adult, it was: "Just cope with the fatigue and pain," until I had a crisis with it about five years ago, when it basically just took over my life. It wasn't that I was bedridden – I was still functioning – but the quality of my life was at the point where I felt: "Why am I even trying to live?" Even so, no-one ever really diagnosed me with anything.

The most frustrating part was that I looked healthy. Although I was extremely tired and in a lot of pain, all the doctors wanted to do was throw drugs like *Lyrica*[2] at me to mask it. I maybe took two pills, then I started doing research on it and decided I just didn't want to become doped up like that. I wanted to be in control of where my pain level was. I tried a lot of alternative things too, like chelation[3] and different IV[4] treatments.

I had cold nodules[5] on my thyroid that had been growing and changing that they thought were cancerous. The growths were pressing on my vocal chords and wind pipe and I couldn't talk properly. So when I was 35, 17 years ago, they took my thyroid out and that's when my whole system just went nuts. After they took my thyroid out, I never was right again. It was extreme, as far as pushing myself all the time went, but I was a lot younger then and I just did it.

After the thyroidectomy I took myself off the thyroxin, because I didn't like it. I

1 GP – general practitioner.

2 *Lyrica* is an anticonvulsant drug used to treat epilepsy, post-herpetic neuralgia, diabetic peripheral neuropathy and fibromyalgia. Two common side effects are dizziness and drowsiness.

3 Chelation is the use of specific oral or intravenous agents to remove heavy metals from the body.

4 IV – intravenous therapy.

5 Cold nodules are non-malignant growths on the thyroid gland.

went onto desiccated thyroid and I've been on that for years now. At the same time, I never had energy – I lived on coffee. I never felt rested when I woke up in the morning. It was general malaise – I didn't feel like a vital person. You could hear it in my voice and see it in my overall personality. When you're in pain all the time, you just can't perform and you can't be yourself. When you're raising a family, you take care of the kids first, then you have to cope with whatever you have left.

I had ongoing muscle and joint pain, aching and restless legs. I always enjoyed sport. With raising three kids, you always have a go, but if I tried to do anything, I physically couldn't. People would say, "Oh, you're just doing too much."

Another thing was that I could not tolerate any heat whatsoever. It progressed to the nerve endings in my hands and feet, so I had this extremely bad burning sensation.

Five years ago, I did a transfer with work and moved from one side of Canada over to where we are now, in the mountains in Whistler Vancouver. I got a call from my daughter who was about to deliver twins. She had two healthy, seven-pound twins, but she lost a lot of blood and then had a blood clot and was critical for two weeks. I still get choked up when I talk about it. Then she had a double pulmonary embolism[6] as well. It was a nightmare.

We got her home from hospital and had these two newborn babies to take care of. My husband and I stayed with her until Christmas and then we had to get back here. I know that was a turning point – my body gave me about two months after we left her and then the fibromyalgia just took over. It started out with tingling in my fingers and feet and I couldn't wear my ski boots. I was so hypersensitive I couldn't touch any fibres. I couldn't touch hair or fabric. I would be cold sensitive, then I would be heat sensitive. I had excruciating joint pain. My wrists were so weak that I couldn't hold the babies in case I dropped them. I couldn't hold hands with my husband. Then my hands would swell. There'd be times when my hands would burn so bad I'd wrap them with cold cloths. I was just so 'hyper' everything. Then the same thing would happen with my feet and ankles, with extreme heat intolerance. There were so many things going on. All through that I thought, "Is this fibromyalgia or what?"

When I had that flare up, I went to a neurologist, but he didn't prescribe me anything. He diagnosed me with carpal tunnel syndrome[7] and that's as far as he went with it. I went to an internist in London, Ontario about the same time. He wouldn't even look at me, because I was taking natural thyroid. He said to me: "Once you get off that crap, then come and see me." This is the top specialist in Ontario. With two rheumatologists it was the same thing. One of

6 Pulmonary embolism is a potentially life-threatening event caused by the blockage of a lung artery, usually by a blood clot, which obstructs the blood supply to the lungs. Symptoms are breathing distress, chest pain, increased heart rate and in severe cases, collapse.

7 Carpal tunnel syndrome – compression of the median nerve travelling through the wrist, causing intermittent numbness of the thumb, index and middle fingers. The numbness and pain often occur at night, waking patients from sleep.

them checked my spine. Maybe I always presented too healthy, I don't know.

The hardest and most disappointing part of the past 20 years was that the specialists and neurologists never put all the dots together for me. They kind of put me under the diagnosis of fibromyalgia, but didn't have a solution for it, or know why I was feeling this way. That's almost as hard to live with than having a drug that doesn't work – it's just so demoralising and hard on you, because you start thinking: "Oh, it's all in my head." I knew it wasn't, because I don't want to be sick. I knew from way back, it was some sort of autoimmune condition, but nobody – neither my rheumatologists nor my neurologists – could put anything together and give me any answers. Because I didn't want to give in to *Lyrica* or any of those really strong drugs, the doctors threw their hands up and said, "Well, what else can we do for you?" I'd go back to my endocrinologist and say that I'd put weight on, and he'd say, "Oh well, just exercise". I'd say that I was exhausted, and he'd say, "Just get out there and do something." Then I realised that doctors couldn't help me much, but I knew there was something wrong with my joints, so I started to look for alternative medicines to try to cope with it.

About three years ago, I had an accident – I fell off the counter and broke my arm. Two months after that I couldn't talk, because of pressure in my chest. I went into a clinic and they diagnosed me with pericarditis,[8] because the doctor there saw fluid around my heart. I was put on 1800mgs of ibuprofen a day for this pericarditis, but wasn't getting any better. That's the most drugs I've ever taken. Then I went to a cardiologist for a follow-up. After all the tests, he said, "I don't think that's what you've got." And I thought, "Here we go again." They were afraid I was going to start bleeding, because the pills were eating my stomach. So I went off all those, then they readily gave me a whole lot of pain medication. I tried it and didn't like the way I felt on it, so I quickly threw it all out. They didn't help the pain and neither did the ibuprofen. I didn't want to get addicted to anything. Then I thought: "Oh my goodness, what am I going to do, because there was no relief. A doctor on one side of the country said I have pericarditis, and a cardiologist on the other side says that I haven't."

Eight months later, I went to my physiotherapist here, to see if she could help relieve some of the pressure. She took one look at my spine and said, "You fell, right?" I said, "Yes, I fell off the counter onto my tailbone." She told me that my T4 and T5[9] were rotated. Within one treatment I had relief. I had all those drugs for a wrong diagnosis, that gave me absolutely no relief. The only thing they looked at was my arm. I went online and saw that classic T4 problems can mimic heart conditions. I listened very carefully to those doctors, because of what I've been through all my life.

While you're coping with all this, the fatigue part goes into the background. A year and a half ago, I started being hypersensitive to light bulbs – electrosensitivities. It didn't have to be very hot, but I couldn't let the sunlight touch my skin. Then I

8 Pericarditis is an inflammation of the fibrous sac that surrounds the heart (pericardium), which often causes chest pain.

9 T4 and T5 – fourth and fifth thoracic vertebrae.

couldn't be too close to the screens in my car. It all just kept changing.

Another thing happened to me again this April,[10] when we'd been out skiing. On the mountains was where I got my stress relief. I was able to let everything else go and just regenerate. We were out there and it was glorious, I'd had a fantastic day, but I'd got sun on my face. I came home and I was bedridden – off work, which is very strange for me. I thought, "Wait, I'm reacting to the sun." Then somebody said, "Have you ever been checked for Lupus?"[11]

You can drive yourself crazy on the internet trying to figure out what's wrong with you, but that's when I got on the internet. Then all of a sudden, LDN[12] popped up. I started reading examples of what people were using it for. Mostly, it was MS,[13] and some for Lupus, but I didn't really think I had Lupus.

From the LDN website, I found a naturopath. The day that I called her, my husband had broken his leg on the mountain. Not that that added a lot of stress, but it was our 35th wedding anniversary. I was at my lowest of low. I thought: "Here we go, I can't go out in the sun, I can't ski and we've got summer coming." I just felt bombarded.

When I called the naturopath (Natalie), she spent an hour on the phone with me and I started on the LDN within two weeks. I felt different with one pill – mentally different. Not physically yet, but I had always had that brain fog going on. I said, "Boy, I'm back." Three years ago I went through one spell where my brain was not connecting. I said to my husband: "I feel like I'm not here. I'm talking, but I'm not here." I don't know the terminology, but there was a disconnecting going on in my brain. When I took that LDN, I thought: "I'm not going to say anything, because what can one pill do?" But I could tell a difference the next day.

We went back to Ontario to see my family, when I hadn't even been on the LDN for a whole month. When my sister asked me how I was feeling, I said, "Well, I don't know. Mentally, I feel better." I didn't want to say anything, then she asked me about my pain. I said, "Well, I'm not sure." Her response was: "Elaine, you just drove 5000 kilometres across the country, in the truck, for four days. You slept in the truck this time." (We didn't bother with hotels – we just laid out in the back of the truck when we stopped over somewhere). She said: "You would never have been able to do that before." In the past, I'd always have to have a soft bed and take a bath. Then she commented that my voice was back. I had energy in my voice. All within a month!

I did have days when I went down. The aching I had learned to live with, and pain in the joints, where sometimes I couldn't turn a door knob, I had learned to live with. But the sensory part in my fingertips and feet, I was afraid would come back. I used to get that 'walking on glass' feeling when I got up in the morning. Now, I'll have it for a couple of seconds, then it eases and doesn't linger. If I had

10 Four months prior to this interview.

11 Lupus is an autoimmune disease, with vague symptoms, making diagnosis difficult. Lupus patients often suffer from sun sensitivity.

12 Low Dose Naltrexone is the off-label prescription of the FDA approved drug *Naltrexone*.

13 MS – multiple sclerosis.

a bad day, I'd think, Uh-oh, I'm going to have bad days from now on. But it's as if my body is working through it. Natalie says that I'm a different person, in my voice and my personality, compared to when she first saw me. She reminded me that I didn't know if I could drive to her clinic for my first visit.

Wanting to do things as naturally as I can kind of allowed me to try LDN, because it's such a low dosage. I thought, "Boy, if it can work at that dosage..." Because, you know, the next thing would have been pot – marijuana. [*laughs*]

I have at least 50 per cent more energy than I had before. I have always needed ten hours of sleep and even then I wanted to sleep a little bit longer. I still don't have the level of energy that I want to have, but I don't feel like I'm pushing myself all the time either. At night time, I feel my joints starting to ache, then the pain disappears. I don't know how to explain it.

I have had some regression with the sensation on my skin. I'm back on bio-identical hormones now. I went off those for a month and I had my hottest month. I couldn't even come close to the windows because of the rays coming through – that's how sensitive I was.

A lot of doctors thought my problems were because of my thyroid, and I've always blamed everything on my thyroid, but I've used the desiccated thyroid and my levels have always stayed good. I think it goes back to autoimmune. My sister has ankylosing spondylitis, my mum has always ached, my grand-mum always ached and called it rheumatism. My other sister was the same, with fibromyalgia – aching and joint pain. She started on LDN too, and within one week, she was able to come off of all her pain meds that she had been on for years!

I kept saying to my husband: "Why can't someone just put these things together and come up with a diagnosis? That's how it should be." Every time I went to a specialist, they'd look at just this one little part, then another specialist would look at another little part. I guess maybe on their own, there just wasn't enough. Then they'd tell me that I looked so healthy. I thought, "If I hear that one more time!"

Now, I know that a lot of other people have the same symptoms that I have. I don't know what this LDN does – something in the brain. It doesn't have side effects and that's all I need to know! I'm just ecstatic with how I'm feeling.

I'm not a morning person, but I would love to be. One thing the LDN has changed is that I get much better quality sleep. I feel more refreshed when I wake up. Before, I would feel ill if I had to get up early. At the very start of taking the LDN, if I woke up, I couldn't get back to sleep, but that didn't last too long. What really bothered me was that after about ten days, I got extreme headaches and I was nauseous. I was afraid I was going to have to quit taking it, but they levelled off after about three weeks. I backed off taking it for a day here and there and then just kind of ramped myself up again.

My naturopath can prescribe LDN for me because in British Colombia there are certain classifications of naturopaths who take extra exams so that they can prescribe. It was passed here about three years ago. She prescribes my hormones too. My sister back East went to try it, but she has to get a doctor to prescribe it. It's really a privilege here in this province to have this service. They're so open to anything you tell them that is helping you, instead of having to go and plead with the doctors who put all those drugs into you that don't do anything.

The craziest thing about it is that my extended health insurance – my 'drug plan'[14] – won't cover the LDN. They booted it back to me because it's not the usual prescribed dose. I thought: "How stupid! I could have been milking you for hundreds and thousands of dollars for all these drugs that the doctors would have given me and this is forty bucks." I don't care – it's so cheap for the relief it's given me, but it just doesn't make any sense.

There are a lot of other people out there who are not seen as really sick, yet they have been living with chronic pain for so long. They don't fit into a category, are undiagnosed and they need help.

We just keep chugging along until a big bump in the road makes us completely crash. That's why I am so glad I found a list of practitioners who prescribe LDN. At that point, I was so weak, I was done. I didn't have any drive in me, so to find that naturopath was just phenomenal.

Harvard educated Bernard Bihari, MD, (1931-2010) discovered the clinical effects of FDA-approved Naltrexone using low doses (Low Dose Naltrexone or LDN). In 1985-86, he conducted a groundbreaking clinical trial on patients with HIV/AIDS. Doctor Bihari says that the immune system normalising effect of the drug application he discovered applies to a wide range of autoimmune diseases.

Research trials can be found at http://www.lowdosenaltrexone.org/ldn_trials.htm

79-minute interview with Doctor Bihari: http://www.youtube.com/watch?v=x54Jc-cr8GT879

14 Health insurance.

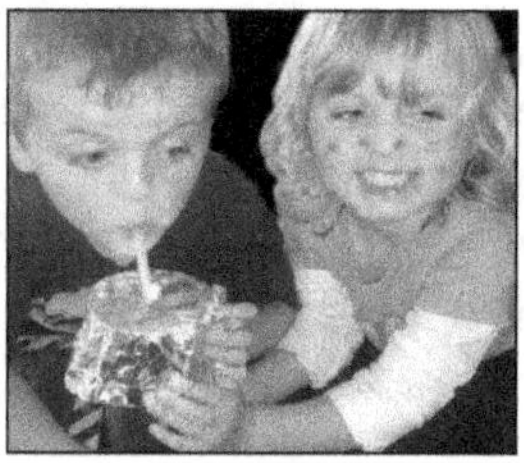

Shamus and Kaitlynn Baldwin

Auckland, New Zealand

Shamus, 7 years, diagnosed with moderate to severe autism at 2 years
Kaitlynn, 5 years, diagnosed with mild autism at 2 years and six months

Interview with Anita Kyle, mother

I have two children with autism. The first one is Shamus, who was diagnosed at two years with moderate to severe autism. The second one, Kaitlynn, was diagnosed with mild autism at two-and-a-half years.

I fell pregnant easily with Shamus. Seven months into my pregnancy, I was in bed crippled with pain. They couldn't figure out what was wrong, but after that weekend I was fine.

I got to eight months of my pregnancy and went to the midwife for my checkup. When she asked me how my baby was moving, I said to her: "Oh, no, the baby hasn't moved for a week." When she asked why I hadn't been to see her, I told her that an older woman at my work said my baby would be settling down getting ready to be born. That night, she sent me to hospital for a scan and called the next morning to say that my baby hadn't grown for a month.

At my insistence with the specialist, I had a C-section[1] and the next night Shamus was born, weighing five pounds and two ounces. His umbilical cord had deteriorated, he was jaundiced, weak and it was borderline for him needing to be transferred to the neonatal unit. I put him on my chest and stayed awake with him all night and we kept him out of the neonatal unit.

Shamus didn't feed well to start with. He was unsettled and wanted to be fed every hour, on the hour. He screamed and screamed until he got food, so it was a rough start. I didn't breastfeed – I didn't really know what I know now.

My husband, Terry, is a stay-at-home dad. I had to work, because his work wasn't stable enough, so there wasn't much option as far as that goes. I had my own business and I went back to work after a couple of weeks of Shamus's birth and Terry was with him full time. Shamus was very small, bloated and refluxy. We bought lots of gripe water, because that's what the midwife told us

1 C-section, or Caesarean section, is a surgical procedure where an incision is made into the uterus to deliver a baby.

to do. I really had no clue what I was doing. When he was six months old, the first meal I gave him was a multigrain baby cereal and he threw it all up. That was the first of many reactions to foods.

He was vaccinated on the 15th of December, when he was 15 months old. By January/February, our medical bills had gone through the roof. Overnight, this kid went radically downhill. He started projectile vomiting up to eight times a day. He had gut issues before his vaccination and he was an unsettled baby, but he didn't projectile vomit until after this vaccination. It would take up to ten days for him to have a bowel motion and then he might have diarrhoea for three days after that.

He started having really big meltdowns. He would leave me with black eyes and bruises down my arms. I could never get him to sleep and it was dire. He might sleep for an hour or two during the day, but the worst thing, was that he never slept between one and five in the morning. He just screamed the house down. We tried calcium, changed his milk formula and kept trying different things, but nobody could give us any answers.

By the time I was pregnant with Kaitlynn, I was aware that I was going to have two babies up at night. In desperation, very, very tired, my husband and I took Shamus to a doctor. She told me that I was an over-anxious mother and I was making him sick. I said to her: "When he projectile vomits and I'm ten kilometres down the road at work, is that my fault too?" Then she realised that I wasn't the stay-at-home parent.

The situation was so horrific that I moved out of the family home for a time and employed a nanny. My husband would get up in the night to him, then sleep during the day while the nanny would look after Shamus. I used to walk Shamus around the neighbourhood in the pram at three o'clock in the morning. Rocking was the only thing that got him to sleep and it was the only thing that we could do. At that stage we didn't know that autistic children like to be rocked.

Financially it was a struggle. We heavily mortgaged our house to keep going, because we didn't know how else to survive. My business was in trouble because I couldn't be focussed enough on it and our huge medical bills were continuing.

By the time Shamus was 18 months, he was craving up to two litres of milk per day. Everyone else's babies around me seemed to be doing things that Shamus wasn't. I kept thinking that he might catch up – *he might catch up*.

We went to a GP[2] who offered me an antidepressant. We saw a paediatrician, who also told me it was my fault. He sent me to have six weeks of counselling for postnatal depression. The nurses and counsellors that I saw told me that I was the most together woman that they had met and that I was just sleep-deprived.

2 GP - general practitioner.

I rang every helpline that I could at all hours of the night, and they kept saying that it was me that was the problem. I was sick of taking him to places and people telling me that it was my fault. Eventually, I went within myself, and thought: "At this rate, my child will be taken off me." I had this big fear that I would lose him.

When we came home from one doctor's visit, I took Shamus out of the truck and he had his first seizure in my arms. I thought to myself: "We're really in trouble now. This child is having seizures and nobody's listening. [*cries*] So I rang the doctor and said: "I've got to bring him back. There's something really wrong," but they wouldn't let me bring him back. Terry took the phone off me and said to them: "That's fine if you don't want to help us." They told me to go to Starship,[3] which is our children's hospital here and then to sit there and wait, but a junior doctors' strike was on, so I didn't take him to the hospital. He couldn't cope with new places and I was six months pregnant, so I stayed up with him all night instead.

When Shamus was almost two years old and I was about six weeks away from giving birth to Kaitlynn, a neighbour of mine, who was helping me, said that I needed to take him to a homeopath. She booked the appointment and told me: "You are going!" She knew what was wrong, but she didn't want to tell me. We were there for an hour and a half. It was the first time somebody listened to me. Shamus was kicking and screaming and Terry was trying to keep him under control. He was trying to get out of the office, because he didn't like being in enclosed spaces. The noise was so horrific that people in the surrounding offices asked: "What's wrong with that child?" The homeopath didn't say that it was autism, but she started me on a gluten-free, dairy-free diet. I was so desperate that I went home, took the kitchen apart and went shopping for products at nine o'clock that night. I didn't understand the concept of good nutrition at that stage, but overnight we went completely gluten and dairy free. Within three days, the projectile vomiting stopped. I thought: "This woman knows something." The homeopath treated him with remedies. I wouldn't say that he was recovering, but he was calmer, although he was still screaming through the night. Then she referred me to a paediatrician who specialises in biomedical treatment[4] for autism.

I went home and googled the paediatrician and saw the word 'autism'. Then I googled 'autism' and Shamus's symptoms ticked every box. It was then that I realised that there really was something wrong with him. It still upsets me all this time later, what we went through and how I had to fight so hard to get an answer.

I couldn't get in to see the paediatrician for six weeks. I knew that I couldn't

---

3 Starship Children's Health is a dedicated paediatric healthcare service and major teaching centre, providing family-centred care to children and young people throughout New Zealand and the South Pacific.

4 Biomedical treatment for autism refers to the process of redressing the anomalies in a patient's biochemistry by using specific nutrients. It is based on the pioneering work of Nobel Prize winner, Linus Pauling, who demonstrated that naturally occurring vitamins, minerals and micronutrients can have a profound impact on health and body functions. Pauling started a discipline called 'Orthomolecular Medicine' based on these principles.

last six weeks and I told them that I was a desperate mother. The receptionist explained that there was a long waiting list. Then a childcare nurse came to our house to check on Kaitlynn just after she was born. Of course, Shamus screamed as soon as he saw her. (We couldn't do things like mow the lawns, or turn on the waste-master, because he was so sensitive to noise.) She said to me: "You've got one just like me – your son has autism." I told her that I was trying to get in to see the paediatrician and burst into tears. She said: "My son goes to this doctor – I'll get you in." She got Shamus in the next Monday and he was diagnosed with 'high to moderate' autism, with a little bit of severity there.

I really didn't know what autism was. I remember going away crying and thinking: "This is the reason I've lost him." He didn't care whether I was there or not. Then I thought: "There is something wrong with him – great." That made me feel relieved, but the other side was: "*Now* what am I going to do?" I still thank that nurse.

The paediatrician prescribed all these supplements and we spent over $500. Little did I know that we were going to spend over $300,000 – that's what we're up to now, five years later. I gave Shamus all the supplements and it was boot camp. She also recommended that I see a naturopath to help me with his diet.

I wasn't even thinking *recovery*. All I wanted was for Shamus to *sleep* – that's all I wanted him to do. The naturopath was away for a few weeks and when I finally got in touch with her, she said, "I'll see you on Friday." I said to her: "No, you will tell me what to do *now*!" So she said to me: "Wean him off the rice milk, go and get some organic beef bones, roast them, boil them and give him the beef broth." In her talks, she still tells everyone about this "one very persistent mother."

I didn't *wean* him off the rice milk – that got thrown out as soon as I got home. I made him the beef stock and fed it to him that night, to go to bed with. We woke up the next morning and I asked my husband: "Did you get up to him in the night?" He said, "No, did you?" We thought he must have died in the night and ran into his room, to see that he was still alive. He hadn't woken up all night. I phoned up the naturopath the next day and told her that *Shamus had slept through the night*. I thought that was the end of it and that he was going to sleep through the night forever. She said: "Now for the bad news. He's not going to sleep for the next six weeks, but we will get him to sleep. But first, he's going to have massive 'die-off'.[5] I didn't know what die-off was. Shamus had an overgrowth of yeast in his gut and also bad gut bacteria.

When I next saw the naturopath, she said: "You're not going to do the gluten-free, dairy-free diet. You're going to do the GAPS[6] diet. It will be the hardest

5 Candida die-off, also known as a Herxheimer response, occurs when yeast in the gut is killed off too quickly and overwhelms the body with toxins that create symptoms caused by the candida being deprived it of its food source. Austrian Dermatologist brothers Jarisch and Karl Herxheimer discovered the phenomenon in 1895.

6 GAPS – *Gut and Psychology Syndrome*, written by Doctor Natasha Campbell-McBride, promotes a Specific Carbohydrate Diet (SCD) based on the work of Doctor Sidney Haas (1870–1964), who pioneered a low-carbohydrate diet to treat coeliac disease. He used it successfully on his patients for over 50 years.

thing you will ever do in your life." She wasn't far wrong. Five years ago there were no cookbooks on coconut flour or almond-meal flour. [*laughs*] There was nothing. I had to look things up on the internet and read books about biomedical food and recovery.

I started trying to cook this special food. I remember carrot cake being thrown up against the wall. I didn't realise that coconut flour absorbed that much moisture, so I was throwing more eggs and oil in – it was a disaster. I was still working full-time, but eventually I got my head around it.

Over the next six weeks, the 'die-off' was so bad that Shamus was getting worse day by day. He was screaming, had the worst temper tantrums, was vomiting and not eating. He looked shocking – he was so tired that he had these big black panda eyes. I called the naturopath and told her that I couldn't even take him out of the house and asked her to come and see him at home, so she did. She didn't tell me at the time, but when she left, she called a specialist overseas, because she had never seen such bad die-off. She wondered if he should stop the diet, but the specialist said to her: "Tell the parents to push through. The worse the die-off is, the better the recovery." So the naturopath came to my home and basically nursed us through it.

When we got to the six-week mark, Shamus started to change – it was just amazing. He looked happier, he was brighter and he wasn't so zoned-out. The changes were small, but we could see them. Instead of screaming for five hours a night, he only screamed for three hours, then two. It took four months to get him to sleep through the night, every night, for one whole week. We would have one good night, and then we might be up for two nights. Then he would sleep for two nights and we'd be up for three nights. But eventually, I could settle him more easily and he'd only scream for half an hour. His screaming always started at one o'clock in the morning.

I kept doing the GAPS diet and then the naturopath said that he needed more fermented foods and asked me to ferment coconut water. I drove all around south Auckland and got lost, ending up in tears, because I couldn't find the place where these young, drinking coconuts were. Finally I found them.

Well, we didn't know what the hell we were doing with these coconuts. Terry went into the backyard and started machete-ing them and we started to ferment them. We didn't know how to ferment, but Shamus was drinking it. We started putting the baby on it too, because the big fear in the back of our minds was wondering what she was going to be like. Over a period of two and a half years, my husband perfected the fermentation of coconut water and now we sell it as our business. That's what we do now for a living.

We were also giving Shamus sauerkraut[7] and all the low-carbohydrate food. He became calmer and went to the toilet better. He seemed more focussed

7 Sauerkraut is fermented or pickled cabbage.

and wasn't beating me and pulling my hair so much. He stopped stimming[8] and flapping as much. He was happier and he started to smile. We'd never seen him smile before.

We had started his treatment in September, but we thought we would have an autistic child forever. So the following January, we moved into a house that had a fenced-in section and a kitchen that looked out onto the garden, so I could see the children and know that they couldn't get out onto the street. I spent so much time cooking, I couldn't only look after the kids. I had to cook all weekend to make enough food to freeze during the week when I was working. We also needed one room at one end of the house for me to sleep in and have Shamus at the other end.

By April, Shamus was sleeping through the night, but I started to feel sick and was having food cravings. I wanted to have sushi three times a day and drink red wine. I'd never touched red wine in my life and yet suddenly I craved it. I was very tired and struggling to get out of bed. I knew that I had been under a lot of stress for a long time, but even though Shamus was sleeping and I was sleeping all night, I still woke up exhausted.

There had been a lump in my breast. I went to my GP soon after Kaitlynn was born and was told it couldn't be breast cancer. I was so desperately tired that I didn't have the brain-power to think to see someone else. Later, I went to another GP and said the lump in my breast was bigger and I had tenderness under my arm. She was the second doctor who told me that it wouldn't be breast cancer, but I knew I wasn't well and booked a mammogram. I was only 40 and had never had a mammogram before. After the mammogram, they did an ultrasound and asked me if I had medical insurance. Then they told me to go and get my husband, because they wanted to do an immediate biopsy.

When I went back to the specialist a few days later, I could tell as soon as I walked into the room by the look on his face that I had breast cancer. He offered to do a partial or full mastectomy. I said that I wanted a full mastectomy, because if he got his margins wrong, I had an autistic child that I had to recover. I told him that my son was misdiagnosed three times and that I didn't trust doctors. I said: "I don't need my breast – it's the least of my worries." He still remembers me from what I said to him that day.

I went back to the factory and got everyone organised, did all the cooking on the weekend and was at the hospital on Monday, ready for my surgery. Once I get my mind set on something I can be very obsessive.

I was very lucky – after the surgery, I found out that there was no lymphatic involvement, so it hadn't spread. I went back to work and took three hours off each Monday so I could have chemotherapy, which I had for four months.

I had been so tired that I never really read the research into why I was doing

8 Stimming means self stimulation, or carrying out a repetitive body movement. Hand-flapping is a common stim in autistic children.

what I was doing for Shamus. Then, with my own healing journey, I was told that I had to take fermented coconut water as well. We went to a talk about fermented foods, I started drinking coconut water kefir[9] and went gluten-free. I told Terry that he had to make more coconut water kefir, because I wanted to take it too.

I started to understand my own background and childhood – there had been huge problems. I had bad learning difficulties, chronic constipation and was hyperactive. I also had dyslexia and dyspraxia. I was expelled from school when I was 12 and left high school at 14 without any qualifications. If it were now, I would have been diagnosed as being on the autistic spectrum. It was then that I began to understand my father. He was an odd, quirky man who probably had Asperger's syndrome.

We were about a year into Shamus's recovery by the time I got over the cancer. I was still very tired and constipated, so I started having intravenous vitamin C and found it really helpful. At my last round of chemo,[10] we started house-hunting. We found our dream house, and we're still there.

When Shamus was three years old, we took him to kindy.[11] He sat under the table and screamed his head off, but he was less zoned out, more engaged and making more eye contact. He was still not speaking and only making sounds. We got him a teacher's aid there.

By this time, Kaitlynn was coming up to one year. We were being guided on what to feed her to try and prevent any autism in her. Our naturopath came to our house one night and tasted some of our coconut kefir and commented that it was better than she could make it. Terry said: "Aha! I've worked out how to get the fermentation right!" Then she asked us to make kefir for her patients, who were having trouble making their own. I looked at her and said: "I'm running a business, doing the GAPS diet, I've got a baby, managing Shamus and you want me to start another business making kefir?" She said, "Yes, I do."

A friend of mine at the time also had cancer, with big sugar cravings, and wanted the kefir as well. She was wealthy and said she would pay me to make it. We were really strapped for cash, so we thought that it would be a bit of extra money. Shamus was spending more time at kindy and we'd put Kaitlynn into daycare, so we had a bit more free time.

We made a few batches of kefir and sold them. Doctors, chiropractors and naturopaths heard about this and started sending people to us to buy it. That was three years ago. My husband and I decided to ditch my fashion business and really give coconut kefir-making a go. We started from our garage, put a fridge and a freezer in and started selling batches of coconut kefir. Terry

9 Kefir is a fermented drink, usually made with milk, using kefir grains, which are a yeast/bacterial fermentation starter. It is claimed to have a wider range of beneficial bacteria than other yoghurts. Traditionally, kefir grains are continually passed on to other members of a community to make their own yoghurt. Kefir grains are able to ferment other liquids as well, such as coconut water and coconut milk.

10 Chemo – chemotherapy.

11 Kindergarten – preschool education.

designed a website for us and we hired a commercial kitchen. The following year, I did my first show. We didn't sell much then, but once I started giving out samples at the next show, the retailers noticed. I told one retailer that I was making the kefir for my autistic children and she asked for 80 bottles. A lot of other retailers followed. I put my fashion business on the market and I said to the Lord: "If you want me to do kefir and help mums who are where I was, when I had no-one to talk to, please show me the way." I didn't think it would sell, but by Christmas Eve, my business was sold.

Shamus didn't like the kefir when I first gave it to him, but I put drops of Stevia[12] in it. A lot of parents come to me and say their child won't take it, so I say to them, "Well don't feed them anything else then." I tell them to put that and their zinc drops in their smoothies, to offer new foods at least 15 times before giving up and to be firm and consistent. One mother came to me and said, "You're very hard core." I said, "Yes, it's been boot camp all the way." My husband is ex-navy and he is just as hard. We love our kids to death and we'll do anything for them. We've gone to hell and back, but we're firm with them. Just because your child has autism, it doesn't mean you let him get away with this, that and everything else. In our house, it's: "That's your food, that's what you get and if you don't eat it, you'll go hungry."

No child will starve themselves. We are very hard like that, but I do make raw food cheese cakes, date and nut balls and special bread, so they get lots of yummy foods. First of all on the GAPS diet, it's not so yummy though. It is a lot of work doing it all.

Since I've been working on the kefir business, it's grown about 90 per cent. We use young drinking coconuts and bring in three-quarters of a container of them each month. It's still not making a full living, but we kept some money from the business sale to help us along. We've also been doing homestays[13] for the last two years to help financially as well. There's nothing I won't do to turn my hand to make a dollar to keep my kids in treatment. This week it cost $1200 for a biomedical visit to the paediatrician, so it was a very expensive week.

We did the GAPS diet with Shamus for three-and-a-half years solidly, and started reintroducing some rice flour about a year ago. We're still 70 per cent GAPS and 30 per cent gluten and dairy-free. He has improved and improved and improved. Gluten and dairy are a no-go with these kids.

When we first started taking him for haircuts, there was no way Shamus would even go into the shop. He wouldn't let anyone touch his head. We would have to get a friend to cut his hair in the bath while he ate cashew nuts. It took about sixteen visits to the hairdressers for him to be able to have a haircut. We had to stand outside the hairdressers for ten visits, then walk into the shop a

12 Stevia is a natural sugar substitute made from the leaves of the plant *Stevia rebaudiana*.

13 Homestays offer travellers and tourists accommodation with a host family.

few times, then sit him in the chair – still no haircut – then, let him play with the scissors. Yesterday, I took him for a haircut and sat in the waiting area and read a magazine while he had his hair cut. Afterwards, the hairdresser offered him a lollipop, but I said no, he couldn't have one because he has autism. He couldn't believe it and asked me what I had done. One of the hairdressers had a friend with two autistic children. I gave her my card and told her to read my story on my website and give me a call if she wanted someone to talk to.

We give Shamus chiropractic treatment, he has Epsom salts baths and he has saunas every third night. We did rounds and rounds of suppositories and he had colonics to deal with his constipation. We could tell he was constipated by his anger and aggression building and you could see dark circles under his eyes. After giving him a colonic, one of the hardest things I have ever done in my life, he would start laughing straight away. The change was just amazing. When the kids get sick, it's off to the homeopath – that's all we ever use.

People cannot believe Shamus is autistic now. A mum came up to me and told me that she took Shamus for athletics and said what a sweetie he was. She wanted to know why his speech was a little bit delayed. When I told her that he had autism, she said that she thought he was misdiagnosed.

Today, he is at a mainstream school and has been assessed as being 'neurotypical'. He has a teacher's aid for four hours a week to help with some reading and writing. Recently, his teacher told me that the progress he has made this year is well beyond a neurotypical child. In another year, she said that he would be completely caught up.

We still do speech therapy. We did a lot of RDI,[14] which I don't recommend to parents when they first start out. I did everything at once. If it was going to help autism, I did it. After my own experience, what I say to parents now is to get the gut right first. "Get the child thinking and in the same world as us, before you start therapy." If children can't think straight, therapy is a waste of money and time.

In my heart of hearts, I always felt with Shamus that if I could heal his gut, I could heal his autism. Knowing my family history and my own gut as well, I just knew his gut was his problem. I still monitor what he eats. When we first did the GAPS diet, he had no fruit and I still don't let him have loads of it. He has the kefir twice a day – my kids have big doses of it.

Tomorrow, we are going on a plane trip to the South Island for the weekend, Shamus and I. That's a big step. I never thought I would be able to do that and I'm not expecting any problems. That's how confident I am with him. When he was six months old, I took him to Sydney. He screamed the whole plane down all the way over there and all the way back. I swore I would never travel with him again, because it was so horrific.

---

14 RDI – Relationship Development Intervention® is a parent-led approach that focuses on teaching children how to develop social skills.

We started to see symptoms in Kaitlynn, and she was diagnosed at two-and-a-half years. She had no fear, like: "I'll just jump off that roof, Mummy." She was behind in her language and Terry was finding it hard to manage her at home, because she was hyperactive. It was: pick up, put down – all over the show. You had to have eyes in the back of your head, because you could lose her in the supermarket, no problem. She had a lot of behavioural issues. I put her into daycare two days a week. Within ten days, the staff took me aside to tell me she was biting children every day and she drew blood on one child. She had the bright red cheeks and bright red ears of allergies. They asked me if I thought she could be on the autistic spectrum. I said, "Oh really? That's a surprise."

So we marched her off to the paediatrician, where she was diagnosed as mildly autistic. There was some speech therapy for a while, but we didn't do any other therapy with her. She was on the GAPS diet with coconut kefir anyway, and we took the phenolic foods[15] out. She needed zinc, magnesium, vitamin C, fish oils and some herbs. We're still tweaking her biomedical plan, because she still has the allergic shiners,[16] so she's still not quite right, but she's on less and less treatment now.

Kaitlynn has just turned five. She's at school with no teacher's aid and is above average. She's doing really well. There are a few behavioural issues with her, but if you didn't know, you would never pick anything up.

I've been really firm about Shamus and Kaitlynn socialising. I don't believe in hiding them away or home-schooling them, because they have to live in the real world. I don't let them become overwrought, but I do believe in pushing the boundaries with them.

When Shamus was first diagnosed with autism, I didn't want to tell anyone. Then I thought: "Well, that's a bit silly, because people are going to realise that he's not quite normal." It was mean to hide him and shield him. I learned that the more I told people, the more understanding and kind people were with him. Now, I'm very up-front with everyone and tell them that my children have autism.

There are lots of ups and downs on the journey – that's how it is with these kids. Kaitlynn's speech is advanced and nobody would know that anything was wrong. When Shamus is tired, sensory problems kick in. If there was a really loud song at school, that would be about the only problem that you would see. It's not just gradual improvement all the time; often it's three steps forward and one back. As you start rebalancing the gut and kill off one bacteria, there might be another bacteria that goes out of control. Sometimes they react to

15 Scientific studies conducted by Doctor Rosemary Waring, PhD, revealed that many children with ADD/ADHD and autism have a deficiency in the enzyme that processes phenols, known as the PST enzyme (phenol sulfotransferase). In the late 1960s, Doctor Benjamin Feingold, MD, discovered that after eliminating all artificial phenols, plus naturally high phenol fruits and vegetables, up to 50% of children with allergies and ADHD significantly improved.

16 Allergic shiners are red rings around eyes caused by allergic reactions to foods.

supplements. Once, a supplement upset Shamus and another one helped his speech really come on. There is a lot of tweaking to do with biomedical treatment. We're probably one of the early, pioneering families. I'm sure in the next 20 years lots more people will do it.

I've got really good recovery for my children, but we're still working on it. The financial aspect of it can be a killer and you wonder where you're going to get the $500 for the next test. That's a strain, but I don't regret one minute of what we've done. I was told that there was no hope for Shamus and that he should be institutionalised. Even my paediatrician recently said to me: "He's just doing so well and has come so far. There really wasn't much hope, was there?" She does biomedical conferences every three months and I'm on a parent panel, speaking as a parent who has recovery. The biomedical conferences are for parents who have just received a diagnosis.

Last week I got a call from a mother: "Are you the kefir lady? Do you have the autistic children? I have an Asperger's boy. Tell me what to do." I get a lot of that.

We're hoping that the kefir business is eventually going to fund us properly and then I can spend time with mothers. I never charge for any of my talks, because I just want to help. I don't want other parents to feel the isolation that I felt. I couldn't take Shamus out and nobody would come to the house and see us because he would scream at them. They felt that they were upsetting him. This mother I spoke to last Sunday sent me a text saying: "It's just being able to speak to another mother who's been there." Unless you've been there, you don't realise how hard it can be.

Shamus has been invited to seven birthday parties this year. When he was in kindy, he never got invited to anything. I ran into an old neighbour the other day, whose daughter is a psychologist, working with autistic children. When I told her my children had recovered, she told me that they must have been misdiagnosed.

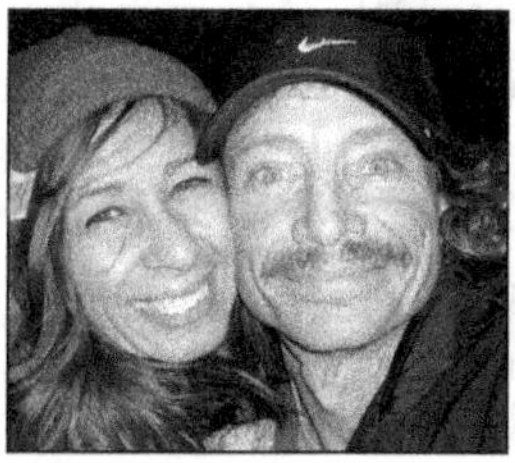

Tom Balk, 57 years

Cambria, California, USA

Diagnosed with hepatitis C at 44 years

I'm a roofing contractor. The labour is intense and I was having strange things happening with my health. My wife at the time was encouraging me to get life insurance. I was also consuming wine – this is wine country and wine was part of my evening diet.

I decided: "Okay, let's shoot for life insurance." They did lab work and to my surprise, there was a letter in the mail informing me that I wasn't a candidate for life insurance. I had tested positive for hepatitis C. Immediately, I went on the internet to find out what that meant and realised that alcohol consumption had to go. That night I stopped drinking entirely.

I went to a doctor who told me that there were six or seven strains of hepatitis C and not to panic. Some strains you can do just fine with and die of old age or other causes. He kept the visit kind of light. When it was time to go back – I can picture it vividly in my mind – he said that my genotype[1] was 1a. I'm like: "Okay, am I fine?" He said: "No, that's one of the worst strains that there is." He immediately told me that I was not in good condition and that he wanted to do a biopsy. I was going to need to see a hepatologist and that sort of thing. He mentioned that there was interferon,[2] that it was a chemotherapy, but he didn't go into detail.

When you find out that you have a critical disease like that, it affects your psyche. Your body can start shutting down with your negative thinking, so of course that was going on. At the same time, you start talking around. I had a small community of church family and people would come up with these remedies. "Oh, do you juice? Do you do this? You should try this and that." Well, basically, next thing I knew, I was juicing five pounds of spinach a night and that's one of the worst things you can do, because it's high in iron. Anybody with a liver disease cannot process iron. The testimony of that is you've got to do your research – you don't just jump into things.

I was struggling, and failing quite quickly. It totally affected me all at once. I had been getting fibromyalgia, which is tissue pain – it's really strange. In the middle

1 Genotype – the genetic make-up of a cell or organism.

2 Interferon alpha is a synthetic form of a substance that some white blood cells make naturally in the body. These blood cells make interferon as an immune response against infection or cancer. Interferon stimulates the immune system by encouraging killer T cells. Side effects include tiredness, lowered white blood cells, flu-like symptoms, nausea, diarrhoea, depression, mood changes and anxiety.

of night I remember having a tough time getting to the restroom and back, so nights were horrible. Even though I had quit drinking alcohol, I was feeling very nauseous, especially after drinking that spinach juice. I wasn't jaundiced, I didn't have cirrhosis, but I had to get up every morning and climb ladders, get on roofs and use my strength to make a living. I didn't have employees and it was hard. A person with liver disease can eat a meal and then have to go lay down or even conk out in the middle of the meal, because as soon as your bad liver is stressed, it starts to shut down. You've got to watch your iron, so you're tired all the time. I found that I needed to eat smaller portions throughout the day, because of the way that my body processed the food. I didn't understand diet and that flour is equally hard on your liver. Not knowing that, my diet wasn't that good.

I ate out at restaurants a lot at that time. I had nausea before I went for the life insurance test, but I would always blame it on the food, that sort of thing. When you're entertaining with wine, like I was every night, that covers up how you're feeling, so the next day you just attribute it to: "Well, maybe I had one glass too many – once again."

For the first couple of months, I still wasn't doing anything right, except not drinking. I ended up noticing at work that I was depressed and was wanting to take naps on people's roofs, because I was out of energy.

The ray of hope came when my ex-wife was handed a magazine of some sort on health, while she was getting her nails done. Somebody said: "Here's an article on a doctor and hepatitis C." In the article, a Doctor Berkson was being interviewed – this was in 2001. He was saying that there were alternative treatments for liver disease, rather than the medical treatments like interferon. He mentioned a triple antioxidant approach to the treatment of hepatitis C [*quotes from the magazine*]:[3]

> *"With the more recently discovered forms of hepatitis, hepatitis C has become a major public health concern in the US. This virus can remain in the body for ten, twenty or even thirty years, slowly damaging the liver, without the patient ever knowing it. In time, as symptoms become evident, as they do in 85 per cent of patients who get the virus, conventional treatment is not very effective. However, pioneering physician Burton Berkson has achieved miraculous results with a therapy involving three antioxidants; 600mgs of Lipoic Acid, 900mgs Silymarin[4] and 400mgs Selenium, taken daily in two or three divided doses. Although doctor Berkson has published his clinical results in international medical journals, his work remains largely ignored."*

I ended up getting these vitamins right away and started taking them. Actually, my ex-wife said, "Here, start taking these." I asked, "What are they?" Then she told me about the article.

3 *An Intergrative Triple Antioxidant Approach to the Treatment of Hepatitis C*, Burt Berkson, MD, PhD *Hepatitis* March/April 2001.

4 Milk thistle (*Silybum marianum*) is a herbal remedy for liver, kidney and gall bladder problems. Scientific studies suggest that silymarin in milk thistle protects the liver from toxins, due to its antioxidant and anti-inflammatory properties. It may also help the liver repair itself. University of Maryland Medical Center http://umm.edu/health/medical/altmed/herb/milk-thistle#ixzz2rLwlXfn8

In three days, I was already feeling better. The fibromyalgia, which was the most significant ill effect that I was getting, started dissipating. Within seven or eight days, it was gone and I was amazed. I said: "Wait a minute – what is this you're giving me? Because it's working."

Soon after that, I went for an appointment with a hepatologist up at Stanford University. We didn't have one locally, so I ended up volunteering to drive to Stanford, which is in San Jose. While I was sitting in the waiting room, I was noticing the expressions on people's faces and it wasn't pretty. It was all gloom and doom. I looked at the literature about hepatitis C – I picked up the article that they had right there. It talked about their interferon therapy and what it involved. But right there on the first page, it said: *"However, if you have Type 1a or 1b, the success rate of treatment with interferon is zero."* I looked at that and went: "Well, that's me."

When it was my turn to meet the hepatologist, she quickly said: "Well, you have Type 1a. We're going to give you interferon, but there's a six month waiting list, so here, I want you to take some *Prozac*."[5] I asked: "The antidepressant?" She said: "Yes – you're going to need it." I said: "You know, I'm a pretty positive person and I don't know that I want to take it. Why are you giving it to me when the literature I just saw outside in the waiting room says that there's a zero per cent success rate?" She looked at me and said: "Well, what else are you going to do?" That was her remark. I said: "Well, it's funny you should ask. I've been taking this 'triple antioxidant'," and she started shaking her head. I said: "Hear me out – I had this fibromyalgia and it's already working and my lab work shows that my liver enzymes are improving." She looked at it, laughed and said: "We're going to put you on a waiting list for the interferon and we'll contact you when it's your turn." It was this feeling of: "You should be happy – it's so popular that you have to wait."

I walked away, perplexed at how everything went down and kept doing the triple antioxidant. Three months later, I got a phone call and a package. It's very well done. They make you feel like there is a support team, almost like: "Yay, it's my turn – where are the balloons?" Then you start reading about the side effects. I started wondering: "Why didn't I take that *Prozac*? This is bad news." I was not schooled in biology, toxins, or chemotherapy – I was too young and it wasn't on my mind. My ex-wife said: "Look at these symptoms – mental illness, suicide, bouts of anger – I've got to live in the same house as somebody with that?" It caused her to dig a little deeper. I wasn't the brains, so I said: "Well, what else would I do?" She said: "Well, you feel better doing the antioxidants. Why don't I call Doctor Berkson in New Mexico and find out if he can take patients?" He did and I thought: "Well, I've had so much success in doing these triple antioxidants – let's take the money and go." I didn't have any hope, really, because anytime I mentioned this stuff, the word 'quackery' came up. People and other doctors that I spoke to used that word a lot.

5 *Prozac* is a SSRI antidepressant drug.

When I went to New Mexico and met with Doctor Berkson, I didn't know how he treated hepatitis C. I just knew I was going to see this doctor that could help. I didn't know he'd written books – I just took it all in. It wasn't fancy, it wasn't a big medical building. But the patients – I saw a man with half a nose who had cancer and I saw another woman who hobbled in after taking an hour to get out of her car, and I'm asking: "Are these liver patients?" I find out that they're cancer patients. Someone struck up a conversation with me and asked me what I was there for. When he told me his story, I started feeling at ease. He said that this doctor doesn't rush his patients. Once you get in there, he wants to hear it all. He said: "He's not your typical doctor." I thought: "Okay, that's the first positive thing." When I met with him, he told me about how he's sort of a rebel, which caused him to go outside of the medical community, even though he's a PhD[6] in microbiology as well as an MD.[7] He told me about the Alpha Lipoic Acid.[8] He looked at my lab work, he looked at everything, and said: "I want you to start taking some vitamins and I want you to change your diet." I said, "Okay, I'll start doing vitamins." Then he introduced me to the room where some people were getting infusions and asked me if I would like to try it and I agreed. I got one treatment that day and flew back home.

After that, I did some more lab work and had a liver biopsy. At that time, my liver inflammation was a three out of four and my fibrosis was at stage two-to-three out of four. Doctor Berkson told me not to get any more biopsies. In biopsies, he says, you're poking an inflamed liver that is already struggling, so the readings can be inaccurate. He shook the sand and he gave me hope. I told him that I had read that interferon doesn't help Type 1a, and he said, "Good for you!" But he didn't push me in to coming back or anything. He gives you the information, then it's up to you what you do with it.

I went home and did some more lab work with my doctor here. He called me in on my personal phone – he'd never done that before. I thought: "A doctor wanting to talk to me instead of seeing him in a scheduled appointment?" There was something he wanted to discuss. I started thinking of all the negatives; that now I have cancer, and I started spiralling down in my head. I was so nervous when I walked into his room and he comes in smiling. He said: "I just looked at your lab work. Everything is balanced – the iron, everything. It's magnificent." Then he said: "So when are you going to start taking the interferon?" I tried to tell him what I was doing, which explained why my lab work was balanced, and he basically said: "You're a fool. That's quackery – I don't want to hear it. When are you going to start taking the interferon?" This is my first experience, I've got a critical disease. I said, "You know what? It

6 PhD – Doctor of Philosophy.

7 MD – medical doctor.

8 Alpha Lipoic Acid is naturally occurring in the body, playing a fundamental role in metabolism. Although known for decades, only recently has it been used as a nutritional supplement and has important therapeutic potential in conditions where oxidative stress is involved. Case studies show lipoic acid used for liver disease was successful in many cases. *Alpha Lipoic Acid in Liver Metabolism and Disease Free Radical Biology and Medicine*, Volume 24, Issue 6, April 1998, Pages 1023–1039.

doesn't help Type 1a. It's confirmed." He said, "What are you telling me?" I said, "I'm not going to take it." He said, "Okay, I'll give you four years and you're a dead man." You can't get ruder than that.

It's important that you know the state of your mental health and to have hope. I enjoy not drinking any more. I have to tell you that my Christianity took a serious step, because I was thinking that if I've got four years left, there's the sad part of saying goodbye to everything you've worked for, and what does it all mean? So I started reading the Bible and I went to a whole new church. My bad marriage – well, she needed a drinking partner, so she took off. That was okay. I went for what I needed, and that was peace of mind. I had a support system, I had a direction and I had hope, even if nothing worked. In that, there was a lot of prayer.

I had a negative attitude that this wasn't going to work, because I had only visited Doctor Berkson once. I ended up going back to see him and he asked me if I wanted to start taking the treatments. He told me that I could get two a day for three days and then go back to California. So I said: "Set me up." I stayed for three days. For the next year and a half, with the stress that I was going through, my lab work was all over the place.

Doctor Berkson told me that when he was an intern that one of the places he worked was a prison and it was his job to tell the prisoners that they had tested positive for AIDS. He wrote an article on this: *Mind Over Matter*[9] – it's in the medical journals. He said that he went to a prisoner who looked muscular, like a poster boy, and was in perfect health. He told him that he had AIDS and saw him, over a period of three months, just wither up and become unrecognisable. Then he got news that this man's diagnosis was wrong and he had to tell him that he didn't have AIDS. The man came back to life before his eyes.

When your mind tells your body that you're going, it'll shut down faster. I found that was very true. I needed to keep going to Doctor Berkson because I was feeling less nauseous, I was starting to eat the right foods and I was feeling better. I remember thinking: "If I could only be 30 per cent of who I used to be, I could still keep working."

One time my ALT[10] was 450 – normal is 10. He asked me: "You were down to around 200 – are you drinking again?" I said, "No." He said: "Are you sure? Because your lab work looks messed up." What I was doing was, as I was feeling better, I was going back to my old diet. I was kinda like: "I'm going to eat pancakes because I'm not going to fall asleep and get nauseous any more and I love pancakes. This guy is making me better so I can go out and go after the wrong foods!"

I was scared. I think I ate nothing but raw vegetables for the next week. When I saw him again in four months for more treatments, my ALT was back down

9 *Mind Over Matter* – Berkson BM. *The Western Journal of Medicine New Mexico Medical Society Newsletter* 161(4), 1994: 2.

10 ALT – Alanine Transaminase, is an enzyme found mainly in the liver and is an indicator of liver inflammation.

to 200 and everything was balanced. So, diet is such an important part. Now, I can tell people: "Hey look, just because you have found a doctor who knows what he's doing and can tell you what to do, you still have to stick to it. If you let it go, that disease is going to take over."

Within six years, I was one hundred per cent. Now at 57, I'm still up there pounding nails and I feel 120 per cent. When I get these treatments, for two months afterwards, I feel like I'm in my twenties. I have the best lab work right now. Last time I had my lab work done, my ALT, AST[11] was I think 47 and maybe 60. When I had this disease 11 years ago, they were in the hundreds. They're better now than they've ever been.

I've met patients who've said: "How old are you? What type do you have?" They had the same type I did, were younger and had cirrhosis. They said to me: "I don't get it. Why have you lasted so long? Type 1a and 1b are deadly."

Most people get to Doctor Berkson when they're jaundiced, when they find out late, so I'm kind of lucky. But he even brings them back. I've seen it over and over. It's just fascinating to go there and see somebody on a Monday come in looking like a green Martian, just as sick as can be and you just smile, because when you leave there that Friday, you know that that they're going to be talking and smiling. Usually, anybody with jaundice who goes there takes Alpha Lipoic Acid for two weeks and they leave there with full colour.

You try to figure out how you got hepatitis C. I've lived a pretty clean life. I'm guessing I got it as a teenager in the early seventies. We all make mistakes in life. I was in the navy at the age of 17 during Vietnam. Needles were shared and I dabbled in the leftover drugs from the sixties. It's not funny, but my generation just bought that hook and that's why it's such an epidemic now. The numbers are huge, yet when you talk to people, they look down and they look around. The number one cause of hepatitis C is the exchange of hypodermic needles, even though I can only remember ten or 12 times. I wasn't a junkie, but I experimented. In the eighties, they were discovering AIDS. I remember thinking: "Oh, I'm glad I missed that – what kind of horrible news that would be to somebody messing around with drugs."

In the late eighties to nineties, when hepatitis C started showing up, they didn't know what it was, so they called it 'non-A, non-B hepatitis.' When I first went up to Stanford, they said that for Type a and Type b not to give up hope, that there may be a drug in the future.

You hear stories of someone who has hepatitis C, took interferon and is now cured. Well, good for them, but I would not go to a toxic chemical, because I have found that in patients where it didn't work, they're really messed up.

There are all these fix-its out there. I drink hydrogen peroxide, 35 per cent

11 AST – Aspartate Transaminase (serum glutamic oxaloacetic transaminase/SGOT) is another enzyme that elevates in liver damage.

food grade – H_2O_2 therapy. I've been drinking it now for 25 years, daily, so I've been oxygenating my blood. I believe that's how I stalled my liver from going into cirrhosis. Doctor Berkson asked, "Why do you drink it?" I said, "Oh, I get energy, it makes me feel good." And he said, "Good!" I asked him, "Is that okay?" He goes: "Sure!" He's not into that, but he thinks it's okay. He treats other things too, not just liver disease – MS,[12] ALS[13] and cancer.

I have met people out here in California and taken them to New Mexico, literally almost carrying them. You know, first you have to threaten them. They look at you and say, "Wow, nobody can do that for me." One guy that I took there had hepatitis C, cirrhosis, he was in bed and had not worked for six months. He'd done interferon twice and it didn't work. I met him at the airport and his son was carrying him. He could walk a few steps then he would have to stop to breathe. He was dancing in three days, saying, "I can't believe this." He got healthy and he was just a new man.

I've watched Doctor Berkson go through different eras of nay-sayers, where nobody wanted to hear about his treatment, or listen to him. He was fine with that – he just kept up his success rate. He published a lot of material[14] and said that he treated patients because he enjoys doing what he does. We were shocked when suddenly the medical profession that shunned him started asking him to speak and applauding him. He got recognised and travelled around the world giving seminars. You can find them on YouTube, so all of his work is now more accepted and respected. He's in demand and he didn't have to die to become famous. It's wonderful to see that. Doctor Berkson's treatment can now be found outside of New Mexico. Doctors are using his studies and his protocol and he's helped people to spread this treatment, so it's not exclusive.

A typical day for me is 50 or 60 vitamins, prescribed to my lab work. It's been 12 years and I feel wonderful.

Acute Hepatitis C Virus (HCV) infection is difficult to detect because of the generally asymptomatic nature of the disease and the marginalization of at-risk populations. Around 25% of patients with acute HCV infection undergo spontaneous clearance. The remaining 75% of patients progress to chronic HCV infection and are subsequently at risk of progression to hepatic fibrosis, cirrhosis and hepatocellular carcinoma. Chronic hepatitis C generally progresses slowly in the initial two decades, but can be accelerated during this time as a result of advancing age and co-factors such as heavy alcohol intake and HIV co-infection.

(Nat Rev Gastroenterol Hepatol. 2013 Sep;10(9):553-62. doi: 10.1038/nrgastro.2013.107. Epub 2013 Jul 2)

The identification of the hepatitis C virus (HCV) in 1989 solved a growing mystery.

12 MS – multiple sclerosis.

13 ALS – Amyotrophic Lateral Sclerosis. Also known as Motor Neurone Disease, Lou Gehrig's Disease.

14 *Alpha Lipoic Acid Breakthrough* by Doctor Burt Berkson.

Large numbers of hepatitis victims had begun to appear, apparently with a virally caused disease. But when examined, these patients tested negative for both hepatitis A and B. The unknown disease was known as non-A, non-B hepatitis. When a test was developed in 1990 to identify individuals infected with hepatitis C, hepatitis C was found to be responsible for the majority of these cases – and it has quickly proved to present a frightening challenge.

In contrast to most other types of hepatitis, 50-85% of hepatitis C infections become chronic and lead to liver disease. Hepatitis C, in combination with hepatitis B, now accounts for 75% of all cases of liver disease around the world. Liver failure due to hepatitis C is a leading cause of liver transplantation in the United States; in all fairness: the majority of these patients have had significant alcohol abuse during a stage of their lives as well.

Since hepatitis C infection is typically mild in its early stages, it is often not diagnosed, or diagnosed in the context of screening of blood donors or testing as part of the application for various types of insurance. HCV is otherwise often not recognized until its chronic stages when it has caused severe liver disease. With a typical cycle of disease from infection to symptomatic liver disease taking as long as 20 years, the true impact of this disease on our growing infected population became more apparent after decades. For this reason, it is often referred to as the "silent epidemic".

It is suspected that there are, at present, more than 4.5 million people in the United States that are infected with hepatitis C, and more than 200 million around the world – making it one of the greatest public health epidemics of our time. We continue to detect new patients with HCV infection and late complications that show up years after the initial event.

Without interventions to treat infected populations and prevent the spread of the disease, the death rate from hepatitis C tends now to surpass that of AIDS. With the impressive control gained in the treatment of HIV infection, HIV-infected patients that have died in the past from a variety of other conditions, including opportunistic infections, outlive this infection, but may well die from the consequences of HCV infection.

(Everett Coop Institute http://www.epidemic.org/thefacts/hepatitisc/silentEpidemic/)

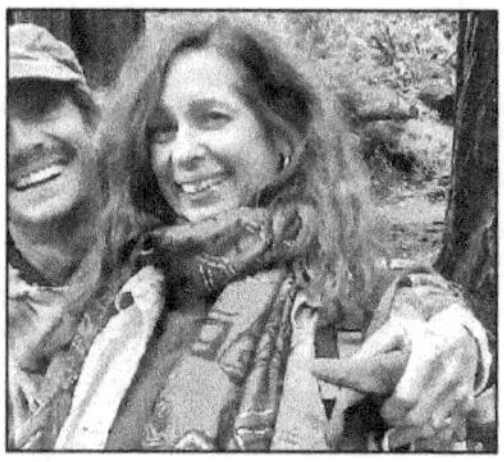

Janet Balk, 52 years

Cambria, California, USA

Diagnosed with hepatitis C at 48 years

I don't remember why I had a blood test taken, but that's when I got diagnosed with hep C (hepatitis C), so I went to see a liver specialist. That doctor actually was pretty nice. He was talking to me about the treatment options, which is interferon.[1] He also was very concerned, because he said that one of the main side effects is suicide, because you get so depressed on this drug. He wanted to make sure that I had some support in my life. I told him, not really, because was a single parent and that's not a thing I wanted to put on my child, so I said: "Would it be agreeable if I tried some alternative drugs first, before going on to interferon?" and he said, "Yes." So for a little while, I did some oxygen treatments, which they gave to me intravenously, but it didn't do anything. I was always scared of the side effect of putting that into my vein, so it was kind of a bummer.

I tried to educate myself with diet. You go to your regular doctor and they do lab tests and their standard answer is to look at certain things and then give you interferon. My doctor was truly concerned about me, and said: "You really need to take interferon," so I was willing to go on that route.

I got the first delivery, which comes in an ice pack and a styrofoam container. I sat down and took out the video tape where they show you how to take it. Then I took out the side effects description and it was, like, four pages wide and long. It was huge, like a poster. I read it and I was, like: "I cannot take this – I'm gonna die, it has such horrible side effects."

I have personally witnessed somebody dying from hep C, and it's horrible to see in the last stages. This person couldn't walk or talk anymore, because ammonia caused by the liver failure goes to your brain. You're mentally all there, but you can't express yourself and you can't do anything for yourself. You start losing weight, you get diabetes and your legs swell up – it's horrible. That person only took a little bit of *Silymarin*,[2] I believe. I know another person who took interferon three times. One time she stopped it because she could only crawl on the floor due to the anxiety attacks. She claims she is virus-free. But anyway,

1 Interferon alpha is a synthetic form of a substance that some white blood cells make naturally in the body. These blood cells make interferon as an immune response against infection or cancer. Interferon stimulates the immune system by encouraging killer T cells. Side-effects include tiredness, lowered white blood cells, flu-like symptoms, nausea, diarrhoea, depression, mood changes and anxiety.

2 Milk thistle (*Silybum marianum*) is a herbal remedy for liver, kidney, and gall bladder problems. Scientific studies suggest that silymarin in milk thistle protects the liver from toxins, due to its antioxidant and anti-inflammatory properties. It may also help the liver repair itself. University of Maryland Medical Center http://umm.edu/health/medical/altmed/herb/milk-thistle#ixzz2rLwlXfn8

I didn't take it.

I went one more time onto the internet and I found Doctor Berkson. I was, like: "Oh wow. Really? He's actually an MD?" You know, you really want hope. So, because I was done with doing oxygen treatments, I called him. At the clinic, they said: "Well, send us your lab work, we'll tell you what lab tests to do and then we'll see whether we'll take you." So I sent my blood test results in. They called me back in a couple of weeks and said they would take me, but I had to wait three months for my first appointment.

Before I started with Doctor Berkson, I had low energy and I was tired all the time, but I don't think I had symptoms where I would have said: "Oh, I have hep C." By nine o'clock in the evening, I would be so pooped that the sooner I could go to bed, the better.

I went out to the clinic in New Mexico – Doctor Berkson is awesome. He does different lab work from other doctors and tailors your supplements to you individually. He also has audited the manufacturers of the tablets, so he only recommends certain brands and not others – he's very specific about this.

After your treatment, you start feeling good almost immediately, within 24 hours. Doctor Berkson really addresses the whole person. He explains everything to you, answers all your questions and gives you such confidence, because he really knows his stuff and he shares it with you, so you can understand what it's all about.

I have probably had hep C for thirty or forty years. The fatigue was pretty substantial, but I didn't have any pain. I can't remember if I had nausea or not. After I had the Alpha Lipoic Acid, it was the best week of my life. I had energy – it was fantastic, and I had hope. It was a relief, oh my gosh.

I went there for a treatment and I came home with a husband! I met Tom there and we went hiking in the desert. I asked him: "What are you going to do today?" He said: "Well there are thunderstorms with lightning, so I'm going hiking out there in the desert." I thought that sounded like fun, so I went with him. That was three years ago.

My lab work is fantastic now. We attempt to go to the clinic three or four times a year. I feel great after the infusions. They give you extra oomph for quite some time. You can also get glutathione treatments there, which Alpha Lipoic Acid is a precursor to.

We don't get rid of the virus, but we do maintain very well. I explain to people that it's a three-legged stool. You take the Alpha Lipoic Acid treatment, you have to have the right diet and you have to have the supplements – that combination. My husband, Tom, had good results, but with diet, it so drastically improved. If you were only to do diet, you couldn't do it, if you were only to take supplements, you couldn't do it. If you were only to do the Alpha Lipoic Acid treatments, you couldn't do it. You have to do the combination. That makes sense.

You shouldn't wait until you're almost dying and then go once. The sooner you do it, the better. You can't raise people from the dead, but even so, Doctor Berkson did it actually, with those mushroom-poisoned people. That is an amazing story. This couple had eaten some salad and there were some raw mushrooms in it that are toxic to the liver. He was supposed to study them dying in the hospital. That's when he phoned a friend of his and found out to give Alpha Lipoic Acid to them and they survived. It's in one of his books.

I wouldn't wait to get treatment. Get the right treatment and go now. I have plenty of energy now.

Acute Hepatitis C Virus (HCV) infection is difficult to detect because of the generally asymptomatic nature of the disease and the marginalization of at-risk populations. Around 25% of patients with acute HCV infection undergo spontaneous clearance. The remaining 75% of patients progress to chronic HCV infection and are subsequently at risk of progression to hepatic fibrosis, cirrhosis and hepatocellular carcinoma. Chronic hepatitis C generally progresses slowly in the initial two decades, but can be accelerated during this time as a result of advancing age and co-factors such as heavy alcohol intake and HIV co-infection.

(Nat Rev Gastroenterol Hepatol. 2013 Sep;10(9):553-62. doi: 10.1038/nrgastro.2013.107. Epub 2013 Jul 2)

The identification of the hepatitis C virus (HCV) in 1989 solved a growing mystery. Large numbers of hepatitis victims had begun to appear, apparently with a virally caused disease. But when examined, these patients tested negative for both hepatitis A and B. The unknown disease was known as non-A, non-B hepatitis. When a test was developed in 1990 to identify individuals infected with hepatitis C, hepatitis C was found to be responsible for the majority of these cases – and it has quickly proved to present a frightening challenge.

In contrast to most other types of hepatitis, 50-85% of hepatitis C infections become chronic and lead to liver disease. Hepatitis C, in combination with hepatitis B, now accounts for 75% of all cases of liver disease around the world. Liver failure due to hepatitis C is a leading cause of liver transplantation in the United States; in all fairness: the majority of these patients have had significant alcohol abuse during a stage of their lives as well.

Since hepatitis C infection is typically mild in its early stages, it is often not diagnosed, or diagnosed in the context of screening of blood donors or testing as part of the application for various types of insurance. HCV is otherwise often not recognized until its chronic stages when it has caused severe liver disease. With a typical cycle of disease from infection to symptomatic liver disease taking as long as 20 years, the true impact of this disease on our growing infected population became more apparent after decades. For this reason, it is often referred to as the "silent epidemic".

It is suspected that there are, at present, more than 4.5 million people in the United States that are infected with hepatitis C, and more than 200 million around the world – making it one of the greatest public health epidemics of our time. We continue to detect new patients with HCV infection and late complications that show up years after the initial event.

Without interventions to treat infected populations and prevent the spread of the disease, the death rate from hepatitis C tends now to surpass that of AIDS. With the impressive control gained in the treatment of HIV infection, HIV-infected patients that have died in the past from a variety of other conditions, including opportunistic infections, outlive this infection, but may well die from the consequences of HCV infection.

(Everett Coop Institute http://www.epidemic.org/thefacts/hepatitisc/silentEpidemic/)

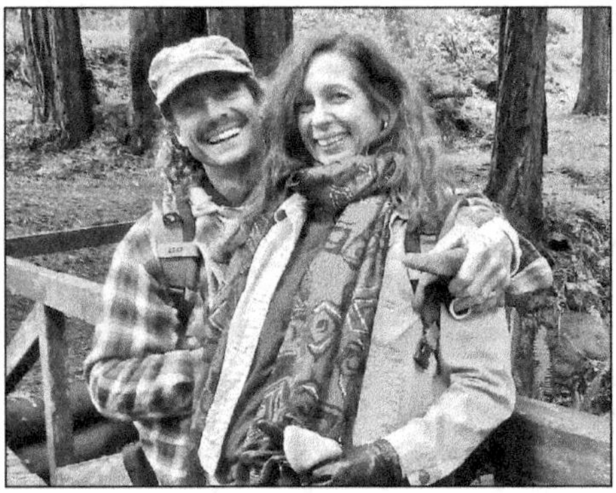

Tom and Janet Balk.

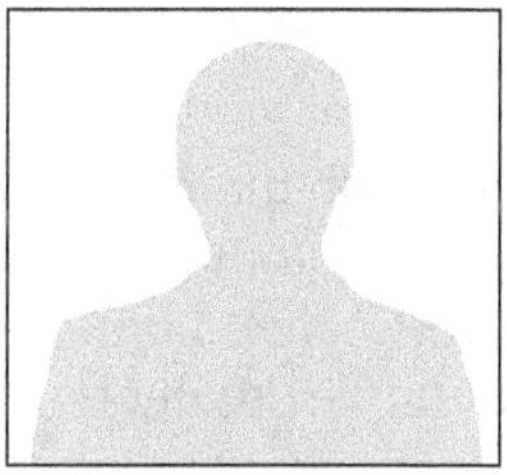

Paula Bambic, 67 years

Los Angeles, California, USA

Diagnosed with breast cancer at 45 years

I never thought that I would ever have cancer. In those days, they said that if it wasn't in your family, you didn't have a problem. As we know now, that's not really true.

My husband and I had been to my cousin's wedding back East and I'd never felt better. I came home and the next day my breasts were a little sore. I felt this lump and I knew that it was not good – I immediately knew that I was in serious trouble. It terrified me at so much at first, that I didn't tell my husband for three days.

I really didn't want to go through the traditional chemo,[1] radiation, surgery and all of that. I just didn't believe in it and I didn't think it was the right thing to do. My husband had been a medical malpractice trial attorney – he always represented patients against hospitals or doctors and had seen horrendous things done to them.

First of all, we did the research to find an oncologist to diagnose me for sure, so we started making the rounds, trying to decide what to do and went to see a number of different oncologists. The first one was absolutely the most brutal, horrible human being I had ever run into in my life. He wanted to put me in the hospital right away and start doing the treatment and we said: "No, we're still in the research stage and we're trying to figure out what to do." He was a big research doctor over at Saint John's in Santa Monica and he looked at my husband and said: "You're going to kill your wife. If it was my wife I'd have her in the hospital right now." None of them ever spoke to me. They spoke to my husband like I wasn't even in the room.

After that, we visited more oncologists and finally found one young man who actually spoke to me, so he's the one we settled on. He did kind of talk us into doing a lumpectomy. I'm saying he talked us into it, because in the first few days you're in a little bit of shock that this is what is happening. In hindsight, I never would have had the surgery. Be that as it may, he was convinced that it was just a teeny tiny little lump about the size of your baby fingernail and that it would be really easy to do a lumpectomy, get in and out and then maybe do a little bit of radiation and then I could go on about my business. I looked

1 Chemo – chemotherapy.

at him and said: "Well, that all sounds great, but I think it's way worse than you're saying. I have a feeling that it's all over my breast." He looked at me like I was crazy.

Most women, if they allow themselves, can be pretty in tune with their bodies. I knew there was trouble here. You have to sign all these papers, that they can basically do whatever they want, no matter what they agree to ahead of time. I said: "Look, I don't care what you find, I don't care what it is – I really don't want a mastectomy." He said, "Yeah, sure, no problem."

The day that I had the surgery, my mother, my husband and my daughter were all in the waiting room. As soon as the doctor opened me up, he completely freaked out, because my entire breast, including the nipple was filled with cancer. So he goes out into the waiting room and says to my husband, "I have to do a mastectomy." My husband said: "You better not. You just don't even want to see this woman upset. If you think she was upset before, you don't want to see this. Just don't do it. Do whatever you have to do, short of a mastectomy." So he took out three quarters of the cancer, and a quarter of the breast tissue, but in reality what I really had was a mini-mastectomy. He sewed me up and that was all he could do.

When I went back for my follow up visit, he said to me: "You have to have four rounds of chemotherapy, you have to have radiation…" and he went on and on and on. That was the only time that I was really upset during the whole process. When we left that office I was in tears and I said that I was never going back there again. Then we proceeded to go on our search for alternative treatments to find another way of treating this.

Everybody was so concerned – I had so many people sending me books and articles and websites and all this sort of stuff. It kind of gets overwhelming. This minister from our church happened to call one Sunday and said: "I think you should look at this Gerson therapy." As soon as he said that, I remembered we had a friend from church who had had cancer years before and had done the treatment and done really, really well, until her family got hold of her and convinced her she should do all the traditional stuff. She was dead within six months.

I knew that I wasn't going to do traditional treatment. If I was going to do anything, I was going to do Gerson. I started reading the book.[2] It all sounds good, in your imagination, and then when you start reading it and seeing what it really entails, you think: "Wow, this is really involved and sounds so complicated," so we continued to look for other methods. Santiago, which is only a couple of hours from here, is kind of a Mecca for alternative therapies, and that's where Gerson's headquarters are.

We went to this one institute, which was basically the Gerson therapy, but cut some corners and made it not so work-intensive. They were also giving

2 *The Gerson Therapy Handbook* by Max Gerson, MD.

tamoxifen.[3] Everyone got all excited – my husband and my mom, who was visiting from back East. On the way home, I started crying, and I said: "You know what honey? I'm not doing this therapy." The whole point of doing an alternative therapy for me is not to do anything more invasive than I've already done and not to do any drugs and chemicals. So I said: "I'm not doing it. Cancel the reservation. I'm doing Gerson – that's it. Please call and make me an appointment. I'm not looking any further. End of story."

And that's what we did. I went down to the Gerson Center in Mexico within a couple of weeks. My husband was managing a law firm at the time in Oakland, just outside of San Francisco, so my mother was my companion down there. Once I decided to do it, I put blinders on and I did exactly what I was told – exactly – and it was an incredible experience. They were cautiously optimistic, but they don't give you any guarantees. Truthfully, there aren't any in life, no matter what, absolutely not, which is something I always tell people, but it looked good. The main thing that they cautioned me about was not to take short-cuts. "Do everything that Doctor Gerson says to do – exactly the way he does it. Just trust in it." After a while, we added acupuncture, Bach Flower remedies and a few things like that, that work right along with it.

The clinic was fabulous and I was there for seven days. They prefer you to be there for two weeks at least, but at the time I could only stay for a week. I always recommend to people when they call me that if they decide to do it, they should definitely go to the clinic if they can, because you're with other people who are going through the same thing and you can talk to them. Charlotte[4] was there – that was great. The first enema (I don't think I'd ever had an enema before) was horrible. You learn how to do the therapy, you learn what the juices are like, and you learn about the diet. You certainly get a taste of what you're in for!

We came home and set up the kitchen. First, my mother did it for me, and then I learned how to do everything that needed to be done. I was very fortunate – this huge group of people from my church came and made juices, did shopping for all the groceries and everything. I had a lot of help and a lot of support – really, really a lot of fabulous support. Even with all of that, it's a very work-intensive therapy. You're doing 13 juices a day and five enemas, then every other day you're taking castor oil, which is kind of brutal. Eventually, we hired someone to help. I was on the therapy for two years solid. I had a few really close friends and an aunt who were just freaking out that I was doing this. What I realised is that people are just worried – they're scared. They're terrified because they think that the medical way is the only way to go. Well, it is the only way to go if you want to die, pretty much. If someone couldn't be supportive, or was being negative about it, my darling husband just wouldn't let them talk to me.

---

3 Tamoxifen is a medication used to treat oestrogen receptor-positive breast cancer.

4 Charlotte Gerson, Doctor Max Gerson's daughter who is a now-retired director of the Gerson Institute.

I had been a strict vegetarian from the time I was 19, and I was 45 when I found the cancer. I wasn't vegan, but I was a strict vegetarian. So to jump to being a vegan, which the therapy is in the beginning, wasn't that radical, except that my whole background is cooking and entertaining. I've had restaurants. So, to cut out all the herbs and spices and have pretty boring food was a real jump for me, but you get used to it.

The therapy cleanses every cell – every part of the body, including the brain, so that can be very emotional. Then you have these healing reactions. I had a high fever and felt sick, but it never lasted more than a few hours. You can take a bunch of aspirin or niacin, but that's all you can really take during those periods of time. Even though I did the therapy for a good solid two years, I only had two or three healing reactions, so I was fortunate. It was probably several months into the therapy before I had any reaction like that.

There were quite a few patients there when I was at the clinic – it's not just for cancer. I couldn't even tell you all the stories I've heard. People who've had brain tumours and were extremely successful, which you don't hear about much in the medical field. Stage four and stage five cancers that people had cures from and were still alive for many years – not just the five years they talk about; 10, 15, 20 years! I remember one young boy who had some sort of autoimmune disease – like the story of the boy in the bubble, who was allergic to everything? His parents had taken him to every place on the planet that could help him, until he got to Gerson.

I had a doctor who I was dealing with at the clinic. Every month I had blood work taken and the results were sent down to the clinic. They would analyse the blood studies and then modify my therapy according to what my blood was saying. There are cancer marker tests that you can take. What mystifies me about the whole medical profession is why don't they do that in the very beginning?

Within 60 days of doing the therapy, I was cancer free. I had no more cancer cells – they didn't show up. I thought: "Ooh, I'm this great anomaly, I don't have to do the therapy forever." They said: "No, no, Paula, this is a good sign, but you still have to do the therapy, because it's a total cleansing and rebuilding of your body so it can heal itself."

It was great that I was cancer free, and it's stayed that way. Charlotte would really like you to stay on the diet forever, but everybody's different. It took me three or four years after I was cured, or in remission, to get back to eating for me, what was a normal life. I was still vegetarian, but I'd have a glass of wine and eat things that Charlotte would prefer I didn't. I went back to wearing make up and colouring my hair – you know, living my life. I truly feel that you have to live your life to whatever's true to you.

Some people are perfectly happy staying on the therapy one hundred per cent of the time. I make it work for me and it's great. I have a couple of juices a day now – the carrot juice and a green drink. Occasionally I skip one, but for the most part I do. I've got my husband drinking celery juice right now because it's good for his blood pressure. I'm a juicer anyway, no matter what.

At first I had checkups every three months, then every six months, then once a year. I still get them about every 18 months, and everything's good. I know people who go back to their doctors after the therapy, but I wasn't willing to put myself through that anymore. When I walked out of that last door after my lumpectomy, I said, "I'm never going back," and I meant that. I've done blood studies and I have had scans. There's a women's health clinic near us, where one of the doctors there invented a new machine that's not as invasive as the PET[5] scan machine, it's just for the breast area. He would test me and I was always fine. That's all I've ever been willing to do. I know I'm fine and I've been fine for over 25 years.

There are a lot of other ways of curing cancer – Gerson is not the only one. I just happen to think that it's one of the most thorough, because it's not just for cancer, it's for almost anything. It's a total body cleansing. From the very beginning I had no faith in the medical system – number one. I had been exposed to lots of alternative ways of living life, eating and healing the body.

Cancer is not a fun thing to experience, but it's not the death sentence we've been trained to believe it is. That's how I feel, especially after going through the whole alternative thing. There are just so many other options out there. You can read so much about other ways of taking care of your body. However, as much as I am against what the medical profession does, I firmly believe that people should have a choice to do whatever they are comfortable with, for their own body. My only suggestion to the whole health field is that they give people an opportunity to make their own choice, instead of telling them what they have to do, to say, "Here, these are your options," instead of being so narrow in their system.

Over the years I've talked to hundreds of people on the phone who have been diagnosed with cancer, called the hotline[6] and are considering Gerson Therapy. Unfortunately, I would say most of them decide not to do it. Most people feel that it's too overwhelming and too much work. They're too frightened to go against their doctors. They're going through those dark moments of the soul when you question everything you're doing. A few are super interested, but for one reason or another can't do it one hundred per cent. I would say: "Incorporate. Do some cleansing with your treatment. If you're going to have radiation, put yourself on a juice protocol and change the way you're eating – at least for this period of time. Look at life from a bigger picture instead of that narrow little box that the powers that be try to fit us into."

---

5 PET – Positron Emission Tomography is an imaging technique in nuclear medicine that produces a three-dimensional image of the body and is widely used in oncology.

6 Gerson Therapy Hotline, run by successfully treated patients.

People really want something else, but in this age they're programmed that the guys in the white coats have the answers. Hey, I wish they did! I wish there was some magic pill that you could take and everything would be wonderful – I'd be at the front of the line. [*laughs*] But that's not the case. We have to do the work — at least that's the way things are now.

I kind of tricked my brain and psychologically made it easier for myself, because two years is a long time. I said: "Look Paula, it took your body 45 years to get into this shape. What's two years to the rest of my life?" That's nothing, when the chances were pretty good that I would make it. I was bound and determined. I was just about to have my first grandchild, I had just married my second husband and I had only been married for seven years. I thought: "Oh my God, I'm married to the perfect man – I'm not ready to go!"

Most people have absolutely no idea that there's anything else out there, but there's a lot out there. Nowadays, a little bit is starting to creep out. You hear it on talk shows and see it on the internet – that's one of the great things about the internet. You might get a lot of nonsense, but there's a whole wealth of information there.

A lot of people say: "Oh, that sounds great, I'm going to go and talk to my doctor." Then I say: "Well, you can do that, but they're not going to support you." There's probably one doctor in ten thousand that support a patient in doing something so completely off the beaten path. That's the way it is right now. It would just be lovely to have people open their minds up to trusting themselves, their intuition and their bodies. Don't give all your power away to somebody in a white coat who you think is in authority. I think that's so important and that's what we cancer survivors have done.

One of the things I tell people when they call the hotline is, "There will be plenty of times when you second-guess yourself." You think: "Oh my God, I'm going against everything that our society is claiming is the only way to cure cancer." Usually those kinds of things happen if you're having a down day, a healing reaction, or you don't feel good for whatever reason. Your brain starts to play tricks on you and makes you doubt what your decision is. That's human nature and you do that, no matter what path you decide to take. What I always did was just pick up the Gerson book and start reading it. When I read it I'd say: "Oh yeah, that's why I'm doing this, this is fine." I'd also talk to people and that would reaffirm the reason I was doing Gerson. There are no guarantees, but you do what they tell you as best you can. That's all we can do.

They don't tell people, but at Gerson they have way over a 70 per cent success rate – there's nowhere near that with the medical profession at this stage.

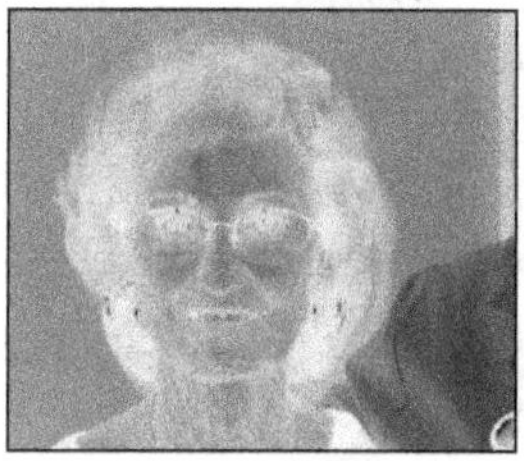

Mary Jo Bean, 77 years

Oklahoma, USA

Diagnosed with liver cirrhosis resulting from hepatitis C at 66 years

I was feeling wonderful – absolutely wonderful. I don't recall feeling any better and I weighed more (I'm a very thin, small person) than I'd ever weighed. My husband had just retired, so we were really looking for a life of travelling and just doing what we wanted to do for a change.

My father had passed away, and then my mother got very ill. In order to keep her out of a nursing home, I went to South Texas, 650 miles from where I live, and took care of her for two years. My husband would come every two weeks to visit me and spend the weekend and then he would come back home, because we had a small ranch and he had to take care of the cattle.

The last year I was down there, I felt myself going down, but my mother was a very difficult person to care for, and I just attributed my feeling so tired and run down to stress and being away from my husband. I finally talked my mother into moving about 50 miles from where we lived, so it would be closer and I could stay at home. That lasted a year and in that year I really, really went down. She was such a controlling and demanding person, it was very, very stressful.

After a month of going 50 miles over there every day to care for her, I physically collapsed and was deathly, deathly ill with horrible, horrible stomach pains. My husband rushed me to the emergency room at the nearest hospital. I was in the hospital two weeks and they ran all sorts of tests. This was in May of 2002, 11 years ago this coming May. The doctors just couldn't understand why I was in so much pain. They finally found out that I did have hepatitis C, but they didn't tell me that I had cirrhosis. They have since told me that if I had not gone through that stressful situation, most likely the hepatitis C would have never reared its ugly head, but the stress caused it to just escalate.

They decided to do an exploratory operation and see what was going on, because all the tests just showed the hepatitis. They got me in the surgery and discovered that the only part of my liver that was functioning was a very, very small part of the left lobe. The rest of it was like wood with cirrhosis. I had stage 4 cirrhosis of the liver. They told my husband and I that I must have had that for 25 to 30 years for it to be that bad. They assumed I got it [hepatitis C] from a blood transfusion, because in the fifties and sixties, I had a lot of blood transfusions, because then I was having surgeries for female problems. Back then they did not check the blood for hepatitis.

So the cirrhosis was caused by the hepatitis C. I was so naïve and so unlearned about all that – I always thought that you could not get cirrhosis unless you were a heavy drinker, and I was not even a social drinker. So I said, "I can't have cirrhosis – I'm not a drinker." And the doctors said: "That's not what this is. This has derived from the hepatitis. It has gotten so bad it is just eating your liver up."

They gave me two to 12 months to live, if I did not go on interferon.[1] Well, I not only didn't know anything about hepatitis and cirrhosis, but I didn't know anything about Interferon either. I was 66 years old at the time and I decided that if I was going to die, I was going to find out all that I could about what was going to kill me. I started doing research. I didn't have a computer at the time, I just had to read what I could and I was still sick as I could be. It was hard to really get it into my head at the times when I would feel like reading, but I did. I read everything and I went to a support group at the biggest hospital in Oklahoma City, which is near where I live, to just talk to people that had the disease and who were on the drug interferon. Everyone that I talked to, even big old healthy looking guys that were six foot one and two that had the disease, said that on that drug, when they took it, they had attempted suicide and that it messed with your mind. A family member had to stay with them at all times to keep them from killing themselves. I thought: "My stars, I don't want to put my husband through that. I'd rather be dead. I'm 66, I've raised my kids, I've had a good life – I'd rather be dead than to put him through that." So I refused to take the interferon. The doctors all just jumped on me every time I went in, that I needed to get on it. And I said: "It's my body, it's my life, it's my money and it's my choice, and I will do what I please and you will not control what I think." I stood my ground and it was a bitter, bitter fight. Every doctor that I saw just approached me with such animosity, because I refused it. They told me how stupid I was, and I said: "I'm not taking it! I'd rather be dead than put my husband through that." They just got angry with me.

Not one time did I pray and ask God to heal me. But I prayed and asked God to give me the wisdom to know what to do, because I didn't know. I knew what I was not going to do, and that was take interferon. But I didn't know what I was going to do. Every day I asked God to give me the wisdom.

I got so weak and I lost so much weight. I went down to about 75 pounds. I couldn't comb my hair, I couldn't dress myself, I couldn't do anything for myself. I felt like such a burden to my husband.

Seven months after my diagnosis (and they had given me two to 12 months to live), I would be in so much pain in my stomach sometimes that I would lay in bed and I'd say: "God, let me go to sleep and not wake up – just let me die in my sleep."

1 Interferon alpha is a synthetic form of a substance that some white blood cells make naturally in the body. These blood cells make interferon as an immune response against infection or cancer. Interferon stimulates the immune system by encouraging killer T cells. Side effects include tiredness, lowered white blood cells, flu-like symptoms, nausea, diarrhoea, depression, mood changes and anxiety.

I was always so active. I loved to be outside, I loved to work in the garden, I loved to paint and decorate, I loved to work with the cattle with my husband. I was very, very active. When my health was good, I got up early in the morning and I would be up until after midnight, just going like a house on fire. Everybody said: "You have more energy than anybody I've ever known." But all of a sudden, I couldn't do anything.

One day, when I was laying on the couch, I looked up at my husband and said: "I feel like such a burden to you. I don't know why God is letting me still live." He assured me that I wasn't a burden and I said: "Well I need to do *something*." So I said to him: "Hand me that stack of trash mail that's sitting over there on the desk and give me the trash can. Maybe I can at least go through the mail and see what's bad and throw it away." So he handed me this stack. You know how in the mail you get a lot of advertisements and pamphlets and stuff that you don't order? That's what was stacked up on the desk. He hands me this stack and he pulls the trash can over there by the couch. I picked up the very first one and the thought came to my mind: "Maybe there's something in here about liver disease." I looked through every page. There wasn't anything in there and I threw it in the trash and I picked up the next one. It was a small little pamphlet from a Doctor Julian Whittaker in California. I had never heard of him. I did not order the little pamphlet, I don't know how it got there – *it was over a year old*. But it was in with that stuff, the magazines and brochures. I picked it up, and instead of opening it on the very first page like I did the other ones, I opened it up in the middle where it's stapled and there on one side in bold letters, it spoke about a doctor in Las Cruces, New Mexico, that was treating liver disease with integrative treatment using Alpha Lipoic Acid (ALA) and having wonderful results. I read that little portion, I think it was about two paragraphs, and it told his phone number and everything, and he had a book out, *The Alpha Lipoic Acid Breakthrough*,[2] and I got cold chills. I felt like this is what I had to do. This is the treatment I'm supposed to take.

I'd never been to Las Cruces, New Mexico, I didn't know anything about it, I didn't know anything about integrative doctors. But I knew in my soul, that's what I had to do. I turned to my husband and I read him this little brochure and I said: "Would you go to Barnes and Noble, and get me this book?" They said that this book was for sale there. And he said: "I sure will," and he drove 60 miles to the Barnes and Noble store and got that book for me and brought it back.

I knew without a doubt in my mind, when I read *The Alpha Lipoic Acid Breakthrough* that Doctor Berkson wrote, that that was exactly the treatment that I had asked God to give me the wisdom to know about. I *knew* it.

I called the clinic and I made an appointment. Usually it was months before you could get in, especially a new patient. This was, I guess, about the middle of November when I called. They had a cancellation and they could get me in

2 *Alpha Lipoic Acid Breakthrough* by Burt Berkson, MD PhD.

by the 10th December. I said, "I'll be there."

By the time that December rolled around, I was so ill that I couldn't even brush my own teeth. We got in the car – it's 700 miles from where we live to Las Cruces – and we started out there to the clinic. We got 70 miles from home, I started crying and I said: "Just turn around and go back, I'm hurting so bad, I cannot make 700 miles, please just turn around. I'll just go home and die." My husband looked at me and he was never ever a man that was hateful, or talked cold, or talked insensitive to me – ever. He was the gentlest, kindest, most sacrificial man to me. And he looked at me, and he was stern. He said: "Just hush. This is our last hope and I'm not stopping until we get there, so just lean that seat back and be quiet." That's the only time in the 58 years that we were married (he has just recently passed) that he ever told me to hush, or spoke to me in that tone. But he did that day.

We drove up to that clinic and it was in the back of a little old Italian restaurant with one door going in it, and I thought: "My stars, what have we got ourselves into?" So did my husband. We thought he had to be a quack to have a tiny office like that. We were expecting a fancy big clinic, and here it is: one little old cubby hole thing in the back of an Italian restaurant! My husband said: "We're here, and we're not going to go back until we see that doctor."

I was so weak, I could not walk without my husband holding me, and I could barely talk above a whisper. We went into a little old teeny tiny waiting room that didn't have room for about seven little chairs. The doctor came in that front door just like we did – he didn't have a back door to sneak in. When the nurse bent over to give an IV,[3] her behind was sticking in somebody else's face – that's how tight a quarters it was.

We went in to see the doctor and he checked all of my records. In those records was that I had been given two to 12 months to live, and he looked at me and he said: "Mrs Bean, let me tell you something: only God knows when you're going to die." I just busted out crying, because every doctor I'd seen had given me no hope. Those words that he told me that day, "Only God knows when you're going to die," gave me hope and something to hold on to.

Then – I do not have any idea why I said it – I heard myself saying: "I would like to have a second opinion." Doctor Berkson looked me in the eye and without hesitation, he said, "Sure, I know a doctor here that would probably see you," and with that he picked up the phone and called a gastroenterologist in Las Cruces by the name of Doctor Padillo. He told Doctor Padillo that he had a 66-year-old lady in his office that would like a second opinion. Doctor Padillo told him to tell me to come in to his office at 7am the next morning and to bring my records. I had never heard of a doctor seeing a patient at 7am, but we were there at seven the next morning. Doctor Padillo looked over my records and he looked at my husband and I, and he said: "Mrs Bean, let me tell you

3 IV – intravenous drip.

something. First of all, you are a very sick woman, and next," and he shook his finger at me, "you are very *wise* to be seeing Doctor Berkson. I have watched him for years, known patients before he saw them and after he treated them, and he knows what he is doing. Go back to Doctor Berkson and do what he says." He asked me a few more questions and stopped and repeated what he had said about me being wise to come to Doctor Berkson. My husband and I got up to leave his office. We had our backs to him going out the door and Doctor Padillo said, "Mrs Bean," I turned around to see him shaking that finger at me again, "did you hear what I said? You are very wise to be going to Doctor Berkson. He will help you". We went to the car and I started crying and I told my husband, "Did you catch what he was saying? I never once prayed and asked God to heal me, I prayed and asked Him for wisdom to know what to do. Doctor Padillo told me three times this morning that I was wise to come to Doctor Berkson. Is that confirmation that God brought me here and planned this or not?" I knew then without a doubt that I was doing exactly what I was supposed to be doing, and God had answered my prayers.

Later that same day, I went back to see Doctor Berkson and I started my vitamin and supplement regimen and the diet that he recommends. I started all of it that day. My system was so bad, that instead of 1000ccs[4] of ALA, I could only take 40ccs. That's all I was able to handle. They start with a low amount and when they give it to you, if you have a reaction, then they know that there's a problem. I stayed two weeks, and the first week I took 40ccs once a day. The next week, they upped it and I was able to take, I think, 200ccs that time.

The first day, after I took the treatment, I went back to the motel and just fell down on the bed and slept like a baby. I had not been able to sleep at night in ages. I just slept and slept and slept and the next day, the same thing. The third day, after my treatment, I felt so replenished, rejuvenated, energised and so much stronger that I asked my husband: "Can you take me to Walmart?" I didn't walk all over the store by any means, I just walked a little ways, but it was such an improvement! It was a drastic improvement.

We stayed two weeks, and when we got home, my husband unloaded our luggage and I started doing laundry. I had not been able to do anything in months. We got home about 4:30 that afternoon, and before I went to bed that night, I had done all of our laundry and dried it, ironed it and put in the closet. That was after two weeks treatment.

The next day, I got up that morning and I couldn't wait to clean my house. My daughter had been coming over to clean it, but she and I didn't clean houses alike and I wanted to do deep cleaning. So I got busy and I dusted and I vacuumed and I mopped. I even climbed up and cleaned all of the ceiling fans. That was the first full day that I was at home.

From the start, I took 600mgs of Alpha Lipoic Acid each day orally and all

4 1000ccs = 1000millilitres, or one litre.

of the vitamins and supplements that he has all of his patients on. You never ever take Alpha Lipoic Acid without B complex, because every time you take the Alpha Lipoic Acid it will deplete your body of B vitamins. It depends on each patient to a degree, but basically the liver patients are all on the same protocol, depending on the issues you have with your health.

I've never been a pill-popper. It was very hard for me to take all of that stuff, because I took most of them three times a day. I would take about ten or 12 at a whack and I could hardly swallow those things. He does not use the tablets, he uses capsules, because he says that your body does not absorb as much of the tablets, or the pills, as we call them here. You will come nearer getting rid of it in body waste, so he recommends capsules only. Some people have lactose or vegetable allergies and stuff like that, so you can get the capsules that hold that powder in different forms. He really, really checks each supplement. The cheap brands – they're so full of fillers and a lot of those fillers come out of China, and that is bad stuff. People say: "Oh, those supplements are so expensive – I'm going to get mine at Walmart or the dollar store or whatever." Well, they can be hurting themselves very, very bad. I'm not on all that stuff now.

Two months later, I went back to Las Cruces and stayed another two weeks, but my husband did not drive me. I drove myself! I took another lady who was as sick as I was when I went the first time, and I took care of her for two weeks. The change was unbelievable.

It was three months before I went back again, and I got to where I went back twice a year. It's very expensive for me to make that trip, because of the travelling, and you have your lodging, your food and then of course your treatment. Our insurance doesn't pay a penny of it. All of that cost comes out of your pocket and it really runs into a lot of money. The IV treatment itself costs $125, then you have about $20 for the B complex shot and they recommend that you take two treatments a day, so that would be $270 a day. Then you have your consultation with the doctor. You have tons and tons of lab work and that is what is so costly.

Doctor Berkson does more lab work than any doctor I've ever heard of, but he explains every single bit of it to you. You know what every lab test is for and what it means. If you're out of line in any way on a test, he knows what you're doing, or what your body's doing, and what's caused that. If you get off of your diet, say your iron content goes flying up, which is a bad thing if you've got liver disease, he knows that you're eating something you're not supposed to. You won't sneak anything by him, I guarantee you that.

The diet that he had me on was six half-cup servings of green vegetables a day and you can eat all kinds of other vegetables. He recommends half a cup of wholegrains a day and no iceberg lettuce or beets, because iceberg lettuce has no food value and beets are so full of iron. I could have most proteins and half a cup of most fruits per day. Fluids: six to eight glasses of filtered water per day, no more than two cups of coffee a day. Avoid all processed food, peanuts in any form, milk by the glass, salty food, soft drinks – especially diet drinks, alcohol, white flour, margarine, sugar, grapefruit and painkillers. He recommends plenty of exercise, rest and 15 minutes of sunshine every day. When he gave me a copy of that, I said: "Gee, in other words, if it's good and I like it, I can't have it." [*laughs*] He's real funny and he laughed at me.

It was so funny, because I always loved almond Hershey's bars. I'd been going, oh, about eight or nine months or something like that, and I was just craving Hershey's Bars something fierce. So I asked him one day when I was there, I said: "Doctor Berkson, do you think it's going to kill me if I ate a Hershey's Bar?" He looked at me and grinned and he said: "Nah, you can have one, once in a while." So I bought one and do you know, I kept it for a year before I ate it. My friend said: "What did you buy the thing for? I thought you were starving for one." I guess it's one of those things that if you can't have it, you want it, and then when you get it, you realise that it's not that good for you and you shouldn't eat it.

At one time, I loved liver. Fried liver and onions, with cream gravy and hot biscuits – I just loved it. Of course, it's full of iron and you can't have it. I'd been going out there [to Las Cruces] a couple of years and I was just craving some liver so bad I thought I'd die if I didn't have it. I called the nurse and I said: "Linda, next time you see Doctor Berkson in the hall, corner him and ask him if I can have a little bit of liver, please?" She laughed at me and she called back and said: "He said that if you thought you was going to die if you didn't get it, go ahead and eat some." Well, I had a piece of liver in the freezer about as big as my hand. I took it out and I salted it and peppered it and floured it and I put it in the skillet with some oil and some onions, and then I thought: "Whoever heard of eating liver without good old cream gravy and hot biscuits?" So I just fixed me a big old biscuit and a big pan of gravy and set out and I made a pig out of myself. I thought I'd die in about 30 minutes. Oh my stars! Well, it was two weeks before I went out there and he walks into the office and he has my file in his hand and he has this big old grin on his face, and he says: "Well dear, how was the liver and onion?" And I said, "Don't ask." And he said, "Jo, how was the liver and onions?" And I said: "Don't ask. I thought I was going to die!" He laughed so hard. He said, "Well, do you want any more?" I said, "No sir, that did it."

He says that every so often you can have something decadent. Don't deprive yourself all the time, but stay within reason and don't make a pig of yourself. He said that if you know that you're going to be going out to dinner with friends and would want to eat something that's not on the diet, then stay on that diet all week, real good. Then on the weekend when you go out to eat, then you can eat something that you're not supposed to. But don't deprive yourself all the time, because that stresses you and that causes you as much problem as anything else. He's very, very easy to work with.

After about eight months, my lab work and all the scans were showing that my liver was rebuilding itself and my liver did not show cirrhosis any more. That tells you the treatment works.

I would have been a liver transplant candidate if I had been younger. You see, I was 66 when I was diagnosed. They're not too helpful in doing that for an old person. [*laughs*] I don't know if I would have gone through it either. Looking back and everything, I felt that I had had a wonderful life. God had been good to me. My husband was one of the greatest guys that ever was, and I just felt that I had been so blessed to have him, and I could not in any way have asked for more. That's just the way that I felt. So I don't think that I would have gone through a transplant. In this country, it is horribly expensive and many insurances won't touch it.

I've had little flare-ups, like when I quit caring for mother. I would have a flare-up sometimes when she would really get on a rampage. Then one of my sisters started doing it. We have some adopted boys that pulled some very, very stressful things, so when I would get in a stressful situation, I would have a flare-up. During my flare-ups, I would get stomach pains and sometimes I would have chest pains, which were not related. It felt like it was the hepatitis C, but my lab numbers didn't go up, so I don't know if it was just a reaction or what. I didn't go get extra treatment then.

Some people can let stress roll off them, like one of my sisters. It just rolls off her like water off a duck's back. She just doesn't let things stress her. I am of a different nature. In between that I would work, except for the times when stress would overwhelm me. I even got on the roof and did roofing when I was 72 years old.

At the same time, my husband got Alzheimer's. For the last five years, I had been his caregiver until he passed away in October 2012. He had a horrible, horrible lung disease. We didn't know he had it until June and he died a horrible death. All of that stress caring for him. I don't know, that was different somehow, I guess because the love was so great. I handled that without one single solitary type of medication, not even when I watched him die. They didn't even give me a medication for nerves or anything. I wanted to always be in control of my faculties, my senses and my emotions with him. But the other things: mother and the boys, stressed me something fierce.

I still have treatment. The last time I was out at the clinic was last May and I got IVs then. It was usually twice a year, or every seven or eight months I would go. I guess I had been going to him for two years when he put me on Low Dose Naltrexone (LDN),[5] the reason being that I was having a lot of problems when I would get up at night to go to the bathroom. My ankles would hurt. They give that for MS[6] and a lot of things and he said, well, maybe the LDN would help

5 Low Dose Naltrexone is the off-label prescription of the FDA approved drug *Naltrexone*.

6 MS – multiple sclerosis.

that – and it did. I'm 77 now and I don't have any joint pain. Also, the LDN is a cancer deterrent, you know. You can take that for $35 and you get 90 pills and you take one at bed time. That's very inexpensive. By the same token, he wants to monitor you. He's not going to give you a prescription if he doesn't see you. I know so many people that are on it for all kinds of things: cancer, Lupus, MS, ALS.[7] You name it and it has helped them, so why would I not take it if I have the opportunity? He's the only doctor that I know around that will give me a prescription. A lot of the doctors, they just do not want to have anything to do with it. They're very fearful.

There's a doctor that practises just seven miles from me and I asked him about getting the ALA and told him how he could order it out of Germany and what have you, and I had the protocol. When I asked him if he would please give it to me, he didn't even want to discuss it, or he'd get kicked out of the clinic. I said: "Look, you can see what it's done for me. Think of the people here, just in this small area, that have liver disease – and that's not all that it treats. It treats all of these other diseases." But he wouldn't discuss it. He said, "No, no, no, it's integrative – uh-uh, uh-uh."

Medical insurance and medical costs here are astronomical – they're horrible. I was in the hospital for four days with one of those gallbladder flare-ups and with chest pain – and it was $29,000. No surgery, just tests. People can't do it.

My daughter didn't go to the doctor with her kidney stones, because she didn't have insurance. She quit her job to come here and help me take care of her daddy and she didn't have any money for medical care. Someone from my support group told me about this stuff called *Chanca Piedra* ('stone crusher' in Spanish) from South America. It is very inexpensive. My daughter had been in bed for three weeks suffering unmercifully and had done everything she could think of. She took *Chanca Piedra* capsules and the next day she could feel that moving around – it was painful. On the third day, she said that she cramped really bad all of a sudden, then she went to the bathroom and it was just like chalk water that she passed out of her kidneys. And that was it – she got better.

I got an email from a man that's been in the hospital for nearly a week, and he's got a $90,000 hospital bill. He has a terminal blood disorder and he doesn't know how he's going to pay it. People are that way all over the country. But ALA can help people. If they can't afford the IVs, they can at least afford the supplements and the vitamins, and they can go on the diet and build their immunity back up.

I have a support group and I am in contact with a lot of people who have read about my situation. They could have a family member, or they themselves have some sort of a terminal or debilitating disease, and they contact me. I send them the recommended diet and the list of the vitamins, supplements, brands and tell them what I was on in the beginning. Then it's up to them to do what they

---

7 ALS – amyotrophic lateral sclerosis, also known as motor neurone disease, or Lou Gehrig's disease.

think. If they don't have the money to go out to Las Cruces, they can at least help themselves that way. I cannot tell them what to do, I'm not about to do that. All I can do is say: "Here's what was wrong with me, here's what I did about it, here's what I took and here's where I'm at now. You draw your own conclusions."

I love the clinic, it just has been my life. I still have ALA twice a year. I don't know what would happen if I didn't have it. It will not hurt you – it builds your immune system. When you get to about 40, your body stops making as much of it as it did. So ALA will benefit anybody who's over 40. It's wonderful. I've had 11 years that I would not have had.

I'm doing fine. Physically, I'm doing great. This last week, I built shelves in the garage – three of them about eight foot long. I carried a bunch of tools – heavy tools and stuff from the shop – and moved a big old stack of lumber. This morning I cleaned house. My house is 2700 square foot and I dusted and vacuumed and mopped and all of that – the whole house.

So many people my age are in a nursing home. I can do everything. I have a huge, huge yard. I can mow it, I can run a weed-eater, I can load the pick-up with hay, I can do whatever I want to. It may take me a little longer, because I have to sit down every once in a while and take a breather. But my goodness, at my age, I'm entitled to take a breather! I drive myself to the doctor, I drive myself wherever I want to go and do whatever I please. People tell me I look 55.

When people asked me: "Did you feel you were sentenced to die, or did you get angry over this diagnosis and resentful?" I said: "No, because after I went to Doctor Berkson and started getting better so fast and everything, I felt that this disease was not a curse, it was a blessing, because it has brought so many people into my life that would never have been there otherwise." It has allowed me to do research on things that I had never dreamed of, and to widen my horizons as far as knowledge goes. Most of all, it has allowed me to help people. That's what we're supposed to do.

Every one of us has a purpose, and I thought for many years that mine was to be a wife and a mother. But I think our purposes change, just like the seasons. So when I was diagnosed, I think God spared me and He allowed me to be so stubborn about refusing the conventional doctor's treatment, because He had a plan for me. He has a plan for all of us.

You feel something that you've never felt before – it's hard to describe. You get in that rut and you know you're in the right place. It's like a stack of dominoes, and really, it blows my mind. The first time that I got a call from someone that I didn't know was from a lady in British Colombia. This lady called me one night, about 11 o'clock. She had heard about me from someplace and gotten my phone number and she called me. I was amazed, I couldn't believe this. Then it seemed like it just snowballed. Now, it's nothing to have people from Taiwan, Japan, Singapore, Hawaii and all these different countries to call me at all hours. I've had men that had heard about me and would call at two in the morning threatening suicide, because they were in so much pain and feeling so hopeless. I had no training to talk to these people; all I have is my heart. But you know what? Sometimes that's all they want. That's all they need, somebody to listen and to care. I talk with them for two hours on the phone in the middle of the night and get them to the place where they're not going to overdose on something and make them feel like they have a purpose in life – that they're worthwhile and they're worth something.

I just am so thankful that it found me and that God led me to it. When I go out there to the clinic and they have me speaking to all of the new patients and everything, I tell them: "Every person that comes in this clinic, in my estimation, has been tapped on the shoulder by God, with something special." He can show us what to do, but He's not going to do it for us. We have to put forth some effort too.

There's nothing more gratifying than reaching out to someone in pain with a disease, and have him grab your hand, and you know in your heart that you've been able to help him just one little bit.

Acute Hepatitis C Virus (HCV) infection is difficult to detect because of the generally asymptomatic nature of the disease and the marginalization of at-risk populations. Around 25% of patients with acute HCV infection undergo spontaneous clearance. The remaining 75% of patients progress to chronic HCV infection and are subsequently at risk of progression to hepatic fibrosis, cirrhosis and hepatocellular carcinoma. Chronic hepatitis C generally progresses slowly in the initial two decades, but can be accelerated during this time as a result of advancing age and co-factors such as heavy alcohol intake and HIV co-infection.

(Nat Rev Gastroenterol Hepatol. 2013 Sep;10(9):553-62. doi: 10.1038/nrgastro.2013.107. Epub 2013 Jul 2)

The identification of the hepatitis C virus (HCV) in 1989 solved a growing mystery. Large numbers of hepatitis victims had begun to appear, apparently with a virally caused disease. But when examined, these patients tested negative for both hepatitis A and B. The unknown disease was known as non-A, non-B hepatitis. When a test was developed in 1990 to identify individuals infected with hepatitis C, hepatitis C was found to be responsible for the majority of these cases – and it has quickly proved to present a frightening challenge.

In contrast to most other types of hepatitis, 50-85% of hepatitis C infections become chronic and lead to liver disease. Hepatitis C, in combination with hepatitis B, now accounts for 75% of all cases of liver disease around the world. Liver failure due to hepatitis C is a leading cause of liver transplantation in the United States; in all fairness: the majority of these patients have had significant alcohol abuse during a stage of their lives as well.

Since hepatitis C infection is typically mild in its early stages, it is often not diagnosed, or diagnosed in the context of screening of blood donors or testing as part of the application for various types of insurance. HCV is otherwise often not recognized until its chronic stages when it has caused severe liver disease. With a typical cycle of disease from infection to symptomatic liver disease taking as long as 20 years, the true impact of this disease on our growing infected population became more apparent after decades. For this reason, it is often referred to as the "silent epidemic".

It is suspected that there are, at present, more than 4.5 million people in the United States that are infected with hepatitis C, and more than 200 million around the world – making it one of the greatest public health epidemics of our time. We continue to detect new patients with HCV infection and late complications that show up years after the initial event.

Without interventions to treat infected populations and prevent the spread of the disease, the death rate from hepatitis C tends now to surpass that of AIDS. With the impressive control gained in the treatment of HIV infection, HIV-infected patients that have died in the past from a variety of other conditions, including opportunistic infections, outlive this infection, but may well die from the consequences of HCV infection.

(Everett Coop Institute http://www.epidemic.org/thefacts/hepatitisc/silentEpidemic/)

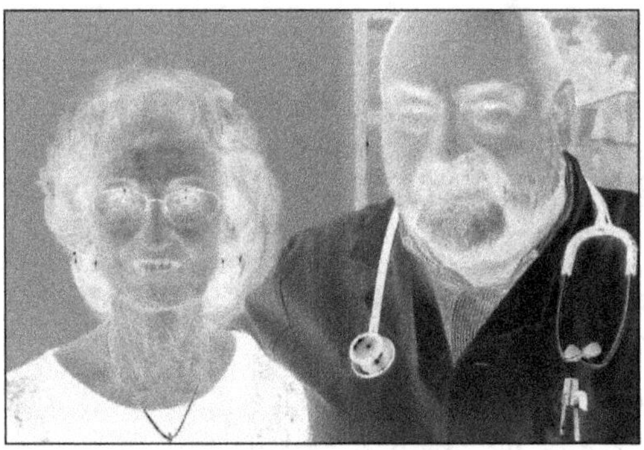

Mary Jo Bean with Doctor Berkson at the Integrative Medical Center, Las Cruces.

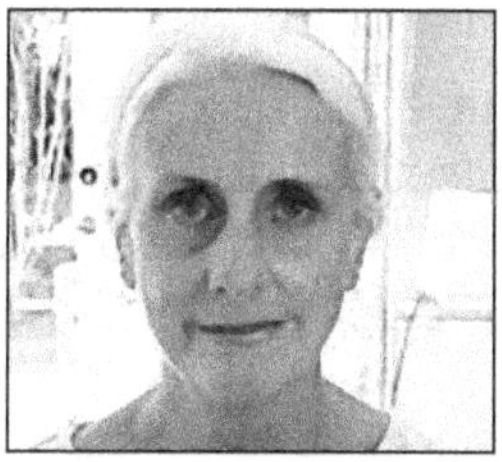

Fairlie Bekker, 53 years

New South Wales, Australia

Life-long allergies

I can remember having problems with allergies from when I was about seven or eight – mostly hay fever, which I really suffered with. When the wind was blowing from the West, my parents had to kept me inside with all the windows and doors shut.

I used to dread the summers. Teachers would send me home from school because my whole being was taken up with dealing with hay fever. I couldn't talk to anyone who tried to speak to me because I was too busy sneezing. My eyes were so swollen and itchy I could barely see out of them – they have always been my biggest problem. I was the most allergic to cats, guinea pigs were bad, also flowers, plants, grass and house dust. I was just a wreck.

Mum and Dad took me to the doctor, who gave me a blue tablet – apparently one of the first antihistamines, which Mum said made me so cranky, she never gave it to me again. [*laughs*] She said I was a really happy, easy-going child, but with one of those tablets I was a horror. Eczema was a problem too – the chemist would mix up this strong-smelling sticky pink cream for me. It worked wonders, but it stunk.

As a child, I was also mucousy on the chest and suffered a lot with chest infections, laryngitis, bronchitis, tonsillitis, and I got a lot of ear infections. When we moved inland to a farm in Nowra, every summer I went through the same thing with my allergies – severe hay fever with rashes on the inside of my arms and behind my knees. They continued right through my childhood until I left home and went to America.

In California, I never suffered once from hay fever in the three and a half years I was there. Not one attack. I didn't suffer from it when I toured around Europe and England either. I didn't have hay fever again until I came home, four years later. As soon I hit the shores of Australia, back came the hay fever. Obviously, it was the fauna or flora or something. I was probably the least reactive when I was living in Wollongong, near the coast.

I did go to a herbalist who told me to stay off dairy. It was then I realised that during the years I'd spent in America, I had very little dairy. My mum was always keen on us having healthy bones, so cream and milk was shoved down us every day, which probably didn't help when I was living at home. Once I went off the dairy, it helped heaps. My symptoms were mostly gone for a few years and after a while I could have little bits of dairy again.

When I was around 25, my hay fever came back and I have had allergies off and on since then. Hiking in the bush in summer would set me off. I had to stay away from cats, guinea pigs and horses. Horses were okay most of the year, except in the summer months when they gave off a lot of dander. I had to be so careful to wash my hands and face if I was near them. Rashes would come and go in any season.

My stomach has always been erratic and uncomfortable. I'd have cramping and diarrhoea, with regular visits to the toilet. I don't know what that was down to. The only time I noticed that it lessened was when I was off dairy products.

I went to get some blood tests from the doctors to see if they could tell me anything about what was going on, but they came back pretty much negative. My doctor would say: "Oh, just keep up with cortisone cream for the rashes, antihistamines for the hay fever, plus the nasal sprays and preservative-free antihistamine eye drops for your itchy eyes."

My allergies made me tired and cranky. Although I was always active, I was often tired and never had much energy. I loved my sports, but I did find that they had to be put on hold a lot of the time, unless I was in the water, where I was fine.

I *still* dreaded summers – as soon as I heard the cicadas I used to panic, because it meant that summer was coming. I would have to try to avoid being out in the hot weather, windy areas, or the bush – summer was usually one big blur.

I seemed to never have really developed any social skills, because I was wrapped up in the way I was feeling a lot of the time. I found it easier to live in my own little world and deal with my own little allergies. My nature is probably withdrawn anyway, but that didn't help. Friends used to get irritated with my sneezing and itchy nose. There were so many things I couldn't do, so I've never been very sociable.

The next stage of my allergy attacks was in my early forties, when rashes started to appear on my hands. For a few years they'd come regularly, and then for a few years they'd disappear again. By now, there were more antihistamines available, so I set myself up with allergy tablets and nasal sprays, so I could pretty much control my life.

When I hit my fifties, the rashes became more regular and I really started to go downhill. I started to feel more and more effects that would actually make me feel ill. Pretty much the whole year I had rashes on my hands, my fingers were swollen nearly all the time and I have been completely covered in a rash each summer. As soon as the warm weather hit, the rashes would spread up my arms, onto my face, the back of my neck and across the back of my shoulders. Not my legs though – they were fine.

As I was getting worse and worse, I went for more and more tests to see if anyone could figure out what was going on, but no-one could come up with any explanation. I tried to get the doctors to give me allergy tests, but the majority of them said they were a waste of time: "They never tell you anything anyhow." Out of the three doctors I asked, not one of them would do allergy tests for me.

When my skin got really, really bad, one doctor thought it could be Lupus[1] and sent me to a dermatologist, who did another series of blood tests and skin biopsies, but she couldn't figure out what it was either, because there was no clear reading – nothing showed up. She was going to put me on immunosuppressants and corticosteroid tablets. I knew corticosteroids were bad for the bones, so I told her that I didn't want to go on them, because my mum had osteoporosis and rheumatoid arthritis. I didn't want to take anything like that. She said: "Well then, we could just start immunosuppressants."

I saw a naturopath, who put me on a homeopathic medicine, which really helped with the hay fever, but the rashes continued. I went away and I thought: "Okay, maybe I should just start taking another food out of my diet. I got serious and I took myself off all wheat, and the rash pretty much vanished for a while.

Then the naturopath gave me some homeopathic Sulphur, which worked wonders. Because the heat has always aggravated my rashes, I have always had to find cool areas or touch something cool. The Sulphur actually took a lot of that burning heat out of me and the rashes settled right down for quite a while. My stomach started to feel better as well. Then all of a sudden, there was another massive flare-up and the Sulphur wasn't helping anymore.

Every time I played tennis, my eyes would flare up terribly. I could feel heat in my eyelids, then they'd start to swell and I'd have to get off the court. After the swelling settled down they looked terrible – they were purple and it looked like I had eye shadow on. It would happen about ten or 15 minutes after I'd been on the court. I got a homeopathic eye-allergy medicine that enabled me to play for 20 minutes. If I took three doses – one before I went onto the court, one during the game and one afterwards, my eyes would still swell up a bit, but I could keep them from getting totally out of hand. Now, if I feel a little bit of itch coming on, even just putting some of those drops on my finger and dabbing it on my eyes, takes the itch and swelling straight out of them. Any time I get itchy, watery, swollen eyes, I use the eye allergy drops and they get back to normal more quickly than using antihistamine drops. It's just amazing. Once, I accidentally put a bit too much on my eyelids and it ran into the corner of my eye and burned like crazy. I thought: "Oh no, more redness in my eyes," but when I went to the mirror, I could see the redness *in my eye* fading. I can't do without that stuff.

Because I was better when I went off dairy, my naturopath mentioned an IgG food sensitivity panel[2] that would test me for 93 foods. It came back that

1 Lupus is an autoimmune disease where the immune system becomes hyperactive and attacks healthy tissue, causing inflammation, swelling and damage to joints, skin, kidneys, blood, heart and lungs.

2 IgG, or Immunoglobulin G Food Sensitivity Panel, is a blood test that identifies sensitivity reactions to a range of foods.

there were 20 foods showing up that I was reacting to, which was one big shock. [*laughs*] The foods you test sensitive to are given a grade of one to four, depending on the level of your reaction. Anything that's a two or over, you have to avoid eating completely for six months. Egg white was really high.

After avoiding the foods that I tested positive for, I felt better and more energetic, but a bit cranky, because I couldn't eat the foods I wanted to! Shopping for food and eating out was a nightmare, but I didn't want to go back to where I had been, so I was pretty careful about what I ate.

Then I started NAET[3] treatments, which involved treating one food at a time: staying off it for a while, and then retesting to see if I was still sensitive to it or not. The treatments themselves were good – not painful at all and relaxing, but the next day they did make me feel pretty tired and cranky. I would be depressed and teary for about a day, pretty much after every treatment. The day after that, I'd feel a little bit better, and then I'd get back to normal after about three days. There's no way I could have handled more than one treatment a week.

We worked our way through the 20 foods over about eight months. We pretty much went through the list, and after about six months, started reintroducing more of the restricted foods a little bit at a time. Peas and corn didn't have an effect on me anymore. Sometimes I'd have a reaction and would need to stay off a particular food for longer, then try it again. Gradually, I wouldn't have any reaction. It was like my immune system was being dulled down.

Now, if I go out to dinner, and someone says, "Okay, this is what there is to eat," I reckon I could eat everything on that plate and not have a major meltdown. I might feel a little bit funny in the stomach the next day, because I had eaten too much of something, but it's a major advantage knowing that my rashes aren't going to flare up.

I have never been free of hay fever and allergic eyes my whole life, except when I'm out of Australia – but now, with the homeopathic treatment, it's gone. I don't know how long the food allergies had been with me – I might have always been sensitive to those foods and just never realised.

Compared to the last few years, when I was a complete mess and looked like a swollen, perspiring, itchy bubble, I haven't had any allergies. I might sneeze three times and think: "Oh no, something's got me," but then there's no more reaction. My eyes might get a little bit itchy, then half an hour later, I feel fine. Nothing has flared up again, and I'm heading into December, which is always my worst time of year. The rashes on my hands still flare up every now and then, but they don't go past my wrists anymore.

It's really been a combination treatment of homeopathy, dietary restriction, supplements and NAET, which have worked wonders on me. I feel like my

3 NAET – Nambudripad's Allergy Elimination Technique is a natural method of effectively treating a wide range of sensitivities and allergies. http://www.naet.com/

immune system has been stabilised and is more balanced. It doesn't just climb onboard and then go overboard like it used to. [*laughs*]

For the past five years, starting at five o'clock in the morning, I would get red cheeks and they would stay bright red until half past nine at night, for no reason at all. Everyone used to ask if I had high blood pressure, or had been drinking! I haven't had that at all in the last few months – my cheeks and body temperature have cooled right down and I'm not red in the face. Now I hate the cold weather and love the heat!

It's been an amazing trip – the hardest part was staying with it. Some people say you can never get over allergies, but I have. If you want something to work, you have to stick with it. If you can even feel a little bit of improvement you've got to keep giving it a go – especially when you're desperate and no-one else has got any answers. It might take a little bit longer, but sometimes it works really quickly, like the homeopathic Sulphur – that was a pretty good reaction straight-off. Some of the other allergies we just had to work at.

Now I don't have reactions or irritability, and I don't have to take medicines for anything. I can enjoy food and enjoy the outdoors. I'm not so scared of summers now and I can go hiking in the bush. It's been life-changing.

If I had gone through normal channels, none of this would have happened – I would have been on immunosuppressants and a series of medicines for the rest of my life.

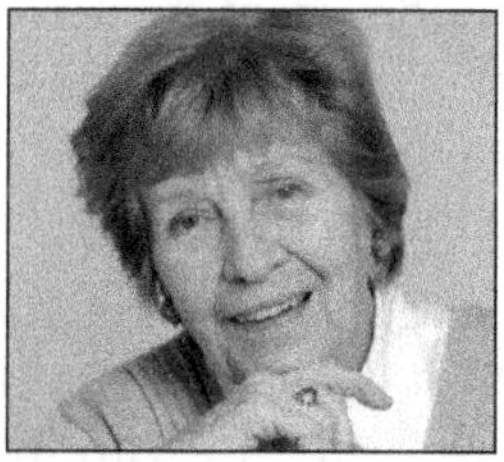

Beata Bishop

London, England

Diagnosed with malignant melanoma in 1979

I was at the peak of my career with the BBC[1] as a feature writer and I had what I considered a very good life. My lifestyle obviously wasn't very good, otherwise I wouldn't have fallen ill. I worked terribly hard. I was a vegetarian and I ate what I had to. There was a lot of stress, but that's normal in journalism. Without stress, you wouldn't have a job anyway.

Then suddenly I had this diagnosis in November 1979, a very long time ago, which absolutely shook me. I was told that I had malignant melanoma and that I had to be operated on immediately, full stop. It was a very small tumour on my right leg, but it was quite ugly. So I had surgery, where an enormous piece of my leg was cut out. Then a skin graft was made from my left thigh, so then I had two useless legs and both hurt like hell. It took me a couple of months to recover sufficiently to walk properly. If you have two bad legs, there isn't a lot that you can do.

My oncology surgeon was very nice, a very humane person, and we got on well. After my operation, he said: "Resume your life where you left it off," which was the worst possible advice he could have given me, because it meant going back to the lifestyle in which I became ill. I was a heavy smoker as well. So I went back to my job and everything was fine. I just had to go back to my oncologist every two months for a check-up, which I did.

Then in early December 1980, just a year after the surgery, he found a lump in my right groin, which was on the same side where the original tumour had been. The atmosphere changed immediately – he became very depressed. He said: "Well, it could be harmless, but perhaps it's a recurrence. If so, we'll have to remove it, but let's wait a few weeks." It was just before Christmas and as you can imagine, I was terribly, terribly frightened.

At the time, melanoma wasn't as well known as it is now. Now, most people know that it's a deadly form of skin cancer. But then, I had to do all my own research to find out what it was all about. Having done that, I knew that once melanoma spreads from the original site, there's practically nothing you can do about it.

1 BBC – British Broadcasting Corporation.

I went back to my oncologist after Christmas and the lump was still there, so he said that he would have to operate, remove all the lymph nodes from the groin and see what else he had to do. I refused a biopsy. I thought: "The first operation didn't solve the problem and the second one would weaken me even more, and what if it spreads further?" So I said, "No," and I wanted to think about it.

I was absolutely determined not to continue with just surgery, because the human body is not like a piece of meat, where you cut off a bit here and a bit there and hope for the best. Then, through the grace of God and with the help of my best friend, we found a link to the Gerson therapy, which is based on nutrition. The idea is to detoxify the body and bring it back to as good a condition as possible, so it can heal itself.

So thinking that this therapy makes sense, I took my life into my own hands – surgery doesn't make sense. What was so convincing in the thinking of Doctor Gerson, who was a highly qualified orthodox doctor by the way (he died in 1959), was that he departed from the conventional thinking about cancer and said that the disease is not a 'thing', namely the tumour. It's a process involving the whole body. The tumour is just a symptom, so if you concentrate on the tumour and don't do anything else, the disease will recur, which is exactly what happened to me. All that chopping off, and if it comes up in a third place, then what? If it gets into the brain, which it very often does, do they cut your head off? So I decided to try this therapy, which sounded crazy to my friends and family. I said: "Sorry, that's what I'm going to do." My bosses at the BBC were incredibly helpful. Afterwards, they told me that they thought I was going to die anyway, so they might just as well be nice to me.

I went to the world's only Gerson clinic[2] in Mexico and I was there for almost two months and underwent this very, very strict therapy. Then I came back to London and continued at home until March 1983, which is exactly 30 years ago. As you can see, I am here and am very well, thank you! That convinced me that the whole official attitude to cancer is deficient, precisely because they don't deal with the process. In cancer, the whole body is involved and if you don't heal the whole body, it will come back. Look at all the cases you hear about in your own circle – friends, relatives, who get the best treatment there is. Then six months, one year or two years later – bang, the cancer comes back and they die very quickly. That's a very sad confirmation of what Doctor Gerson discovered.

I discovered that I had diabetes at that time, but I didn't know about it until a doctor in London had my blood and urine test done. He gave me the news that I had early stage diabetes type 2, which was quite a shock.

I knew that I had incipient arthritis in my right hand, which I inherited from my mother, because she too had it. My fingers were already getting a bit distorted and deformed. When I went to the Gerson clinic I was examined and

2 *The Gerson Clinic* http://gerson.org/gerpress/gerson-health-centre

questioned, and I mentioned the diabetes and asked what they were going to do about that, and the Gerson doctor said: "Nothing, it will go." I thought she was stark raving mad, but after three weeks on the intensive therapy, I had no diabetes and my hands had no arthritis in them.

When I say intensive therapy, I mean it. The therapy consists of a very strict diet, which is vegan for the first six weeks. Only organic food is consumed – nothing else. You have 13 glasses of freshly made juice, on the hour, every hour of the day. On the intensive, you have three very good meals plus the 13 glasses of juice that have to be made freshly and drunk immediately. You can't make a gallon and put it in the fridge, which makes it a very labour-intensive therapy as you can imagine. The detoxification is done by coffee enemas, about which most people say: "What?" In the beginning, there are five coffee enemas a day, to detoxify the liver. Every other day there is castor oil, which was a dreadful part of my childhood [*chuckles*], but you get used to that too. So what you're doing is on the one hand you build up the body with the juices and the food, and on the other hand you remove all the toxins, so that the immune system comes back to life. That's all. If you didn't have a depleted non-functional immune system, you wouldn't have cancer. Then the body begins to heal itself, but you have to be very patient. It's not like popping a pill and you're okay.

Way back in 1981, in the very first lecture to patients that I heard, the medical director of the Gerson clinic in Mexico said, "The Gerson therapy is not for everybody." No truer word ever was spoken, because some people just look at it and say, "No, I can't do it." A lot who start it, after the first two weeks genuinely can't continue, because you can't do it on your own – you need help. Then there are some people who persevere and they either recover or they don't. It's not a miracle cure.

There are cases where the Gerson therapy can't help, because the disease is too far gone, or people have had a lot of chemotherapy, which puts a lot of extra poisons into the body and they simply can't cope, so I want to emphasise that this is simply not a miracle cure.

Some experts, who are excellent in their own field of medicine but know absolutely nothing about the potential of nutrition, may declare that you are terminal when you are not. You are really sick, but if you step on the gas and do it properly, it's possible to turn the disease around.

After my return home, blood tests were done every four to six weeks in London. No further tumours appeared anywhere, which with melanoma is remarkable. I remember in Mexico, an American lady in the room next to mine who also had melanoma, had 50 tumours. Once it starts spreading, it just goes like wildfire. The tumour in my groin just sat there, doing nothing, which was good. I was feeling better and I was looking really well. If you have cancer you can have a sort of grey skin, which I had when I got to Mexico. Now my skin was pink and healthy and my eyes were clear. I looked a damned sight more healthy than my friends who came to visit me, which was quite funny – I was supposed to be dying and they were supposed to be healthy. So I knew that the therapy was doing something good and my energy was up. That is the critical moment: you must not think that because you feel and look good that you are cured – you are not. You are just 'well'. Until your liver, which is important for your immune system, is totally detoxified and reconstructed, as it were, you are not cured.

At the end of the first year I realised I was going to get well. That's when I started writing my book, at the beginning of the second year, because I thought: "I must do something with all this energy." The therapy is tapered off as you appear better, on the basis of the blood tests and how you feel. It's going back to the basis of ordinary good medicine – look at the patient and ask the patient how he or she feels. After all, you know how you feel. I felt very well and I was very happy that I could go down from 13 juices to 11, then down to ten, and cut down on the enemas from five to four. It was fantastic.

By the time two years and three months were up, in March 1983, I stopped the therapy as such and began 'maintenance', which I've been doing ever since. Maintenance is sticking to a very good organic vegetarian diet, but having some animal protein, like a small piece of fish or chicken, and not eating anything with four legs. No stupid habits like smoking, drinking or taking drugs. I used to smoke heavily and I drank a little, but I never took drugs. Now I make a couple of juices every day. I bought a beautiful new juicer, which is quite fun. And I make sure that I have enough rest – I sleep at least seven hours a night. That's maintenance.

The lump in my groin never went down and it became very hard. My wonderful London doctor and I called it: "Little Rock". Eventually I had a scan, which showed that it was a small round thing sitting on a stalk, not attached to other tissue. That's interesting in itself, because normally tumours attach themselves to the surrounding tissue. This just sat there like a cauliflower. I consulted Charlotte Gerson[3] and asked her if I should have it out and she said: "Yes." So I went to Mexico again. They don't do any surgery at the Gerson clinic, so they took me to another hospital where I had the operation. It was quite easy – they just had to snip the stalk. It was then taken to the lab to discover what was inside, which was fascinating. There was a very thick outside layer that was calcified – almost bullet-proof. At the kernel of this "Little Rock" there were some active melanoma cells, but imprisoned, so they couldn't get out. But the therapy couldn't get in either, because of the terribly tough outside layer. I thought it was very funny – like having a whole lot of criminals in your house and they can't get out, but you can't get in, because of the armour plating. So I was nicely stitched up again. I have a very discreet mark on my groin and that was the end of "Little Rock".

I am not the only Gerson patient whose encapsulated tumour was just sitting on

3 Charlotte Gerson, Doctor Max Gerson's daughter, is now in her 92nd year and in good health. She founded the Gerson Institute in San Diego, California in the late 1970s. She has retired as the institute's director, but still plays an active role in its work.

a stalk. There were several others that were also simply snipped and removed. That's rather clever, isn't it? There are several possibilities of how the Gerson therapy gets rid of tumours. One is that the body reabsorbs the tumour and it disappears of its own accord, so there is no need to remove it. Other people have encapsulated tumours and say, "No thanks" to any more surgery – "I'll just live with it" and it's perfectly okay. Then there are others, like me, who say: "Let's get rid of it." I know of one lady who had an encapsulated tumour deep in her abdomen that was removed the same way as mine. Once it's encapsulated, it's quite safe, you see.

Here in Britain, cancer specialists tell us by the end of the 2020s, every second person will have cancer in their lifetime, as if it were an act of God, which it isn't. What makes me very angry is this acceptance that all of us are getting sicker and sicker at a time when enormous sums are spent on healthcare. It's the modern lifestyle and the consumer society that make people sick, but they just accept it. Cancer doesn't come from outer space – you didn't catch it from your neighbour. You did it to yourself due to your lifestyle, which your body can't cope with. There is also the issue of environmental toxicity, but that all comes together with the stress, plus the insane business of being so busy that you can't sleep or eat properly. Unless we change this whole lifestyle of bad living, yes, every second person will get cancer. Okay, I'm off my soap box now!

Doctor Gerson's approach seems more logical than just slicing bits off, poisoning the cancer with chemotherapy or burning it with radiation. In the end, those things don't help. I want to emphasise that his huge discovery was that cancer is not a thing, namely the tumour – it's a process. Unless you deal with the process, you're in big trouble. This is what convinced me. It wasn't faith, it was logic – simple logic.

I wanted to repay my debt to Doctor Gerson's memory and I thought the best way to do it is to give information to help people to go on this therapy. The first Gerson clinic opened just before I fell ill in 1978, but there is now a Gerson Health Centre in Hungary,[4] which I helped to set up. It is the world's first and only accredited Gerson facility outside Mexico, so now people who are in Europe can go to Hungary, which is much nearer. I go there twice a year to work with patients. I'm not a doctor, I don't give advice. If people ask me, I give information – that's all.

I couldn't go back to the BBC. They had to retire me on medical grounds, because they couldn't wait for me for two years, so they had to fill my job, which was a great loss. Before becoming ill, I had trained as a counsellor and psychotherapist. After I recovered, I decided to change direction and follow that career, which I did. I built up my practice and was very busy and I still do some writing. Of course, I am deeply involved with helping my colleagues at the centre in Hungary, which is extremely successful.

4 The Gerson Health Centre, Hungary http://gersontherapy.eu/therapy/gerson_therapy

Over the years, I wrote my book *A Time to Heal*,[5] which was first published in 1985. Since then it has been republished in English four times and translated into nine languages. I developed a lovely friendship with Charlotte Gerson, which is one of the treasures of my life. Together we wrote a book, which is called *Healing the Gerson Way*.[6] I wrote it for and with her and that is also all over the place in different languages, so people can find out about the therapy. Then if they want to do it, they do it, and if they don't, they don't. We have to make our own choices, you know? It's risky, but nothing ventured, nothing gained.

5 *A Time to Heal: Food As Medicine – The Way to Heal Incurable Cancer* by Beata Bishop.

6 *Healing the Gerson Way: Defeating Cancer and Other Chronic Diseases* by Beata Bishop and Charlotte Gerson.

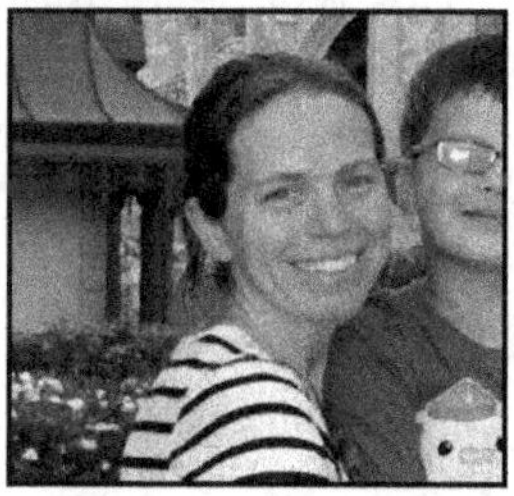

Melissa Cabral, 35 years

Dighton, Massachusetts, USA

Clostridium difficile after antibiotics for root canal treatment at 34 years

I was a happily married mother with two young children. At the time I got sick, my daughter was one year old and my son was three. We went out a lot and were very active. Then I needed a root canal and they gave me an antibiotic before it was done. The dentist did tell me to take it with a probiotic. I'm a pharmacist actually and I didn't take that advice of taking a probiotic, because I thought: "Oh, things like that never happen to me."

I finished the antibiotic and then about a week later, I came down at work, all of a sudden, with severe diarrhoea, nausea and vomiting. I had had diarrhoea for a while off and on, so the doctors just thought it was due to me not having a gall bladder, so I thought it was just a flare-up of that.

It was a Friday night – I made it home from work, to go promptly into the bathroom. I was vomiting and had diarrhoea all at the same time. I didn't get any sleep that night and I spent the whole day on Saturday between the bed and the bathroom. Sunday, the same thing – I couldn't hold anything down or in. At one point, my son found me sleeping on the floor in the bathroom and he yelled: "Daddy, Mommy's on the floor." By that time, I was so weak I couldn't get from the toilet back to the bed. My husband would bring me some toast and I would vomit it up, so finally I thought maybe it was more than just the gallbladder diarrhoea, so he brought me to the ER on that day. We figured it was just a stomach virus or something and they would give me fluids and send me home. They couldn't get an IV[1] line started, I was so dehydrated, so they did a CAT[2] scan without any contrast. My whole colon was inflamed from beginning to end. They weren't sure if it was an inflammatory disease, like Crohn's disease, or colitis. They thought it could be infectious colitis, so they needed a stool sample, which I had no problem producing! That came back positive for *Clostridium difficile (C. diff)*, both the antigen and toxin. I guess a small percentage of the population are actually positive for the antigen and just carry *C. diff* around and are asymptomatic. But the toxin was positive too, and that's what causes all the damage in the colon.

1 IV – intravenous drip.

2 CAT scan, also known as a CT scan or Computed Axial Tomography, is a diagnostic medical imaging procedure that examines cross sections of the body allowing a three dimensional view of specific areas.

So they admitted me and I ended up being there for eight days. I got worse before I got better. The nurses had to gown up and wear gloves whenever they would come into my room, and I had a 'Contact Precaution' sign on my door way down at the end of the hall so that no-one else risked catching it. It's very contagious and it can stay on hard surfaces for a long time. It was embarrassing.

In the middle of the stay, I was so weak I couldn't answer my cell phone in my locker. The nurses wanted me to call them when I had to go to the bathroom, but when I had to go, I couldn't wait for a nurse to come all the way down to the isolation room, then take me to the bathroom. It was horrible. I was so weak, I couldn't do anything, and I really thought I wasn't going to go home and see my children anymore and I started to get emotional. I was so sick. Even with being on IV fluids, I was so dehydrated, my potassium and magnesium were still dropping. They were giving me lots of supplements intravenously. Finally, around the seventh day, I begged them to let me try some solid food, because I thought if I had some solid food, some of the nausea would go away, and my headache would go away. I hadn't had coffee in so long, I had a caffeine-withdrawal headache.

At the same time, my son was admitted to the children's hospital, so I just needed to get out of the hospital and go home so that my kids could see that I was alright. On the eighth day, I was able to go home, but I was really, really weak. It took a lot out of me. This was last summer. The whole summer I couldn't do anything. I stayed in the house and went to the doctors for more medicine, or to the ER for IV fluids. It went on and on and on – constant antibiotics, but they just weren't working.

I left the hospital in mid-July. It was summer. My kids were home, but I couldn't do anything with them. I didn't work all last summer. I tried going back to work, but it was hard, because I would always have to run to the bathroom and it's not really convenient if I'm counselling a patient or trying to give a flu shot. It took a long time for me to build up enough stamina to stand up for eight or 12 hours at a time. My husband took a lot [of time] off of work, because I didn't have any energy. I had to go to the bathroom double-digits times a day. I was useless – I couldn't do anything. I was afraid to go out, because I needed to know where every bathroom was. I couldn't drive, because I was needing to go to the bathroom. I had to have iron infusions, because I became so anaemic from losing so much and not absorbing any iron. I was really weak and very pale. I lost a lot of weight, about 20 pounds, and was in rough shape.

Ironically, when I was in the hospital, my brother sent me an email about this new treatment for *C. diff* and it was a faecal transplant and I thought that was the most disgusting thing I'd ever heard of. I said that I will never, ever, ever do that, because that's absolutely disgusting. But when I got out of the hospital, the *C. diff* would just not go away. Lots of money was spent on antibiotics and in doctors' offices and in the ER until finally my gastroenterologist said: "You need to go see this doctor who does faecal transplants." She'd been telling me for a while that I needed to have this done. They made the appointment for me and I went and saw her. She was the most wonderful doctor, and she said: "Yes, you need to have this done, quickly," and got me in early.

I would probably have died or needed a bag or something if I didn't have a faecal transplant. I was so grossed out about it, but after four months, I knew it was what I had to do. So I saw the doctor.

My husband was actually going to be my donor. They test the donor stool very thoroughly and it turned out that he was one of those few people who are an asymptomatic *C. diff* carrier, so he couldn't be my donor. So I had to start over and I asked my mom. She passed fine, so she was my donor.

I had to do a bowel prep, which I don't think I really needed, because I went to the bathroom so much anyway, but I did the bowel prep. As the donor, my mother just had to take a mild laxative the night before, so she could produce a sample the next morning. My mom came over with her sample the next morning. She wanted to make sure that they had enough, so she brought two containers! The doctor said it was the best textured poop she had ever seen. [*laughs*]

My husband drove me to the clinic and we handed over the poop. The worst part was starting an IV, because I was just so constantly dehydrated. They finally got an IV in, then it's just like a regular colonoscopy. I'd had colonoscopies before, but for this one I was so worked up and nervous and had so many emotions. The medicines didn't knock me out – I was watching the whole thing. The doctor finally asked the nurse: "How much did you give her?" She said: "100." I was still awake, and as I'm a pharmacist, I said: "A hundred of what?" She said: "Fentanyl."[3] I said: "Oh wow, but I'm still just wide awake, watching." I was so nervous and I was just so sick of being sick. I remember it was a little painful, because I could still feel the colonoscopy. At one point, the doctor said: "Alright Melissa, here it comes." As gross as it sounds, I could see on the screen all this brown liquid going in. After I knew that it was in me, that was when I finally just let myself relax and fall asleep. The nurse was joking: "Now you're going to take a nap on me?"

The doctor takes the sample, mixes it with saline, strains it. Maybe about 60 or 100ccs go in and then they want you to hold it in for about an hour. You have to take *Imodium*[4] or *Lomotil*[5] beforehand, so you don't go to the bathroom. I was able to hold it for about 45 minutes. I remember waking up – they have your feet up in the air, so that gravity kind of keeps it in. The whole thing took about 20 minutes.

It was a Monday in the week of Thanksgiving.[6] By Thanksgiving on Thursday, I still hadn't had a bowel movement, after having had diarrhoea every single day at least 15 times, since July – it worked that fast, the very next day. I wished I had done it a lot, lot sooner. It really is huge. So many things – bacteria good and bad are in your gut. It's amazing, I have my mom's poop in me, and now

3 Fentanyl is an opioid/narcotic analgesic.

4 *Imodium* (loperamide) – medication for diarrhoea that slows digestion.

5 *Lomotil* – atropinediphenoxylate – anti-diarrhoea medication.

6 In the USA, Thanksgiving is held on the fourth Thursday of November.

I'm *C. diff* free. I haven't tested positive in any of my *C. diff* follow through. The next day, I was actually fine, but within two weeks or so I could eat and finally build up some energy and put some meat back on my bones. Then I started having normal movements again. I had totally forgotten what a normal bowel movement was like.

My first instinct, when my brother sent me that email describing faecal transplants when I was in the hospital, even as sick as I was to say, "No way. That's absolutely the most disgusting thing", but it really wasn't. It was not the slightest bit disgusting at all and it was so quick and easy. It saved my life, so if anyone is suffering and thinks it's gross, it's definitely worth it. I wish that it was offered sooner for patients suffering from recurrent *C. diff*, rather than putting them through vancomycin, *flagyl* and *dificid* and all these expensive antibiotics that sometimes their insurances won't pay for, and they're expensive. Most insurances will cover a colonoscopy if that's how it's billed.

This all happened right before the FDA[7] stepped in and banned faecal transplants. Now, they've reversed their ruling, but it was right before all that happened. I wish more doctors would do it, but there aren't a lot. I don't know if they think it's too risky, if they're afraid their patients will be disgusted by it, or if they're disgusted by it. I have no idea. If a doctor tells a patient that it's experimental and the patient signs, then they can do it, but there are still a lot of doctors who won't do it. But it's effective and quick and easy. It probably should be offered to people more as a first line of treatment rather than antibiotic after antibiotic. The doctor who did mine was really passionate about it – she's fabulous. I should have done it a lot sooner than I did. I could have had more time with my children and saved a lot of time and money from being in the hospital and on antibiotics.

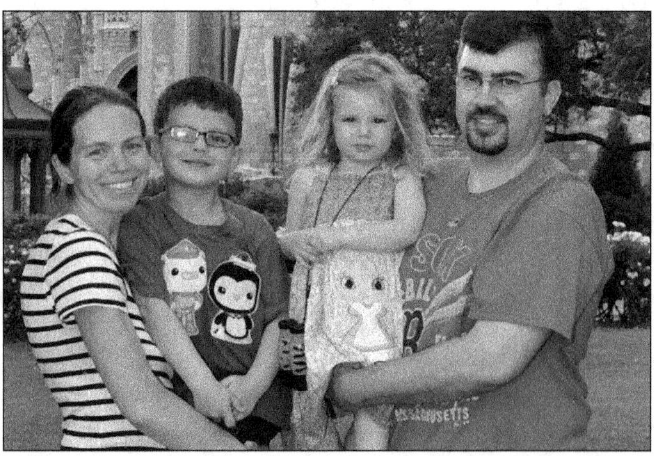

Melissa Cabral with her husband and two children at Disneyland.

7 FDA – US Food and Drug Administration is an agency of the United States Department of Health and Human Services, responsible for protecting and promoting public health.

Clostridium Difficile, *or* 'C. diff', *is a bacterium that can cause symptoms ranging from diarrhoea to life-threatening inflammation of the colon. Illness from* C. diff *typically occurs after use of antibiotic medications. However, studies show increasing rates of* C. diff *infection among people traditionally not considered high risk, such as younger and healthy individuals without a history of antibiotic use or exposure to health care facilities.*

Each year, more than a half million people get sick from C. diff, *and in recent years, infections have become more frequent, severe and difficult to treat. (Mayo Clinic http://www.mayoclinic.org/)*

Clostridium difficile *causes diarrhoea linked to 14,000 American deaths each year. (Centers for Disease Control http://www.cdc.gov/hai/organisms/cdiff/cdiff_infect.html)*

'Sophia', 56 years

New South Wales, Australia

Diagnosed with Lyme disease six years after symptoms first developed

In 2006, when I was in my late forties, I moved back to Australia from Mexico with my children after 15 years of being away. We were fortunate to have a great home in rural New South Wales and I established a fabulous studio where I was going to pursue my passion for ceramics.

My symptoms began subtly, with a weird tightening over half of my face and a muscle spasm, which left my face feeling frozen. Then one day, while working in my studio doing turpentine washes over my work – stupidly without a mask – half of my face went totally numb. It felt like I had been affected by the turpentine, which was probably true, but I was not prepared for the downhill spiral that followed. I walked out of my studio that day and have been unable to return.

The numbness and tingling in my face continued and I became very chemically sensitive. It developed into a mild Bell's palsy[1] with visible muscle weakness in the right side of my face, from my cheek to my eye. I began to have trouble speaking, thinking, and developed a constant buzzing, vibrating sensation in my head. It felt and sounded like champagne bubbles moving from my cheek to my brow. I had a constant headache, which felt like someone was sitting over my eye and I found myself having to hold my eye open. At times my head felt like a bowling ball that my neck couldn't support. I had a taste of metal in my mouth and it felt like my words were totally slurred. My right cheek was constantly flushed and burning, so I was sure that the problem was in my cheek. A GP[2] ordered a CAT[3] scan to rule out a brain tumour. It showed nothing except a mucus retention cyst in my sinus, which doctors assured me would cause no symptoms, although to me, it seemed quite a coincidence that was where I felt my problem lay.

My symptoms continued, constantly and fluctuating, without anyone knowing of any cause. About three months later, I developed a rash of small blisters over my torso and upper legs, which lasted a few weeks, but my doctor didn't

---

1 Bell's palsy – one-sided facial paralysis caused by a dysfunction of the facial nerve. While the cause can be unknown, it occurs in patients with a brain tumour, stroke, myaesthenia gravis and Lyme disease.

2 GP – general practitioner.

3 CAT scan, also known as a CT scan or Computed Axial Tomography, is a diagnostic medical imaging procedure that examines cross sections of the body allowing a three dimensional view of specific areas.

know what it was. I also had one numb finger and toe.

By early 2008, my symptoms became more pronounced. I felt as if I was being poisoned. I had had no alcohol for over a year, but constantly felt hungover. The noise, vibrations and pain in my head were always there. I felt like there was a knife sticking in my neck and poison was being injected into the top of my spine, which then spread through my brain. Certainly not fun! Even with this feeling, there weren't any measurable symptoms, except the facial weakness and flushing on one side. I thought I was going crazy. I had one episode where I had no control over my arms and almost collapsed in the shower. My GP thought it was a panic attack, but looking back it was probably a mild seizure. It took me five days to recover from that – I felt like I'd been hit by a bulldozer.

From that time, everything seemed to fall apart and my symptoms spread to the rest of my body. I started getting weakness in one leg. Sometimes it wouldn't work and I couldn't stand up. There were days when my legs felt unattached to my body, and others when they just felt really weak. Balance became an issue, so that climbing stairs or a ladder was difficult or impossible. My hands and elbows became sore to touch and my arms felt like they were going to fall off if I let them hang, so I would walk with my arms crossed in front of me. At times I felt like someone was tying straps around my legs, head and torso. I had electric shock sensations all over my body and weird muscle spasms where my arms would just shoot out involuntarily.

There would be weeks when I could hardly hold my head up. I had no strength in my voice, so carrying on a conversation was totally exhausting. A dentist decided TMJ[4] was the problem so he gave me a plate to wear, which made it so much worse. One day, I accidentally dropped my plate on the driveway and ran over it with my car. Probably the best scenario, but another very expensive exercise. Then an ear, nose and throat specialist suggested I had 'globus'[5] and recommended speech therapy so that I could learn to talk, with no explanation as to why I had lost that ability after 50 years of doing that pretty well!

Those symptoms rotated for years. After seeing neurologists, ENTs[6] and dentists, having MRIs[7] and CAT scans, nobody found anything, so there was no treatment. I was functioning, but doing day to day chores really took such a huge conscious effort, yet I simply had to do them.

I found a toxicologist who tested me for all sorts of things, which revealed that I had extremely low vitamin D and magnesium. He put me on really high doses of magnesium, which made a huge difference within days – it was magical. I never got spasms or the electric shock feeling again, but we weren't coming up with any explanation for my other symptoms.

4 TMJ – temporomandibular joint dysfunction is an umbrella term used to describe pain and other symptoms felt in the jaw when chewing.

5 Globus, or globus hystericus, is a feeling of a lump or foreign body in the throat thought to be psychological in origin.

6 ENT – ear, nose and throat specialist.

7 MRI – magnetic resonance imaging is a medical imaging technique used in radiology to investigate the anatomy and function of the body, using magnetic fields and radio waves to form images of the body.

I had some pretty derogatory responses from people along the way, basically saying that there was nothing wrong with me and that I needed psychological help. I went to psychologists, but they didn't respond to me in the same way. One of the eye doctors I went to, who was also a neurologist, told me that I should sit up straight, put goanna oil on my neck, wear my glasses all the time and I would be fine. [*laughs*]

An integrative GP picked up a mild encephalitis and treated me with antibiotics and herbs for neurological inflammation. He warned me at the time that treating bacterial or parasitic inflammation in the brain can cause a worsening of symptoms, because neurotoxins are released as the organism dies. I took the antibiotics for six days and nothing happened, so I assumed the diagnosis was wrong. Once again, I thought that I really was going crazy.

Three weeks later though, half of my face and eye swelled up. I was disoriented and had incredible headaches, but I didn't connect these symptoms with the antibiotic treatment. I returned to my GP (not the integrative one) and another MRI was done. It was clear – the cyst in my cheek had *gone*. No-one associated the antibiotics, the visual inflammation and the cyst disappearing together. If that connection had been made, the next three years of my life may have been very different.

I continued in a downhill spiral, with the multiple, fluctuating and migrating symptoms. Sometimes I felt almost normal, which may have been a result of the antibiotics and herbs, but then I would have another low period. The vision in my right eye would come and go, but the vibrating and pulsing had now spread to my torso and legs. Also, my heart was doing some pretty crazy things.

My asthma became extremely bad. Some days just walking across the room was an issue. I was having up to 17 double hits of *Ventolin*[8] a day. Although steroid inhalers helped my breathing, they made the noises and pulsing in my head worse, so I refused to take them. I also had what I now know to be air hunger – not so much asthma, but feeling a lack of air. I would walk into a room and feel like someone had vacuumed out all the air and I could not be in a room where the heating was on. The experts at the asthma clinic did not ask me once why my breathing was getting rapidly worse. Steroid medication was their only option, and if I wasn't going to take that medication, they were not interested in me.

I did try and continue to do some exercise – walking, swimming and tennis – because if I didn't keep moving, I would seize up. Sitting for any length of time was an issue. On good days, I'd go for walks and almost break into a jog. Other days, I would shuffle. Sometimes I couldn't lift my arms above my head or hold a cup, let alone run around a tennis court! I would try to swim, but there were weeks at a time when just the water pressure on my hands and

8 *Ventolin* (salbutamol) is a prescription medication used via a puffer to dilate the bronchi in the lungs to improve the lung capacity.

feet was too painful.

I've always pretty much believed in mind over matter, so when the doctors couldn't find anything, I did think that it was just me, but by mid-2012, I was pretty desperate. I was given *Endep*, the antidepressant, in a low dose for my fibromyalgia pain and to help me sleep. Within three days of taking that, the shaking and buzzing in my head were so much worse. They were keeping me awake to the point where I was pretty much ready to end it all, so I took myself off it. My doctor said: "Oh well, if you can't take that, we can't do anything for you."

After that, I had another rash – this time on my back, accompanied with severe abdominal pain and numbness around my torso, which was diagnosed as Herpes Type 1. Then, I lost more feeling in my legs and began to have bladder issues. One day, when I got into a hydrotherapy pool where I went regularly for exercise, I couldn't feel the warmth of the water on my legs. My left hand and my right knee were swelling for no reason and my toes were all numb, so walking barefoot was a challenge. I had waves of nausea, pain and weakness. My concentration was about nil. I had not read a book – partly because holding one was an effort, but also because I found it really hard to follow a plot. Making a decision was almost impossible. I know menopause can cause similar issues, but my brain-fog was extreme. While driving, at times I would forget where I was going and I was constantly forgetting where I had parked my car.

Soon after that, a concerned friend asked me if I had heard of Lyme disease. She knew someone who had been bitten by a tick in India, became really sick and was told she might have early onset Parkinson's disease. She insisted on having her blood sent to the States[9] and it came back positive for Lyme disease. A lot of her symptoms were similar to mine, especially the shaking and the strobe light feeling, so I looked at Lyme disease again.

A bacterial infection like Lyme disease seemed to be the only real explanation for my multiple and fluctuating symptoms. I'd already had an ELISA[10] test, but the result was negative, so I tried to dismiss Lyme disease as a possibility. I saw on the Australian Lyme Disease website that there was a protest on in Sydney that week, so I went along to learn more. There, I heard stories of people who had been in wheelchairs and recovered. Some didn't look so unwell but their symptoms overlapped with many of mine.

I was put in contact with a Lyme literate doctor in Sydney. By the time I got an appointment a few weeks later, I really was in bad shape. It was as if I had a brick wall shutting out access to half my brain and I couldn't access information. Words would come out backwards and back-to-front. I had pain all over, yet I couldn't work out what hurt. It wasn't muscular and it wasn't my joints – it was everything in between. I was taking painkillers just to get through the day.

9 The States – United States of America.

10 ELISA (enzyme-linked immunosorbent assay) – antibody test that measures the body's response to a specific bacterial infection, such as *Borrelia burgdorferi* in Lyme disease.

When I walked into the doctor's office and told her what had been going on for the past six years, she seemed pretty sure it was a bacterial infection that was undermining my health and recommended the American blood tests to test for Lyme disease.

I was ready to do just about anything. My blood was sent to the US and tested by the IGeneX Lab[11] in California. I tested positive to the IgG and IgM[12] antibodies that develop against the *Borrelia burgdorferi* bacterium.[13] These tests met both the IGeneX and CDC[14] criteria. Because of these positive results, I had to have the Western Blot[15] done. I also tested positive for *Babesia*, which is a co-infection[16] of Lyme disease.

So finally, in November 2012, I had a diagnosis from a Sydney GP of suspected chronic Lyme disease. It was such a relief. Until that time, I hadn't even thought about the tick bite I had on my stomach back in 2006, while I was visiting friends at Clareville in the northern beaches of Sydney. The timing seemed right and the pieces all fell into place.

Now with a diagnosis, I was prepared to do what was needed to regain my health. Always one to denounce the use of antibiotics, I took a cocktail of oral and intramuscular antibiotics for six months in combination with herbs and a strict diet. After a couple of months of antibiotics, I felt so much better and continued to improve over the next year.

The treatment protocols certainly worked. I had no real issues with the antibiotics, except I became extremely sun and light-sensitive on the doxycycline[17] to the extent I blistered and felt like I was on fire for days. I also had Herxheimer[18] responses, but they passed.

I would now say I am a pretty fit and normal 56-year-old. I have my brain back and my body works again. My creativity and physical strength have returned. Once again, I can work as a designer and enjoy my life. I will not say my health is perfect. I still have mild buzzing and shaking in my head and the weakness and pain does seem to return from time to time, but I am so very much better. I now know that it does not all need to be downhill from the age of 50! A few months ago, I did a ten-day walk along the Camino de Compostelo in France, and then went on to Morocco. I returned feeling *scarily well*. For the five years between 2007 and 2012, that trip would certainly not have been an option.

Back in 2006, I had looked to mainstream medicine, as I knew I was in serious need of help. It took a lot of time, money and energy to receive the help I

11 IGeneX, Inc www.igenex.com/

12 The IgG and IgM antibody test for *Borrelia burgdorferi* can also detect antibodies to other spiral bacteria, so if the test is positive, an additional Western Blot test is often required to confirm the presence of specific antibodies to the bacterium that causes Lyme disease.

13 *Borrelia burgdorferi* is the main bacterium that causes the symptoms of Lyme disease.

14 CDC – Centers for Disease Control and Prevention in the US focuses on many diseases, in particular, infectious disease.

15 The Western Blot is a widely used test used to detect specific proteins in a sample of tissue. Compared to ELISA, Western blotting has higher specificity.

16 Ticks can carry infections in addition to *Borrelia*, which are called 'co-infections'.

17 Doxycyline is a tetracyline antibiotic.

18 The Jarisch-Herxheimer reaction is a response to endotoxins released by the death of harmful organisms within the body.

required. I am seriously disillusioned by so many in the medical profession I encountered along the way and the inability of the so-called 'specialists' and 'experts' to look at patients as a whole or to really even listen to what we say. I went around in circles for years. From the beginning, I had said that I believed I had an infection or a parasite and that chemicals had caused me some harm. I did not know about Lyme disease and I couldn't put it all together. I believe that was their job, and they failed me in that. So many were so dismissive of my symptoms. I left so many doctor's visits in tears, feeling so unheard.

I can only assume my Lyme diagnosis was correct. Lyme disease, or borreliosis, is controversial in Australia and I haven't yet been fully tested for it here. My case may not be typical, as I lived in Mexico for many years and travelled and hiked in the States, where Lyme disease is epidemic. I did become very ill in 1995 while I was at a beach in Mexico. They had warned us there were animals in the trees that can make you go mad. My Spanish at the time was not good enough to understand the word for 'tick' nor the significance of that advice! However, there was also the tick bite at Clareville in 2005, and my health decline began in 2006. In my case, the jury is open as to which tick-bite did the damage, but from 1995 to 2006 I was in perfect health. They do say the *Borrelia* infection can lay dormant in the body and only appears when the immune system is compromised and I believe my trigger was chemical exposure.

The thing about Lyme disease symptoms is that they move – the bacteria can get anywhere in your body. My Lyme-literate doctor in Sydney asked me if I remembered a monthly cycle in my symptoms. I never put it down to a monthly cycle, but I certainly knew my symptoms would come and go in waves. I'd feel okay for a few days and think: "There's nothing wrong with me." Then there'd be another downward spiral and I'd think: "What have I done that's made it worse, because I haven't changed anything?"

It took six years for me to have the Lyme bacteria *Borrelia burgdorferi* recognised. I must have seen at least 20 doctors and alternative health practitioners, including three neurologists, three ENTs,[19] allergists, kinesiologists and more. I had multiple CT scans, MRIs and hundreds of blood tests. I was tested and poked to exclude MS,[20] fibromyalgia, myasthenia gravis, a brain tumour, spinal stenosis, arthritis, shingles, chronic fatigue, allergies, sinusitis, TMJ, rotator cuff injury and severe chronic asthma. The list seemed to be endless and the diagnosis nil. No doctor would look at me as a whole. I kept saying: "What's going on in my head and my cheek?" I knew that my symptoms were all connected and there was something in my system that was underlining everything, but no specialist would look beyond their box. So, I went round in circles for all those years. It was a waste of time, money and my life.

I feel embarrassed to think of what I have spent on my health. I went from

19 ENT – ear, nose and throat specialist.

20 MS – multiple sclerosis.

a really healthy mother of two, who had lived, worked and raised a family between Mexico and Australia, had home births, hardly visited a doctor, relied on herbs and homeopathy when needed, to a person I didn't recognise. I was crawling into doctor's surgeries almost begging them to find something wrong with me. I was not prepared to take medication until I knew what was being treated, so doctors decided they couldn't help me. No-one seemed to think it was unusual for a previously healthy person to suddenly have so many fluctuating symptoms. No-one really listened to me when I said all my symptoms were related and that the cyst that was clearly visible on an MRI was at least part of the problem! Each specialist looked only at their specific area. One particularly helpful doctor suggested that if it was something serious, I would be already dead. Others just dismissed me with: "You're over 50 and this is how it will be from here on in." My family suggested I was lazy and didn't want to work. My kids laughed and said I was just getting old. Most people commented on how healthy I looked. If only they could have understood what an effort it was to appear normal.

I did raise the question about Lyme disease with a few doctors along the way. They were all totally uninformed and dismissive of the idea. If they did not believe it was here in Australia, they knew I had lived abroad where it is common, but they still not did not consider it as a possible cause of my varied and fluctuating symptoms, so they weren't interested in testing me for it. I now know I wasn't crazy and there was a reason for my deteriorating health. More importantly, I now know that it isn't normal to feel poisoned and be in constant pain. You can have a life after 50!

There shouldn't be so much intrigue. So many people's lives are being screwed up. They are told they have MS and the steroids they're being given are just making them worse. Doctors need to start looking for causes of mysterious illnesses and not just offer a band-aid for symptoms. If a bacterial infection such as *Borrelia* is undermining a person's health, they can recover with antibiotics and get better.

Ten years ago, Newcastle University said that we had Lyme disease here in Australia. I am now part of the Sydney University Research Programme into tick-borne illness in Australia. Hopefully, there will be some positive outcomes, which will help future generations of Australians. Of all those people who remain undiagnosed, or misdiagnosed, some lucky ones can return to wellness.

I talk about my experience a lot, because I think people need to know how common Lyme disease really is. I feel thankful to all those who finally led me towards a diagnosis and recovery. My advice to others is: "Listen to your body and to your heart." Something in my long-winded story may sound familiar to you.

I feel blessed to have a second chance. I share my story in the hope it may help others in a journey to recovery. Awareness is empowering.

It is common for people who have contracted Lyme disease to experience a long road to diagnosis. This is due to symptoms being interpreted as the neurological disorders multiple sclerosis and Parkinson's disease, or as being psychosomatic.

> *"Lyme disease, transmitted by the bite of a tick, is prevalent across the United States and throughout the world. Lyme disease is a clinical diagnosis and is caused by a spiral-shaped bacteria (spirochete) called* Borrelia Burgdorferi, *which can cause infection of multiple organs and produce a wide range of symptoms. Fewer than fifty per cent of patients with Lyme disease recall a tick bite or any rash. A "Bull's Eye" rash is considered classic, but atypical forms of this rash are seen far more commonly.*
>
> *The ELISA screening tests miss thirty-five per cent of culture-proven Lyme disease, with only sixty-five per cent sensitivity. By definition, a screening test should have at least ninety-five per cent sensitivity.*
>
> *The Western blot test should be performed by a laboratory that reads and reports all of the bands related to* Borrelia burgdorferi. *There are five sub species of* Borrelia burgdorferi, *over 100 strains in the US and 300 strains worldwide. Testing of other tick-transmitted organisms such as* Babesia, Anaplasma, Ehrlichia *and* Bartonella *should also be performed.*
>
> *Evidence indicates that active ongoing spirochetal infection, with or without other tick borne co-infections, is the cause of the persistent symptoms in chronic Lyme disease. Most cases of chronic Lyme disease require an extended course of antibiotic therapy to achieve symptomatic relief. The return of symptoms and evidence of the continued presence of* Borrelia burgdorferi *indicates the need for further treatment. Many patients with chronic Lyme disease require prolonged treatment until they are symptom free. There are no tests currently available to prove that the organism is eradicated, or that the patient with chronic Lyme disease is cured.*
>
> *Like syphilis in the 19th Century, Lyme disease has been called the 'Great Imitator' and should be considered in the differential diagnosis of rheumatologic and neurologic conditions as well as Chronic Fatigue Syndrome, fibromyalgia, somatization disorder and any difficult-to-diagnose multi-system illness."*

(International Lyme and Associated Diseases Society (ILADS): http://www.ilads.org/)

ILADS is a nonprofit, international, multi-disciplinary medical society, dedicated to the diagnosis and appropriate treatment of Lyme and its associated diseases.

Under Our Skin, *a 2008 documentary, is a multiple award-winning and Oscar-short-listed film about the Lyme disease epidemic, informing people around the world who are undiagnosed or misdiagnosed. A sequel,* Under Our Skin: Emergence, *was released in 2014.*

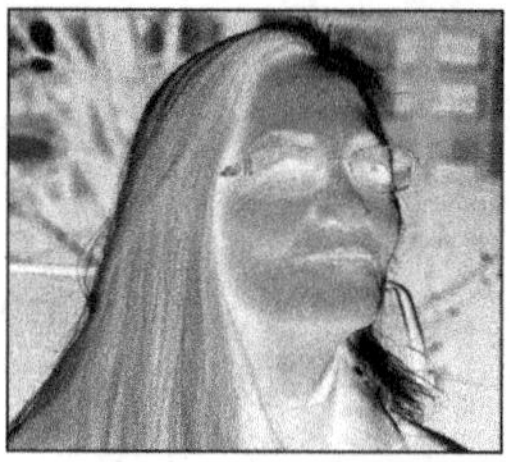

Sarah Ann Cooper, 72 years

Littleton, Colorado, USA

Diagnosed with pancreatic cancer at 59 years

I went in for an annual physical. I had an explosive bowel – that's the way I would put it. Every time I ate, I would have to run to the bathroom. I had lost about 20 pounds in weight over a three or four month period of time. For my age at that time, which was 59, I was eating everything I always ate, so that was a big surprise. Those were the two warning signs that caused my doctor to do some other investigations. She wanted me to do a chest X-ray because I had past bronchial problems.

We did the X-ray and I knew something was wrong, because it took a little while. She said: "It appears that the bottom third of your chest is flat." I was shocked, because I was feeling so wonderful, other than the two things that I mentioned. The holidays were coming up and I was planning Christmas and everything like that. I have three children and at that time, had three grandchildren. I had asked her: "Well, what does that mean?" She said: "I'd like to get a CAT[1] scan of your chest and I would also like to include in that your intestines and your colon – we can do it all at once." So I went in and they did the CAT scan. I hadn't gotten home and my doctor called me. She said: "I need to see you in my office tomorrow." I said: "It's getting close to my anniversary, can I put it off?" She said: "No, I really need to see you." By this time we knew each other and I was being stubborn, so I said: "Janet, I'm not coming in tomorrow unless you tell me what's wrong, because obviously something's wrong with the CAT scan." I thought maybe she was going to say that I had something like emphysema. She said: "Well, if you put it that way, you have a tumour in your pancreas." I thought: "Okay, pancreas." My mind was going one hundred miles an hour to figure out what your pancreas is and what does that have to do with losing weight and everything else. I knew a tumour could be cancerous and so I agreed to go in and see her the next day.

I went in and she said that she believed that from the CAT scan it was cancerous, and wanted to send me immediately to a surgeon. I went in to see the surgeon. He

1 CAT scan, also known as a CT scan, or Computed Axial Tomography is a diagnostic medical imaging procedure that examines cross sections of the body allowing a three dimensional view of specific areas.

said that he would like to do a 'Whipple'[2] surgery. I said: "Okay, I want to understand everything that you're telling me. I want to know what that entails and I want to know exactly what the prognosis is and how long I will be in hospital." I made him go into a whole lot of detail and of course the Whipple surgery is very complex. I didn't know how complex until he started telling me. Then I said: "Wait, we're not going to schedule surgery right now. I want to give this some thought. I want to find out what's going on. Can't we make sure that it is a cancerous tumour?" They said they could, but didn't see any need for it, and I said, "Well I do."

They sent me to another surgeon, right after the first of the year. He said that he'd like to schedule surgery. Then I got to thinking about it and I really felt in my spirit that it was not the thing for me to do, because of the extensive surgery. They take out part of your stomach and your duodenum and all of your pancreas. I asked them if they could just take out the pancreas, because I could see the size of the tumour. It was a 3.2cm tumour and the pancreas is about 4cm and so I knew that it had taken up a good portion of the head of the pancreas. They said, no, they had to do the radical surgery.

I said to them: "Okay, schedule the surgery. Now I'm going to go on a trip with my husband." We went to Mexico, stayed at this wonderful place and enjoyed ten days there. That was absolutely fantastic, just doing nothing but walking on the beach, listening to songs and everything. I was doing a lot of praying. I got back and I called them and said: "I'm cancelling the surgery." They said: "Do you know what you're doing?" I said that yes, I did, and then they said: "Okay then, let's do a biopsy and make sure what it is." I thought: "If I'm not having surgery, why am I doing a biopsy?" But something just told me to go ahead and have the biopsy. They sent it from Kaiser Hospital to the Mayo Clinic and both of them confirmed that it was a carcinoma, so I had to face the fact that it was cancerous. I gave it a lot of thought. They told me that if I did not have surgery, I had three to six months to live. They gave me a percentage of how many people make it through the surgery and another percentage of the recovery time at home, then the chemo[3] and the radiation. Then I said: "Okay, after all that, if I've passed everything and done really well, how long is my life extension?" They said that it was very rare for pancreatic patients to live beyond 15 to 18 months. And I said: "Well, I feel fine, and I'm not having surgery."

At that point, I started looking into all kinds of alternative medicine – herbs, vitamins and things along that line that would build my immune system and help me. What made me think of this was about ten years prior, I got ill and they could not find out what it was and thought it was all kinds of things. A very good friend of mine's husband, who had been into alternative

2 The Whipple procedure (named after Allen Whipple, a Columbia University surgeon who first performed the operation in 1935) involves removal of the "head" (wide part) of the pancreas, the duodenum (first part of the small intestine), a portion of the common bile duct, gallbladder and sometimes part of the stomach. The remaining intestine, bile duct and pancreas are then reconnected.

3 Chemo – chemotherapy.

medicine for about thirty years, gave me some simple pills to take morning and afternoon. After two weeks I was over it. But really, what influenced me to make the decision I made, was that I knew I had two choices. I had to either get my body healed, better than I was, or at least extend my life. I knew what my chances were the one way and how sick I would be during that period of time. I thought: "If I've only got 15 to 18 months to live, maybe I can extend it with alternative medicine and get my body back. If that's the case then I might as well enjoy that time instead of being sick in bed." It was really a choice that made sense to me.

I realised that I had seen so many people who had cancer and what they went through with traditional medicine. My own sister went the traditional route with breast cancer. They claim that if the cancer is arrested after five years that you're 'cancer clean', I think is the term they use. But 12 years after her chemo, surgery and radiation, it came back. I thought, "I've seen so much of that." For me, it wasn't hard, because I do follow what I feel. This wall came up and said to me: "This is not for you." So there was no choice for me.

On my path, I was taking all sorts of things that I could read and find out about. My immune system got run down and that was a problem. I can't tell you how many books I read – in the two years, I probably read a hundred books. I got books from every doctor that had ever written anything on cancer. There was very little on alternative medicine back in 2000 – it was just not something you talked about. At that time, a lot of people thought that it was all quackery – anybody who got into that was kind of weird or whatever. Now I think it's changed greatly, but still it's not totally accepted.

I went to a Cherokee medicine man to see if he had something from way back. I read Hulda Clarke,[4] who was a famous nurse a long time ago. I spoke with Doctor Kelley,[5] who was one of the first who had success with cancer, especially pancreatic cancer. In my searching, things kept popping up for me. I went to the healthfood store and would look through their volumes. I started with things that made sense to me. I know that we have to build our body back up, so I started with that. Then I heard about a Rife machine[6] that uses sound frequencies. One man I called about it was hesitant to speak to me. People hesitate to talk to you because they're afraid. They don't want to cause any problems with the AMA[7] to be honest about it. He told me his wife used the Rife machine to treat breast cancer. Then he said: "Oh, by the way, have you heard about the trial they're doing on pancreatic cancer in New York?" I said that I didn't want one of

4 Hulda Clarke (1928-2009) was a naturopath who authored several books. She believed that eliminating parasites, bacteria and viruses from the body and removing pollutants from the diet and environment would cure all diseases.

5 William Kelley (1925-2005) was an orthodontist who developed pancreatic cancer in 1962. He formulated his own cancer cure, survived and wrote his book *One Answer to Cancer* available at www.drkelley.com/CANLIVER55.html

6 Royal Raymond Rife (1888-1971) was an American inventor who claimed that cancer was caused by bacteria. During the 1920s, he developed a microscope that could detect living microbes by their vibratory rates. His Rife Frequency Generator generates radio waves with precisely the same frequency, causing the offending bacteria to die. His therapy was, and remains, highly controversial, but many people claim it has cured their cancers.

7 AMA – American Medical Association.

those tests where you can get a placebo, because I wanted to do my own thing with alternative medicine. He said: "Oh no, it's alternative medicine basically versing a new type of chemotherapy." He said that the gentleman's name was Doctor Gonzalez.

So I called New York and his office put me in touch with his associates. I had to go through an intensive 'filtering out' process including my biopsy report. They saw that it had been done by two pathologists that concluded that I definitely had pancreatic cancer, so that was no problem. The reason they chose pancreatic cancer for the trial test was because they knew that most people don't live past two years. I had to send in all kinds of blood samples. My doctor was wonderful in helping me through this process. We got everything together and I flew up to New York and met with the head surgeon at the Colombia Presbyterian Hospital to get the 'okay', because the National Cancer Institute was financing and overseeing this trial. Colombia Presbyterian Hospital was the place that was using the chemo for pancreatic cancer, although I didn't know that at the time. He walked in and said: "Mrs Cooper, why can't you have surgery?" And I said: "I can have surgery, but I refused it." And he said: "Oh, we've got a problem. We can't accept you in the programme if you can have the conventional process." That's when it kind of cemented in my head that I didn't have the choice I wanted to have. I said: "I'm making the choice, I know exactly what I'm doing, I'm 59 years old and I'm not going to have surgery. I own my own businesses and I am aware of what you're telling me. I would love to be in the trial test." All the medicine of course was taken care of, paid for, but I didn't say that. And he said: "I'm sorry."[8]

I was crushed. Absolutely crushed. I cried all the way back to my hotel room. The poor cab driver didn't know what to do with me. I got into my hotel room and Doctor Isaacs[9] called me and said: "Anne, I am so sorry. I don't know what to say. There's nothing I can do." I asked her if there was any way I could be in the trial test and she said: "No, not with them paying for the alternative medicine that you would need to be on and that's 150 pills a day. Do you still want to be on the programme?" I said: "Yes, I do." She told me that if I was willing to pay for my protocol, she would only charge me a minimal fee for her services. So I got in a cab and went to her office and got started on the alternative protocol. It's called the 'Isaacs-Gonzalez Enzyme Therapy'. That was when I really got into the alternative medicine.

It's a lot of cleanses of your liver. There were juices you had to take, two or three a day that were basically vegetables. They gave you a couple of different things that you could put in your juices, but I stayed with carrot juice, because I didn't care for the mixture. I used to get carrots that were organic from the healthfood store. They would come in great big bags and I would go and pick them up. You have to do coffee enemas every day. They had me on a pretty

8 *What Went Wrong* is a book by Doctor Gonzalez on the details of the New York Presbyterian Hospital trial.

9 Doctor Isaacs is a partner in Doctor Gonzalez's practice.

much vegetarian diet, which helped me keep my weight down, so I never regained all of the weight I lost. Knock on wood, I never spent a day in bed.

I was on the programme for about three years. It takes getting used to, but we waste a lot of time. When you're on the programme, you're allocating your time to that, instead of maybe watching a TV programme. I was not working at the time, so that made it a little easier. It's setting your mind to it. If you can get in your mind that this is going to make you live, you allocate the time. The pills are really very simple. Once a month you have to put all your pills in a packet. I was on 60 enzymes a day – ten tablets six times a day, or every four hours, wherever you go. Getting up in the middle of the night was a little problem, but you put them in packets and you just swallow. I got to the point where I pretended I was eating a steak – swallowing a pepper steak or a cherry pie or something!

If you have a positive attitude that this is what you're going to have to do, then it can be fun, and you do it. That attitude is really important. Don't get me wrong though, I would have lows. Early on, I'd think, "What am I doing?" But if I really looked, there was always something that I could see that made it really worth it. We have beautiful snows in Colorado – if it was just waking up in the morning to a beautiful snow and seeing the sun glow off it, or if it was spring and seeing the first flowers and the first trees budding out.

About a month after I started my treatment, my symptoms stopped, although it was gradual. I wasn't going to the bathroom all the time and I started gaining weight.

We did the treatment in stages over the years. I was on 160 pills, then I was on 120. I feel like I'm healed. At five years, the medical profession would have said I was cured. I guess some place along the line, that was the same with the alternative therapies, only I realise that we had to keep up with some of the things, because I just needed them. They're just common sense things, like vitamin B and folic acid and all kinds of minerals.

I can honestly say that on my path, I knew God was with me, without a shadow of doubt, giving me little signs. Not in a booming voice saying: "Ann, thou shalt be healed," or something like that. But one time, I was kind of down and I decided I wasn't going to go to church that Sunday. It wasn't that I was feeling that much worse or anything, but my mind was that much worse. Just like we all get down, but then I thought: "I'm going, *I'm going*." I didn't know it, but they had a guest speaker who had come all the way from South Africa. Of course, we believe the words being said in a sermon. Not very often, they are for people in the congregation. He was sort of like Billy Graham.[10] He was well-known and had a tremendous amount of people in South Africa who camped out in tents to come and see him. He was speaking and talking about God being the head of the Kingdom and he stopped right in the middle of it and he said: "There are two people in this congregation who have been told

10 Billy Graham is an evangelist known for his dynamic delivery of the Christian gospel.

by their doctors that they will die. The Lord just said that you will not and one of you has pancreatic cancer." What is it? 35, 40 thousand people are diagnosed with pancreatic cancer a year, so it's not one of the real biggies as far as volume is concerned. Those little things, like hearing something on the TV or the radio, or from a friend or even a stranger, were encouragement. If you have a positiveness about you, they want to say something to you.

I went to Disney World with my eldest daughter and my grandson, and I went to New Mexico with my other daughter and her two sons, and I went to California with my son. They weren't expensive – they were road trips where you stop where you can and things along that line. But it's enjoying life. If you're going to succeed, I would say that 50, 60 per cent of it is the attitude that you approach it all with.

Since this time, which is 12 and a half years ago, I have talked to a lot of cancer patients who have been sent to me. People think if they get the cancer out, then it will be gone and it will be over. But it's never over. I realised that with the alternative medicine: if it succeeded for me, I would be on a path that I could utilise for the rest of my life. We should know that we did not get sick overnight. It comes on gradually over time with the wrong diet, the wrong air, the wrong water – whatever it is. Our body can't get well just by cutting something out, because it's a total body. It's not just that organ.

I still do my cleanses occasionally, I still do my coffee enemas and I still take a limited amount of pills. As the years went on, they would change the number of pills and the times I had to take them. Periodically, I still take all of those things. It's good for me. Now, I don't have any juices, but I know I should. You know, all of us need to be taking some enzymes if we're over 50 just to stay in good health. I believe everybody should be able to do what they want to do and not have to walk with a walker. If we take care of ourselves there's no reason that we can't.

I had a total trunk CAT scan done three weeks ago. I hadn't had one for six years, because I don't want the radiation in my body. I don't want to do things that will hurt me. At first, I had CAT scans every six months, then nine and 18 months. The tumour is still there. It is still carcinoma, but evidently it is encased, crystallised or whatever, so it's not doing anything. It has shrunk a little bit, but not enough for anyone to go: "Oh wow!" There's nothing wrong with me any place else. I just celebrated my 72nd birthday in April. When I meet them, people can't believe my age.

I'm going to Atlanta in September and we're having the first faith-based alternative medicine retreat ever in the United States. We're going to talk to people who have been diagnosed with cancer and get them to tell their whole story. I'm absolutely excited beyond all means. We will have MDs[11] and research people who are well known across the United States, giving talks. It's

11 MD – medical doctor.

called 'Healing Strong'.[12] A group of ex-cancer patients, people just like me, put it together. It's for cancer patients, but anyone with a degenerative disease, or something they have to live with for the rest of their life, can attend.

If you're given a life-threatening diagnosis, you have to take control of your own life and be responsible to yourself. We all should be able to know what the doctors are doing to us. They give you pills and you don't even know what they're for, and you can have a negative reaction. I'm not saying don't trust doctors, I'm saying know what they are giving you, because they have so many patients and they're busy. They can't be on the top of their ladder all the time, so we need to take responsibility for what's being done to us.

Is every healing a miracle? No, it's not. Sometimes you have to walk the path so that you learn the lessons that you need to learn, so you come out stronger. Everybody says: "You're so strong, Ann," and I think, "I'm not strong at all." Just like everybody else, I've got fears and concerns and worries and children's problems and grandchildren's problems. I have lived long enough to see my only granddaughter born. She is ten now and she's named after me – at least the Sarah part of it. We spent so many wonderful days going to lakes and things while this was all going on. It makes you really want to live the life that you have, instead of wasting it. Everyone approaches things in a different way.

I'm planning on the future, but living day by day. This year, I hope to finish my book about my experiences. Just one ordinary life who happened to hear about other ways to handle cancer. At this time, I want to title it: "Ask, Seek, Knock."

I was fortunate to find wonderful people – doctors, writers, talk show hosts, friends and family who believed as I do and encouraged me along the way.

12 *Healing Strong* http://www.healingstrong.com

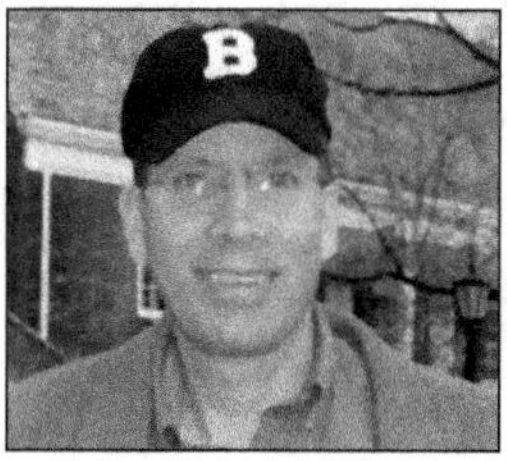

David Emerson, 52 years

Cleveland, Ohio, USA

Diagnosed with multiple myeloma at 34 years

I had experienced for a period of months, literally, a pain in my neck and ignored it like all good young people. Eventually, I began noticing other deficits, and the pain became severe enough that I went to an outpatient clinic. I was x-rayed and a mass was determined to be present in my fifth cervical vertebrae. I went under the knife a couple of days later at University Hospitals here at Cleveland Ohio and was diagnosed with multiple myeloma.[1] At the time it was a single plasmacytoma,[2] which is a fancy term for a single tumour site. I underwent stabilisation of the tumour site with local radiation, and was told that there was a chance that the cancer might not become full-blown multiple myeloma.

About 12 months later, I experienced a relapse, which meant that the single plasmacytoma was now in a number of sites. I began a course of more aggressive conventional therapies – five rounds of a chemo[3] cocktail called VAD (*Vincristine*, *Adriamycin* and *Dexamethasone*), two rounds of something called *Cytoxan* and then a peripheral blood stem cell transplant in December 1995. I came out of the hospital in what was referred to as: "Very good partial remission." Months later, I underwent another relapse, had more local radiation and went into remission again.

Then I had another relapse. I had undergone such a tremendous amount of chemotherapy and radiotherapy that my oncologist basically said: "There's nothing more that we can do for you." It was September 1997 and I was 36 years old. So what do you do? You start looking around. The internet was a fragment of what it is today, but my wife was quite computer literate. It was her that turned to the internet and began searching. Somehow, she stumbled onto the patient website of the Burzynski Research Institute.[4] If you don't have a mortgage and you don't have kids… I didn't have the same responsibilities that most people have to cope with and I didn't think about the long term side of it. So, between being young and sort of foolish, and: "I can't die," to: "I'm scared," and then: "Okay, we've got some money to spend, and then I'll die."

I didn't feel comfortable going to places like Tijuana or Germany – there's

1 Multiple myeloma is a rare form of cancer of the bone marrow.

2 Plasmacytoma is cancer usually found in soft tissue.

3 Chemo – chemotherapy.

4 *Burzynski Research Institute* www.burzynskiresearch.com

expense and there are time issues. So in November of 1997, I began antineoplaston therapy. Within four months, my tumours began to shrink. It's difficult to really pinpoint the time I went into complete remission, but after about 17 months (ten months of liquid, intravenous therapy and then another seven months of a dry form in capsules), my tumours were continuing to shrink and my bone pain was receding. By April 1999, I was in complete remission.

Antineoplaston therapy is referred to as a chemotherapy and is quite similar to traditional chemotherapy, but the big difference is that it's non-toxic. The administration is almost identical – a piece of plastic and metal is sutured in under your skin over your right chest – the same as the port that I had put in for my VAD therapy two years before.

The main drawback of antineoplaston therapy is that there's quite a lot of the stuff. In my case, there were two ten-hour infusions daily, so you have this tube sticking into you, and you walk around with a bag hanging, like you see on the medical shows. I had a handy-pack and a programmable pump, so every day I punched in how much I weighed and the bags dumped into me throughout the ten hours. Then I switched them for the next ten-hour infusion. It's a lot of liquid, so I'd wake up once or twice during the night to go to the bathroom. It's also quite high in sodium, which can be a problem if you're older and have high blood pressure. I was in my mid-thirties and it was comparatively easy for me. Having four hours off every day was great. I could take a shower and work out a little bit and it was great. That felt terrific.

All the therapy was distributed on an outpatient basis. We're from Cleveland Ohio and the treatment is in Houston, so we had a hotel room there. Every morning for three weeks, we'd drive over to the clinic. A part of the therapy is that they teach you really how to be your own administrator, but they want to watch you for the first week that you're on the therapy.

I don't remember specific side effects, but my wife, who was with me from the very beginning of my time spent at the clinic, remembers vividly that I experienced headaches. After undergoing toxic chemotherapy and radiation though, the side effects I was experiencing were child's play – they were nothing. A few headaches are nothing compared to the nausea and other side effects that I had been through. I experienced a variety of what I refer to as late stage side effects, all from my conventional toxic chemotherapy and radiation therapy. I have some nerve damage in my feet, which you can notice when I walk.

There are costs involved, but I tell people that, really, you know what direction you're going in after three or four months, when I was definitely feeling better. It was all about bone pain in my case. I felt better moving, walking and lying in bed. After about three months, my lesions were shrinking. At the end of the therapy, I felt much better and I was pronounced to be in complete remission.

Multiple myeloma is usually considered an incurable form of cancer, meaning that everyone relapses. It's usually pretty easy to reach some stage of remission.

You can go in and out, in and out, so I worried that in a year or two I would come out of remission, but that was in 1999 and it's 2012 now and I'm still in remission, knock on wood! The American Cancer Society counts the entire cancer picture and considers you cured if you're still alive five years from the point of your diagnosis, no matter what condition you're in! That might be different in different countries, I don't know.

I would love to be able to say that in choosing antineoplaston therapy, it was some form of courage or something. In fact, really it was fear. My wife and I were recently married and we didn't have any kids at the time. Other than the bone pain, I felt okay. I was in pretty good condition, but had stopped playing basketball with friends of mine. I cut down sport during the bone marrow transplant – that's quite a taxing therapy – but up until then I was fine. I was 37, and it was inconceivable to me that a doctor could turn to me and sort of imply that I should go home and die.

You don't write a cheque for all the money at once. You spend a few thousand here and there, then you start to feel better. Then it dawned on me that my tumours were shrinking; it was working. That year, from November 1997 and all through 1998, I felt better and it was pretty exciting – things were starting to look up. 1996 and 1997 were awful years – they were dark days. I was apprehensive about the long term, but at least for right then and there, things were good.

My son was born in 1998 – that was certainly a wonderful experience. The only trouble I had at that point was, I began to worry that he would never remember me. There were side effects from the initial chemotherapy that were beginning to take hold. I had cataract surgery on both eyes and I began to experience neuropathy from nerve damage from the effects of my early treatment. By 2001-2002, my myeloma continued to stay in complete remission. That was a good thing! There are a couple of different blood tests that I do every six months and I remain in the normal range.

I tried chemotherapy, it didn't work – fine. I was on to something else. But then you wake up one morning and your eyes or something are going wrong, or your legs aren't working, or you're beginning to experience numbness; these things can happen. Chemotherapy and radiation really are awful stuff. No-one should ever rely on their oncologist to fully tell them what's probably going to happen. There were some great things, like my son being born, and there were some not so great things – the late stage, long term side effects.

As a cancer survivor, it doesn't take much to get me worried. It's always been about bone pain in the past. Since the antineoplaston therapy, I've never had the same bone pain. You wake up one morning and you have an ache or a pain somewhere. Where a normal 52-year-old would just kind of grumble and stretch, I wonder if that's myeloma and my cancer has returned. The issue that invariably comes up is what happens if you ever do relapse? I know that antineoplaston therapy is there, especially the oral form. To be honest, I'm not crazy about doing the liquid form of antineoplaston therapy again, having to prepare the bag every day. But I do know that the therapy worked. The capsule form is much easier to administer even though they're big old horse pills and there were a lot of them. Six times a day I would take ten capsules, then you've got to go to a drinking fountain and you've got to sit there and wolf down these things. But that's a breeze compared to the alternative.

I learn about cancer stuff all the time. I would say that I know enough now to want to mix in detoxification strategies or other general immune boosting therapies. They're not too cheap, but a lot less expensive than antineoplaston therapy. That's another reason for managing my website, *People Beating Cancer.*

Having undergone so much toxic therapy, it's not just a case of having another myeloma relapse – there's a very real chance of a secondary cancer. In fact, a friend of mine who really taught me about myeloma and who was diagnosed a year or two before I was, is now in hospital with leukaemia.

In 2004, I decided to start The Galen Foundation,[5] which is a website with stories of People Beating Cancer on it. The Galen Foundation is a 501(c)(3)[6] non-profit organisation with a mission to inform, educate and support cancer survivors and caregivers. I cancer coach on the internet through PeopleBeatingCancer.org. Though I specialise in multiple myeloma, I work with all cancers. Knowledge is power, as they say!

That's really what I do now. I sit and I do research and I run the website. It's good when patients are exposed to a spectrum of therapies. I find the study of cancer, like alternative therapies, interesting. I spend the day reading studies and articles on various topics. My goal is not to take a position, but to get a conversation going. Through the website, I can speak to the end-stage people who don't have many options. Personally, I can't imagine not trying some of these therapies, as outlandish as they may sound. Why wouldn't you try any number of them? If a patient's cancer is stage one or two, that's one thing. But if it's end stage, that's another story.

My wife is the primary breadwinner in our family. I drive my son around to football practice and things like that. That's what I enjoy.

Multiple myeloma is a rare blood cancer similar to lymphoma and leukaemia. Symptoms include bone pain, anaemia, bleeding, bruising and lowered immunity. Treatments include chemotherapy, radiotherapy, stem cell therapy and immunotherapy. There is no cure for multiple myeloma, but treatment can prolong life for up to ten years. The length of survival depends on when the myeloma was diagnosed.

(American Cancer Society http://www.cancer.org/)

5 *Galen Foundation* http://peoplebeatingcancer.org/galen-foundation

6 A 501(c)(3) is a tax-exempt nonprofit organization in the United States.

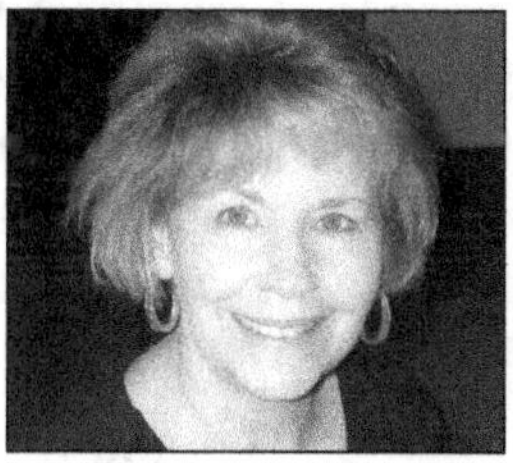

Wanda Flick, 68 years

Lexington, Kentucky, USA

Diagnosed with breast cancer at 46 years

I was in my second marriage when I started having panic attacks. My husband and I both had children. They were mostly grown, but he had one young son whose life was very out of control – that was my perception. Ten years prior to that, I had raised my children as a single mom.

This 'out of control' feeling triggered my heart racing. I could not get anything to stop my heart pounding. It kept me awake, so I was not sleeping at night. I didn't know what was wrong with me, but I knew that what was happening within my body was not good. I just knew something was not right and I was seeking answers.

I had a lightbulb moment when I turned on the TV right in the middle of an interview with a lady who had cancer. The interviewer asked her: "And you had no symptoms?" And she said, "No, only weakness." I knew at that moment what was wrong with me. When I told my husband that, his response was ballistic, because he had lost his first wife to cancer – now here's a second wife diagnosed with cancer. There were a lot of different dynamics going on.

I had a mammogram in September of 1991 that suggested some suspicious activity, but I didn't pay much attention to it, because I'd already had two benign tumours. One was removed in the seventies and the other one in 1986, so I thought: "Oh, it's just more of that, so I won't do anything about it." Then in April of 1992, I went for a biopsy and that's when they found the cancer. It was one of the first needle biopsies done in my area. I was diagnosed with invasive ductal carcinoma with micro-calcifications that were spread throughout my breast – metastatic breast cancer, so it was life-threatening.

Within a few days after I was diagnosed, the surgeon and doctor recommended a radical mastectomy, with follow-up radiation. I went home and prayed. They [the doctors] kept sending me cards about how concerned they were about me, but I never answered any of them. They are very scared for you.

That weekend I found out about Doctor Gonzalez. I learned about him through a friend of my daughter's who had Hodgkin's disease. She was a patient of his for 14 years and had great success with his treatment, so my daughter insisted that I call this lady. When I called and listened to her, it made absolute sense to me – your body will heal itself if you give it the right support.

I thought: "They want to cut off a part of my body, but they haven't checked to see if I have cancer in any other part." It didn't make any sense to me, how you can cut off a part of the body and cure a disease. It's in the interior of your body that things develop. I knew that changing the interior atmosphere of my body was crucial, so I determined that this was the route I wanted to go. Dealing with what was going on with me emotionally was key for me, so I knew that this was a way to work out my healing.

All this caused me to make the call to Doctor Gonzalez, who accepted me as a patient. I told him that I had a trip planned to go and see my mother. He said: "That's fine. If you have cancer, it's been coming for a very long time and it will take some time to get over it. We'll just make the appointment for a month later."

Before I saw him, Doctor Gonzalez ordered a bone scan, a liver scan and a chest X-ray. The cancer was not in my lymphatic system, it was just confined to my breast. He also ordered blood tests and asked for a sample of my hair, which he said showed more accurate results than blood.

You do the programme for ten or 15 days on the supplements, then you have a five-day break. During the five-day break, you do either a 'liver flush', the 'clean sweep' (which is cleaning out the colon) or the 'purge'. Those are the three detoxes[1] that I did – you do one of them a month. I was taking 157 supplements every day, juicing four times a day, and having two coffee enemas a day. I did that for years.

I did not reveal to my mother or my father, who both live in different states, that I had cancer. I knew if I told them, their reaction to me doing this programme might be difficult for me to deal with. I waited a good six months or more before I made a trip again to see them, when I took all my stuff with me – my juicer, my supplements, gallons of purified water and all my food. Of course, they wondered what in the world I was doing, but by that time I was able to tell them how well I was doing on the programme.

The programme was my life for a long time. Because it takes so much time, focus and attention, I really did not have the physical strength to maintain other functions in my life. I mean, we're talking round-the-clock enzymes timed an hour away from your meals, juicing 60 pounds of carrots every two weeks, two coffee enemas every day and eating organic food.

At the height of my weakness, I didn't have enough inner strength even to have a conversation on the phone. It was all I could do to just do my programme. I worried about my strength and energy ever returning and I didn't think they would – I thought I would just have do a lot of resting for the rest of my life. I believe what was happening is that with all the massive support of enzymes and vitamin supplements, my body was working so hard that it was a drag on my energy. If I had a book lying on my lap, it felt like it weighed a ton. Not

1 Detox – detoxification is the elimination of unwanted toxic material from the body.

everyone experiences it the same way, so I don't see it as a negative. I wanted to make sure it was going to work, so I did it religiously. I could literally feel this movement within my body that was working to overcome the cancer. I was determined to do it right, because it was my life. It took an enormous amount of attention, but it was worth it. It *is* worth it.

After I got past the intensity of the programme, my life began to resume somewhat again and I felt like I had a way to live. I developed a lifestyle of healthy eating, learning how to manage stress and defuse negative emotions. It was a huge education and it took years before I was able go back and resume a normal life. When I first went back to my aerobic class, I literally cried.

Every three months I sent in a hair sample to Doctor Gonzalez, which showed nutritional deficiencies and excesses of heavy metals in every system of my body. Through that, he monitored my progress. He also determines your cancer rate through the hair sample. I started off with a cancer rate of 27, which was quite high. Within 18 months, I was down to to a ten, which he said was "safe". When your cancer number gets down to ten or under, that's normal. That has been maintained, except when I went to see him this past May. I hadn't been to see him for four years and my rate was up two points. That's the only time it's gone up in 22 years.

Can I say that there isn't a single cancer cell in my body? I don't know. The cancer rate can potentially go back up if I decided I wanted to eat a bunch of sugar (if I could even tolerate it), but my lifestyle has to be maintained so that my immune system can deal with cancer cells.

Once, after I did one of the purges, where you use grapefruits, lemons and oranges, tears were just pouring out of me. I called Doctor Gonzalez and said: "I don't know what's wrong with me, I cannot stop crying." He said: "You're too alkaline. Take two tablespoons of apple cider vinegar and a glass of water with a little honey," and boy, my acidity level balanced right out and the tears stopped. The purge throws your body into an alkaline state. Once you learn to know your body it's wonderful, because it will send you a signal that something's not right.

To this day, I can call Doctor Gonzalez any time I have a question and he is absolutely available. He will call me back the same day, after he has finished with all his patients, without fail.

There were emotional things I was going through, though. Parallel to my recovery from cancer, I was going through a recovery from infantile incest from the age of six months to five years, so I was processing two tracks of healing.

I had known about this healing path – I'd been to seminars that talked about repressed memories, so nine months into the nutritional program, things that were pressing for resolution began to come up to my conscious level. It was just like pressing a tape recorder button on rewind – I discovered what had happened to me from six months to five years, which until now had been mercifully repressed. As these memories came back into my conscious mind, it made my whole life make sense. My husband witnessed it, because I asked him to come and be with me during this time.

There were 12 days of memories coming back. I guess most people would call it a complete breakdown. It was a shattering of my false self that I had erected to just survive. Doctor Gonzalez explained that my brain was now getting enough nutrients to recall and my body was healing enough to be able to handle this information.

Some people find it very difficult to believe, but I don't, because I experienced it. Even in the womb there is a knowing. I knew that while I was in my mother's womb that there was an abortion attack against me and I had a healing experience around that.

When I was six months old, my father began to orally molest me. I was raised in a very sheltered, strict religious home and was very naïve – even as an adult I did not know that that could happen. When it came back into my conscious mind, I thought I was going to choke to death. I could smell and feel what was happening to me.

It's very important to be cognisant of the connection between trauma and the way your body expresses it. The fear that was in me prior to my cancer was the emotions coming up due to the abuse of my past. I had had fear and rage with me all my life. Once those memories came back, I had a recovery path that lasted a good ten years, alongside the cancer. The fear was crippling, yet once the memories came up, there was no fear in that realm anymore.

The recovery work for the emotional healing was more difficult than just following the health regimen that I had, because the path was not as clear. It was discernible, but difficult. Doctor Gonzalez's program is right there in front of you and you know exactly what to do every day. With the emotional path, there are ups and downs, peaks and valleys. Now I look back and I say: "That was pretty massive, it's just not your ordinary day." I had about two hours a day that I could really be very active – the rest of the time I was just doing the programme. A conversation like this I couldn't have had, because it took too much strength.

I went to a therapy centre out in California, where I was diagnosed with major depression, with only a fair prognosis, but I was determined to get well. I knew that I could recover and face down all the things of my past. I was healing both physically, emotionally and spiritually from the abuse, alongside the cancer. That's an important piece for me, because people sometimes try to focus only on the physical and don't take a look inside to say: "What is triggering this overwhelming loss of life here?"

While I was at the therapy centre, they took all my supplements away and I had to literally fight to get them back. It was good for me to have to fight, because I had been such a victim.

For a very long time I couldn't even talk about these things because I still had so much emotion. Now, I can tell it just as a fact, because I'm healed from the effects of it. I went through 12 days of those things and I discovered exactly what had happened to me. It was a relief to know why I was in a second marriage and why I had always had relationships with men that I didn't understand. My whole life was like a puzzle and it came together with my emotional recovery and being on the nutritional program. It is very empowering for me to be able to say this.

My marriage did not survive. It was four years into my second marriage that I got the cancer diagnosis and we were married for a little over ten years. We had an enormous number of challenges to deal with in our blended family. I realise now that our response to what happens to us is more important than what happens to us.

Once my energy began to come up, oh my goodness. I think I probably have the energy now that I had in my early forties before the cancer, where I had energy all day and I still do. Being on a nutritional programme like I've been on reverses not just your inner health – it helps your ageing process. Your skin is healthy, your hair is healthy. I'm 68, but most people wouldn't believe it. That's not because of who I am – when you do the right things for your body, you maintain your health.

After I went through the change of life, I did have a problem with energy and took some hormones. I believed I didn't need to keep taking them and so I stopped them, but lately I found out that I needed them again. Five days after being on bio-identical hormones, my energy shot up again. It was wonderful and I'm still on those. I have more energy than most people my age.

I didn't have another mammogram. I believe that the radiation and the pressure of mammograms are harmful, so I've never had another one and I never will. I did not go back to my primary care physician. All these 20 years, I think I've had the need for an antibiotic maybe four times for something I just couldn't overcome.

Now I do the detoxes occasionally, rather than one a month. I still do the coffee enemas, because I feel better when I have them. I got so detoxified at one time that I couldn't tolerate anyone with aftershave or perfume coming into my home. I'm still sensitive to odours, but not nearly as much as I was. I still can't tolerate a newly painted room, or fresh varnishes, but I've learned to live that way.

Right after I was diagnosed, I had a confrontation with God. He kind of pulled me up by my shirt collar and looked at me right in the face and said: "Do-not-fear." It was like a Daddy that would say: "Don't you dare do this." It was strong and it reached my core. I had to face the fear down and know that the fear itself would be overwhelming, so I didn't fear, I didn't. Fear will take you down quicker than cancer itself. I had to get a hold of that very early.

I do have a strong faith in God. I knew that He made my body and if I followed principles of good food, supplements, cleaning out my whole system, all my negative thinking and emotions, that it would be life-giving. If I hadn't had a faith in God and believed that something more than my own will was at work, I don't think I would have overcome my cancer. I also knew if I did this programme I was going to be fine. I didn't have fear of the cancer because I knew that I was being healed. I knew I was going to live.

Each person has to have the courage to explore rather than just accept what is currently said through the traditional means of doctoring. It does take a revelation though – it takes something like: "This makes sense to me." People have to listen to their body and listen to what their own spirit is trying to say to them. There's so much truth in it. When you hear truth, it settles inside you.

Our bodies are wonderful and I'm so grateful for that. We have to listen to what's happening and ask: "What is driving this? Why am I doing what I'm doing?" It's wonderful to recover in your body, soul and spirit. It's just wonderful.

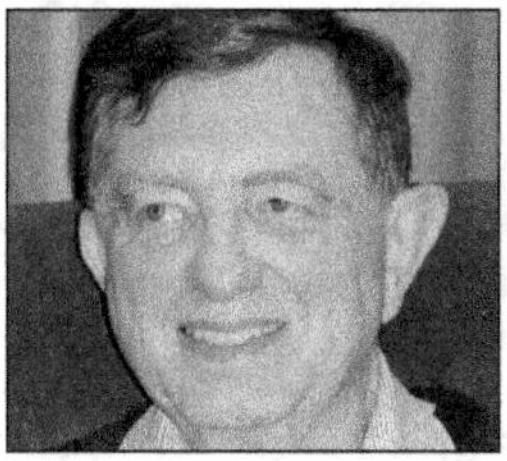

Philip Flournoy, 79 years

West Chester, Pennsylvania, USA

Diagnosed with prostate cancer at 71 years

I had received word from my uncle that he had prostate cancer and was going to have radiation treatments. He refused the surgery because he wanted to continue to have a relationship with his new wife. What disturbed me, was that he was the fourth blood relative of mine to be suffering from prostate cancer at around the same time. (He's four years older than me.) One of my cousins had a radical prostatectomy. They took his prostate out and he was having a lot of side effects. He had to wear diapers and they told him it would probably be a year before he could look forward to better things.

So I went to my urologist. I had been doing that for five years or so, because I had an enlarged prostate and my PSA[1] had moved up above four. It was about six and a half, but my urologist thought that it was okay, because my prostate is – I don't know about the units, but a normal prostate is about 20 in size and mine is 100, so it was five times the normal size for somebody my age. I understand that's not a Guinness Book of Records number. That number would be owned by Tip O'Neill, Speaker of the House of Representatives while Ronald Reagan was President. He passed away in 1994. I remember him saying his prostate was 220 – the largest on record. Anyway, mine was large enough that I was going to urologists and having PSA tests every six months. So I went to him and I said: "I want mine biopsied." And he said: "We can't really do a biopsy, because there's no concern about cancer. We don't expect you to have any trouble and insurance is not going to pay for it." Then I said: "Well, I want a biopsy anyway, because I want to be able to sleep at night. With four relatives who are roughly my age having trouble, it's coming at me from both my mother and father's side." I insisted. After the biopsy, my doctor came to me and said: "I'm really surprised that you do have cancer and I think we should operate." Then he sent me to my general practitioner (GP) for a physical, because I hadn't had one for a number of years. At the physical, my GP said: "You're fine for surgery, but who's doing the surgery?" I told him who, and he said: "I wouldn't do that, because he's only done two of these robotic surgeries that he's now doing and neither of them worked out well. If you're going to have surgery, I would recommend going to a more reliable place." He recommended

1 PSA – Prostate Specific Antigen is a screening blood test to detect possible prostate cancer.

that I go to one of the leading hospitals in the treatment of prostate cancers. They didn't repeat the biopsy, but I took the samples with me and they said it was Gleason 6,[2] so it's relatively early and it is a type that is not aggressive. I said: "Well, when can we do the operation?" They said: "We will not operate on you because you're over 70. It ruins our record to operate on people over 70. We're very proud of our record, but people over 70 don't do well with surgery of any kind."

I was sleeping at night, but I didn't like the word cancer and I didn't want to do nothing. I went to the radiologist at the local hospital and he said that he would do radiation treatments. He thought we should do them right away. "Let's not wait, let's do it right away, let's catch it early, that way we'd have more success." My urologist would have liked to operate, but I wasn't anxious to be the third patient.

Then an amazing thing happened. The day I returned from the hospital, I got a newsletter from a Doctor Julian Whitaker. I had never heard of him before. Right on the front page, he said: "If I had prostate cancer, this is what I would do." I thought: "Rather than do nothing, which the hospital says I should do, maybe I'll do what Doctor Whitaker says." The three things were: get your vitamin D level up to 80 or 90. I'm not sure what the units are. The second thing he said was to take a modified citrus pectin powder, which has been shown to shrink tumours in prostate cancer and breast cancer, plus limit the spread of the disease. Then he said that the third thing he would do is take Low Dose Naltrexone (LDN).[3]

I had taken *Naltrexone* when I was with a pharmaceutical company in the 1970s. I used to work as a research manager there and they developed *Naltrexone* with another well-known pharmaceutical company. I had nothing to do with developing that drug, but we were often asked to sign up for drugs when they were testing them. They gave us LDN during the flu season to prevent us from getting the flu. If it would help me escape the flu every year, I was willing to do it. They knew at the time the main function of that drug, if you're taking it low-dose, would be to boost your immune system. They wanted to market it for cancer and all kinds of things, but the company said: "No, we can't do that. We have drugs for cancer. We get $50,000 a month for these drugs. That's what chemo costs these days. We can't go in there with this drug – it might knock out a bunch of drugs we already have."

What the drug companies do here is when the patent is beginning to run out, they come out with the next drug, which they claim to be a little bit better than the last one. You know, 'this one kept you alive for four months, this one will keep you alive for six months.' Then they can start their patent running all over again.

Because I was familiar with the drug, I knew I could tolerate it. The other

2 Gleason Grade is a pathology grading for common prostate cancers from 1 to 10. 2-5 is slow growing, 5-7 is moderately aggressive.

3 Low Dose Naltrexone is the off-label prescription of the FDA approved drug *Naltrexone*.

thing was that I knew there would be no harmful side effects. So why not do something? If it doesn't work for me, I always can go back to the urologist and say: "Okay, you can operate." Maybe this would give him time to learn how to do the surgery. [*laughs*]

The other two things I could do on my own, but for the *Naltrexone* I had to have a prescription, so I asked my urologist for one. He said: "I've never heard of it and I'm not going to stick my neck out – you'll have to ask somebody else." So I went to my GP and he said: "We have a policy here of not writing prescriptions for any use that is not approved by the Food and Drug Administration." Then I went to another doctor that I see for my eyes and we're really good friends. I thought that he would certainly write it, but he said: "Phil, I can't do that. If it was something to treat your eyes, I might do it, but I can't do this."

So I called a holistic integrative physician that I had used when I lived in Raleigh about 15 years earlier and he said: "Phil, I will write you the prescription, no problem. I have my mother on it right now. If you give me your telephone number, I will call in the prescription to the best pharmacy in the world for that drug. It's called Skip's pharmacy and it's in Florida. They will call you, get your details, and you'll have your medicine tomorrow." So that's what happened. He told me to take 4.5mg daily, which is a very small amount. Drug addicts take 50-200mg a day, depending on how bad their problem is. He said: "Take it just before you go to bed and it should do the job for you. Call me every six months and I'll renew the prescription. I'll charge you 50-60 dollars for the phone call." Then he said: "I'd like to see you personally every two years. We're in different states and the licensing people might get mad at me if I don't see you." We did that for a while, but the trips from here to North Carolina for somebody who's 79 years old are getting pretty bad, so this year I moved to a local holistic doctor who also writes the prescription for me.

With *Naltrexone*, a lot of people start low, by taking 1mg and work up. Some say they can't sleep when they first take it, otherwise there are few side effects. I took 4.5mg. After that first dose, as soon as my head hit the pillow that night, I was gone for nine hours. My wife said I didn't move. Ever since then, I have been going to sleep instantly. I have never in my life had that experience. I would always lay there for half an hour, toss and turn and get comfortable and that kind of thing. It's been like that ever since I started taking it eight years ago.

Let me tell you some things that happened along the way. My vitamin D level was 19 when the cancer was discovered. Within about two years, we managed to get it to 93, which is when the doctor wanted me to stop. I take ten thousand units per day and my vitamin D level remains above 90.

The doctor I was getting the LDN from ordered a batch of tests and he said to take a natural killer cell test[4] before I started the first dose. Before I started the

4 Natural Killer, or NK cells, are lymphocytes that provide rapid responses to virally infected cells and respond to tumour formation.

LDN, my levels were 70 per microlitre. I've kept track of them on a chart until 2011 and now they're 440. If you put a straight line on there, the whole time I've been on the LDN they've been creeping up.

Everything was looking good – the cancer wasn't running away. I got my vitamin D level up and my natural killer cell level up. My PSA was 6.4 when I started and after about 18 months or so, it dropped down to two.

I was having rectal exams plus a PSA test every six months and they were saying: "Well, we can't feel any cancer and with the PSA dropping like this we think the cancer is in remission." I had a repeat biopsy that I can easily remember, because it was 11/11/2011. And it happened to be 11am when they took the sample! After being on the drug for five years, the biopsy was clean. There was no cancer. As I'm a scientist, I said: "That's a sampling problem, you're grabbing samples and you could have missed the area where the cancer was." Originally they took 12 samples, so they took extra samples on the worst area, but they found nothing.

I don't like to use the word 'cure' because I don't think LDN cures anything. I think what it does is it boosts your immune system and that's what takes care of health problems, so you can't really claim that LDN does anything as far as curing things goes. It's your body that cures the cancer. That's why the drug is used by so many people for so many different things. The doctors will say that it's impossible for one drug to cure all those things that are claimed, but the drug isn't curing anything – that's what they're missing. The drug is just making your immune system work better and also helping people with Crohn's disease, MS,[5] Alzheimer's, autism and rheumatoid arthritis. There are so many uses for this drug. I think if I stay on the LDN and keep my immune system healthy, I will live a long life, free of cancer. It's a lot like diabetes, you can live with it if you have the right diet and the right exercise, but it's always there.

About ten years ago, I had 13 teeth crowned at one sitting. They wanted to do it all at once and it took six hours, with *Novocaine*[6] every 15 minutes. Towards the end, my throat closed off, and they had to put a tube in, so I could breathe. Later, I was having difficulty swallowing, so I had ultrasounds that found three nodules on my thyroid – caused by the *Novocaine*, I was told. They suggested we do nothing except follow it. Another case of doing nothing, but I couldn't swallow. So I went to my ear, nose and throat doctor and he said: "With your permission, I'll stick a needle in the one in the front and see what we can do with it." He decided that it was a cyst and he removed the contents. I still had the other two nodules, but I could swallow. He sent it off to be analysed and they said it was nothing but cyst-like fluid with cells in it. I stopped worrying about it and didn't do anything and I didn't even go back to the endocrinologist – he used to want to check them every six months.

---

5 MS – multiple sclerosis.

6 *Novocaine* is an injectable local anaesthetic.

I'm having hearing problems and a couple of months ago I went to a doctor who had done surgery on my ears 30 years ago. He felt my thyroid and he said: "You have a growth on your thyroid. I'm not doing anything until you get rid of that." So I went to the endocrinologist that he wanted me to go to and they did a biopsy. They came back and said that I had a two inch in diameter tumour on my thyroid, but it was completely dead. All the cells inside that they sampled were dead cells. There is no evidence of any live cells in the samples that were sent to them. Since I didn't know I had it, it didn't bother me. What they said is that it was probably malignant, but it had died for some reason. I personally think that the LDN not only stopped my prostate cancer, but also a thyroid cancer I didn't even know I had.

I'm one of these people who develops colon polyps – it's a genetic thing. My sons both have a problem that way too. They couldn't remove one of my polyps during the colonoscopy, because it was two inches in size. It was not cancer, but pre-cancerous. To get it out, they had to remove 18 inches of my colon. They said if they hadn't removed it, I would have developed colon cancer. After that I had colonoscopies every three years and they needed to take out little polyps every time. After I started taking the LDN – no more polyps. They would go in there and there was absolutely nothing, so they said: "We don't need to do any colonoscopies anymore, because for some reason, you have stopped making polyps."

At this point, I am very healthy. I feel great. It might be the vitamin D, the citrus pectin, the LDN, or a combination of all three. I get up every morning with a ton of energy and I'm still going at midnight. I take care of my five-acre property. I cut all the grass, pull the weeds and prune the shrubs – you know the routine. I feel almost like I'm back in my thirties. At 79, it's hard for anybody to believe, but I'm as strong as I was then.

The side effects from this treatment have been amazing for me. The first thing was the sleep that I mentioned. The second thing is that I haven't been sick in eight years – I've not had a sniffle. My wife gets a cold two or three times a year. I have four grandkids and every time they come in here one of them is sick. She catches something and I don't. She sleeps on my shoulder when she's sick and I still don't get it. No flu, no colds for eight years.

When I used to go out in the yard to cut grass, I would sneeze my head off because of the pollens. I took some drugs to try to help with the allergies, but not anymore. For the past eight years, I don't even worry about it. My allergies have just disappeared.

Another thing, which is hard to put your finger on, is that my attitude to life is different. I'm very happy. I wake up every morning raring to go. I guess I'm saying that the LDN is acting like an antidepressant. It's making me feel great and ready to go. It gives me energy. Before, I wasn't depressed to the extent that I took any medication, but I used to worry about things and they would keep me awake at night. Now it's almost as if they run off my back, I think because I'm sleeping so well.

Some years ago, I made a list of the drugs that other people might need to take, but if they took this drug, they wouldn't have to take them. That's: sleeping pills, antidepressants, antivirals, energy boosters, antihistamines and chemotherapy.

The last time I had my natural killer cells measured, the lab wanted another sample. They said: "The numbers are so high they're off our charts. We've never had anybody in here with numbers so high." They wanted to be sure that they hadn't contaminated the sample. I gave another blood sample and they got an even higher number. In that particular lab, it was the highest number they'd ever seen.

Naltrexone has done all this and it costs me US$15 a month and I don't take anything else. My wife doesn't take anything either, so it may not be the *Naltrexone*. She fixes everything from scratch in the way of food. We're not vegetarians, but almost. We eat a little chicken and fish, but primarily we eat raw vegetables and raw fruit. I work out every day with vigorous exercise for about ten minutes. My weight is 155 pounds and I'm six feet two, so my BMI is below 20. I think everything that's good in my life is due to the LDN. You can't go through life but one way. I don't know what would have happened if I hadn't done this. I caused all of this to happen because I looked at my uncles and cousins and said: "They're going through hell and they're having a lot of bad side effects and I don't want that." On the other hand, I didn't want the cancer to get away.

My urologist told me one day: "I've learned more from you about cancer than I did in med school. If I get prostate cancer, I'm going to follow you and have you help me through it." I said: "Well, why don't you give your patients LDN?" He said: "No, I'm a surgeon. I'm trained as a surgeon. I have kids in college, I have student loans to pay off, I have office staff to pay and I do surgery. I don't do LDN." This is a common attitude of the doctors here, or that one anyway. I have not found very many doctors who will even listen to me. They said the Food and Drug Administration has to put their stamp of approval on it before we can touch it. It has to do with their liability insurance, their group medical practices and a lot of political things. The doctors who use it are thinking outside the box and taking a chance. The doctor in Raleigh who prescribed it for me the first time lost his licence. Not because of the LDN, but for doing something that was not approved by the Food and Drug Administration. He tried oxygen treatments – ozone right in the bloodstream with a woman who had stage IV cancer. She had been told she had a couple of months to live. He said: "This is the only thing I know that can take care of you at this point." She died and her husband sued him, saying he was using ozone treatment which was not approved by the Food and Drug Administration. He had wanted her to use chemo, but she refused and went with the ozone. He got his license back a couple of years later. These are people who are willing to take risks with their own business in order to help people.

A friend of 40 years who was my first stockbroker heard me say I had prostate cancer. When his PSA went to 16 and was told he had prostate cancer, he called me and said: "Phil, I don't want to do the surgery, chemo and radiation – what did you do?" I told him and he said: "Let me write down the name of that Low Dose Naltrexone and I'll see if my doctor will give it to me." He went to his doctor and she said: "I've never heard of it, but looking at it on the internet, it probably couldn't hurt you, so I'll write the prescription for you." His PSA dropped to below two in about six months. They have done a repeat biopsy and his cancer is gone. We talk once a month or so and he's doing really well. He took 4.5mgs the first night like I did and slept beautifully. He has not been sick since he went on it five years ago.

My case is not a miracle for me that wouldn't work for somebody else, because I know it worked for him. I have helped a number of people on the website go on the programme that I did. They haven't stayed in touch with me, so I don't know how they're doing, but I assume they're doing okay. It chews me up to see the miracles that happen every day on that website – it's amazing. Some people say they can't take it and it doesn't work for them.

There's a class reunion from my high school in a week or so and the class secretary asked me about coming down and talking to them about my experiences with cancer, because so many of my classmates are dying of cancer. I can't get away, but I started telling her my story and I said: "You can tell them that they can call me or you can give my email address to anyone that's interested and tell them about my success." Then she started asking me about Crohn's disease, pancreatic cancer and a number of other things and her relatives started to call me. There's a 20-year-old second cousin who had to drop out of college because of Crohn's disease. I think something like 85 per cent of people treated with Low Dose Naltrexone have gone into remission. So I'm doing a little bit to help people.

People don't necessarily have to choose one method of treatment over another. The LDN will boost your immune system and it's not going to interfere with the chemo or radiation. The only thing it interferes with is opium-based drugs, so if you're not taking these painkillers, then you can take LDN. There's evidence that you won't have as many bad side effects from chemo. One woman said that she didn't lose any hair and the doctor was surprised because all of his other patients lost their hair. She didn't have an upset stomach and the others were having nausea and all kinds of problems.

I didn't actually make a decision about which way to go myself – the hospital I went to sort of made it for me. I didn't have to hurry to make a decision – I could live with the cancer a little bit longer. Doctor Whitaker's newsletter, I felt, was almost like a message from heaven. Even though I knew about the drug, I wouldn't have gone on it if I hadn't seen his leaflet.

When I told my urologist that I was going to get the prescription from a doctor in Raleigh who practiced integrative medicine, he said: "Well have you checked him out on quackdoctors.com?" I said: "What's that?" He said: "In the medical profession we have a website that you can go to and it will keep you from going to quacks, because there are a lot of quacks in the medical profession. You ought to check that website to see if the doctor you're dealing with is on that website." I went there and yes, the doctor I mentioned was on that website. But the number one 'quack' doctor on the top spot on the website was Doctor Whitaker. So I went back to the urologist and thanked him for giving me the website, because, I said: "That's the place to find the really good doctors."

Harvard educated Bernard Bihari, MD (1931-2010), discovered the clinical effects of FDA-approved Naltrexone *using low doses (Low Dose Naltrexone or LDN). In 1985-86, he conducted a groundbreaking clinical trial on patients with HIV/AIDS. Doctor Bihari says that the immune system normalising effect of the drug application he discovered applies to a wide range of autoimmune diseases.*

Research trials can be found at http://www.lowdosenaltrexone.org/ldn_trials.htm

79-minute interview with Doctor Bihari: http://www.youtube.com/watch?v=x54Jc-cr8GT879

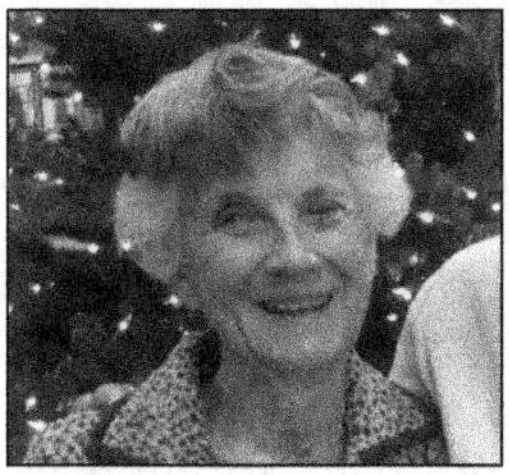

Joyce Forsythe, 76 years

Dover, New Hampshire, USA

Diagnosed with mantle cell non-Hodgkin's lymphoma at 68 years

My husband Pete and I lived in New York in the early seventies. My internist was Robert Atkins, the famous cardiologist who advocated a high protein, low carbohydrate diet. I followed his way of eating a lot of meat and eggs and I felt wonderful. He promoted taking a five-hour glucose tolerance test to find out how I handled sugar. I discovered that I was pre-diabetic, and hypoglycaemic (low blood sugar). So I had my husband buy a second refrigerator, put it in our pantry and put a lock on it, so I couldn't get to his cookies and chocolate milk. That way I stayed away from sweets and other high-glycaemic, processed foods quite well and I have not had a headache since 1973. I felt like steel. I worked several jobs and travelled a lot. We had apartment buildings that we rented to students, so I was extremely busy cleaning apartments and renting them.

Pete and I began dating in ninth grade and got married at the end of our first year of college at the University of Michigan. As soon as we finished college, we had a son (the day after my last exam!) Then we had a daughter. We figured that we had replaced ourselves on the earth, so if there were children who needed families, we would adopt kids with special needs who were not being adopted by other people. We adopted three kids (not related), so we ended up with five kids – I was a very busy person.

I have a Masters in social work and I'm a retired psychotherapist. Pete was a lawyer. In 1967, we started The North American Council on Adoptable Children made up of lay people mostly – couples who were willing to adopt these kids. Its headquarters is in Minneapolis, Minnesota. Our motto was: "Concerned about the children who wait." That organisation went national, then we started another organisation called Court Appointed Special Advocates (CASA) all in our living room. CASA worked with judges and used hundreds of thousands of volunteers around the country in the courts to help locate kids who needed to get into adoptive families. That organisation went national too. Now it's headquartered in Seattle, Washington.

The other agency I started was in an 80-year-old farmer's house outside of Ann Arbor, Michigan. He wanted to donate his farmhouse and land to help children. We named this new, specialised agency after the farmer, Spaulding for Children, and put two social workers in his home with him. No kids were brought into the house – social workers would go out and find homes for kids in other agencies who were really hard to place. One of the first kids they placed was a baby whose bio-mother had taken thalidomide during pregnancy, so was born with no arms or legs.

I wasn't working at the farm – I was helping to find money to pay the workers. The parents who adopted the children were to pay nothing, because they were helping by adopting. They would raise the child and get them through college after that. That agency was duplicated in a number of different states around the country. Four years ago, we were invited back for their 30th anniversary, videotaped to tell the history of the Spaulding for Children agency. That agency is now located next to metropolitan airport in Detroit. The budget for one year is 11 million dollars. They are the main adoption resource centre of the United States now. It shows other agencies how to get the job done and has helped many kids find adoptive homes.

I was busy at that time sending out newsletters, speaking engagements and working with Wayne County Court in Detroit with a judge named James Lincoln. He was the president of the Juvenile and Family Court Judges Association for the whole of America. I talked him into letting me put Junior League women volunteers in his court to dig out the kids who were stuck in foster homes and institutions. Then, maybe other courts around the country would be willing to do this, because the agencies were full of these kids.

When we tried to adopt a child, we had been married a long time and we had a big house. We were very stable, but it took us four years, 11 adoption agencies and 22 social workers, *studying* us, before we got three kids – kids who had been waiting for years to find a family and were moved from one temporary place to another. That's the trouble that families like us were having. So that's kind of my background.

Then we moved to New York, where my husband got a job with a foundation, so he would have money to help support some of these projects. I was at home with the children and going to social work school at New York University. There was a very good radio programme on nutrition by Carlton Fredericks, PhD, that ran for about 20 years. When he died, Robert Atkins took it over, and so I listened to *him* every day. From Atkins, I learned to be very careful about sugar and processed carbohydrates, and that's when I felt like steel. I was about 36 and I felt like I had the answer to being very healthy. My cholesterol was unbelievably good. I had so much energy, never a headache, but I didn't know about the importance of pH.[1]

When we retired 20 years ago, we moved to Dover, New Hampshire. My doctor here called me 'Methuselah'. The bible says that Methuselah lived for 900 years. I was taking no drugs and I hadn't had an aspirin since I started

1 pH means literally 'power of hydrogen' and refers to the acid/alkaline balance of aqueous solutions. Below 7.0 is acidic, and above 7.0 alkaline. In this case, the reference is to the pH level of body fluids, namely blood and urine.

with Robert Atkins in 1973.

We bought 11 multi-family student rental buildings. We were working long days rehabilitating the buildings and cleaning up after students, which meant the use of toxic materials.

In July of 2005, I went to the doctor for my annual physical. A week before that, I was lying in bed watching television and noticed that one side of my belly button was a little more firm than the other side. I didn't feel any bump, so I thought when I go to the doctor, I'll ask her about that. I went through the physical and she said: "You're fine, I will see you next year." Then I asked her: "I'd like you to put me back on the table and push on my stomach again, because one side feels more firm than the other." When she pressed harder, she exclaimed: "Oh, my gosh, you have an enormous mass in there."

I was sent immediately to the Dover New Hampshire Cancer Centre. They did a bunch of blood tests, a PET[2] scan, a CAT[3] scan and a bone marrow test.

I was sent from the cancer centre to the Dana-Farber Cancer Institute in Boston, which is a teaching hospital under the auspices of Harvard Medical School. Our eldest daughter is an associate professor and physician at Harvard Medical School. She learned a lot of nutrition from me as she grew up – that's why she became a physician. My cancer was diagnosed as 'mantle cell non-Hodgkin's lymphoma' – an unusual form and I needed a lymphoma specialist who had treated other such cases.

I was told I needed to have four chemo[4] drugs through a port implanted near my shoulder. One was a trial drug which might put this in remission, but in six months or so, the lymphoma would come back and I would need different chemo drugs. My husband was with me – he came to every appointment. I respectfully listened to the doctor, thanked him and told him that I would discuss it with my husband and give him a call the next day to let him know if I wanted to take the chemo.

We walked outside the door of the office and I said: "You know Pete, I'm not going to take the chemo. I'm going to use Doctor Max Gerson's nutritional therapy." He said: "I figured you would." So we stopped on the way home, bought a lot of organic food and I bought Charlotte Gerson's first book.[5] It cost me $17 and I did the treatment here at home, in the kitchen.

When I told my oncologist that I was going to turn down the chemotherapy and use a nutritional approach, he emphasised that I had stage four cancer, which was very life threatening.

I started the Gerson therapy immediately and felt fine. When Pete and I made

2 PET Positron Emission Tomography – a nuclear medical imaging technique that produces a three-dimensional image of the body to assess the metabolic activity of tissues. It is used to identify cancer cells and their possible spread through the body.

3 CAT scan, also known as a CT scan, or Computed Axial Tomography is a diagnostic medical imaging procedure that examines cross sections of the body allowing a three dimensional view of specific areas.

4 Chemo – chemotherapy.

5 *The Gerson Therapy – The Proven Nutritional Program for Cancer and Other Illnesses* by Charlotte Gerson and Morton Walker.

my first green juice, I gagged on the first sip – then I said: "It's better than chemo" and drank it, never again to mind the taste of the red cabbage, Granny Smith apple, green pepper, red chard and romaine lettuce! I also called the Gerson Institute to find out if there was a physician near me in New Hampshire who might be familiar with Gerson Therapy, who I could turn to if I had any questions. They had a list of Gerson-licensed naturopaths I could choose from, so I chose Bonnie Marsh, a naturopath in California. I could call toll-free or email her and didn't have to see her in person. The first month cost me $350. I could talk to her or email her as often as I needed. Other months that I used her cost $200. I consulted her for four different months, when I had a particular question. Of course, insurance does not cover such medical bills.

I did the 13 fresh vegetable juices and five coffee enemas every day, stayed strictly with the recommended nutritional supplements and I felt fine during the whole treatment. I had no pain and I had nothing that I could tell was wrong with me.

My oncologist at Dana-Farber wanted to biopsy my spleen. It's very vascular – if they stuck a needle in it, I might bleed to death. So they wanted to take my spleen out carefully, and biopsy it 'out'. They found that it weighed five pounds and was about the size of a football. I thought that it would go down in size, but mantle cell lymphoma is uncommon and it would be good to know as much as I could about it. I would have preferred not to, but I thought: "If they want to take it out, I'll let them take it out."

I was a member of a large landlord organisation here in Dover and the secretary who did the minutes of meetings had just had a baby. The night before I had to go down to Boston to have the operation, I typed up the minutes and photocopied 200 of them for her. Before I did the newsletters, I went up on the fourth floor of our house, which overlooks a large river flowing upstream from Portsmouth, New Hampshire. We built our house here, four stories high, with a widow's walk on top so you can see the night lights of Portsmouth and boats going up and down the river. I wanted to get a coat of wrought iron paint on the railing, so I painted it, took the newsletters to the post office and dropped them in the mail box at midnight. I had to leave at about 4.30 in the morning for my operation. That's how sick I was. How can you be sick with a Stage IV cancer, not know it and not feel bad?

It was getting time for me to go to Naples in Florida, where we go for six months out of the year. I was having CAT scans and blood tests done every four months. I went to the Dana-Farber hospital and asked for the name of an oncologist in Florida in case I needed one while I was down there. The oncologist looked at my test results and said: "This is absolutely fantastic. I don't think you're going to need an oncologist in Florida."

When I got down to Florida, I got a letter from the Dana-Farber oncologist who said: "Keep doing what you're doing, the chemotherapy would not have cured your cancer anyway." He said that it was a terminal cancer and that people don't usually live longer than about three years. I was still feeling great. Of course, we didn't go to any restaurants – we ate at home. [*laughs*]

At the five-year point, the local oncologist called me in and said: "Your cancer has been gone now for quite a while. We have not been able to find any cancer, and so you don't have to keep coming back." I was healthy and the CAT scans and blood markers were good. The local oncologist then said that she would like to see me every year, at no charge. She just wanted to follow me because she was interested and she cared. She commented that had I taken the chemo, she didn't think I would still be alive.

I've had a perfectly healthy eight years since being diagnosed. Gerson therapy has been a lot of hard work. I have eaten organically and vegetarian – no meat or eggs. I gave up all animal products except no-fat, plain, organic yogurt, which I have with orange juice and cold-pressed flaxseed oil. Later, I was able to add wild salmon once a week. I'm off Gerson now and living more normally, but try to stay as close to it as possible, even when I'm at a restaurant or somebody else's house for dinner.

We have a very busy social life in Florida. It's not fair to my husband, so I have not turned down all of our social invitations. When you go to a restaurant and order a big salad, it's vegetables with pesticides, and the dressings are not made with the right kind of oil. Their water is not the distilled water that I always drink – it's water with chlorine and fluoride.

I get scolded by friends for wasting my money on organic food. "It's no better than other food and the people selling organic are lying to you. It's foolishness." [*laughs*] I think they just forget I ever had cancer, because I never looked sick. A group of friends, who are about ten years younger than we are, often talk about all their aches and pains and drugs. One of their daughters works for Merck, the drug company, so they really believe in drugs. They think I'm terrible for not taking drugs, but I don't take any – ever.

The same week I was diagnosed with cancer, a friend from our church, 20 years younger than I, was diagnosed with non-Hodgkin's lymphoma. Her husband was the mayor of the town north of us and a chemistry professor. I gathered my Gerson books and loaned them to her. She returned them a few days later, saying she was going to do what her oncologist recommended. She stopped attending church, but her husband kept going, so he told me how she had many blood transfusions, surgery and a variety of chemotherapy treatments. It appeared for a while her cancer was in remission, but it came back and different chemo drugs were used. I recently telephoned them to see how she was doing. Her husband answered the phone and told me that she had died a couple of years ago – an awful death at home under the care of a hospice.

I have always had an enormous amount of energy. I go to bed at about 11.30 at night and I wake up at five without an alarm, read, work at the computer and I'm wide awake. I never take any naps. As a child I was always healthy. My mother gave me a teaspoon of cod liver oil every day, and I licked the spoon – I liked it! Maybe that gave me a good foundation, I don't know.

My licence to be a clinical social work psychotherapist came from the Education Department at New York University in Albany – the same place that Doctor Gerson got his medical license. He wrote a book called: *A Cancer Therapy – The Results of 50 Cases*. He would be called up to the licensing department to have his license revoked, so he took his 'terminal' patients who had been given up on by the Mayo Clinic, Sloan Kettering Cancer Centre and other places, and they brought their medical records with them. Doctor Gerson would show their records to the licensing department and then they would not revoke his license. But they would still say: "We want you back in six months for another hearing." It touched my heart, because he was licensed by the same body that licensed me.

On Nutrition

• Oils

Doctor Gerson learned from Johanna Budwig, nominated for the Nobel Prize in medicine seven times, that cold-pressed flaxseed is very healing, especially when combined with no-fat, plain, organic yogurt. He says not to heat any oils, because the molecular structure changes. I switched to Udo Erasmus's oils at around the four-year point. It has all three essential fatty acids, omega 3, 6 and 9 in the right ratios. His book is called *Fats that Heal, Fats that Kill*.

• Acid/Alkaline levels

When I was first diagnosed, I had a pH of 5.0 – so acidic, I was asking for cancer. At that level, it steals calcium and other minerals from the bones. The osteoporosis epidemic is due to our eating acidic foods like meat. After being on the Gerson therapy for just a couple of weeks, my pH reading rose to well above 7.0.

• Bone density

I've been thrilled with the results of my bone density tests since starting Gerson therapy. Doctor Gerson said not to take calcium supplements. I've had three bone density tests over these last eight years. Each test shows my bones are better than the previous one. My internist thought that it was strange, when I wasn't taking calcium supplements, so she did an overnight test. She said: "You are making new bone as fast as you are sloughing off the bad. Whatever you're doing, that's the thing to do."

Many of my friends take biphosphonates to improve their bones, statin drugs for high cholesterol, blood pressure medicines and allergy medications.

• Sugar metabolism

Doctor Atkins says: "The most important test you will ever have is a five-hour glucose tolerance test, but your doctor will fight you and not want you to take it." I called my doctor, who was a good friend, and said: "I want you to order for me a glucose tolerance test." He said: "You don't need it – there's nothing wrong with you." Well, I occasionally had a headache, my heart would sometimes flutter, I would feel weak and nauseated if I didn't have breakfast. He said: "No, no, you don't need it – and they use a real big needle, so it hurts a lot and the test is very expensive." (About $80 and paid for by my insurance.) Finally, I said: "Look Larry, if you don't order it for me, I will call another doctor and get it, because I want that test."

I went in for the test, and I went in alone, but it's better if you take someone with you, because you might go crazy in that lab. They gave me a very sweet coke and then took a blood test every half hour for three hours. The sugar in the blood should rise and fall back down to the fasting level at about three hours, and stay there for the next two hours. After about an hour, I was throwing up into the waste basket in the waiting room, had a headache and was perspiring terribly. I got home, went to bed and stayed there for three days, very sick. Larry called me on the third day and said: "I just got your glucose tolerance test back and you're fine! I told you there was nothing wrong with you." I said: Larry, I've been so sick for three days – I'm just now coming out of it." He said: "Well, there's a flu bug going around – you must have caught it at the lab."

Doctor Atkins said: "Don't believe your doctor – get a copy of the lab report yourself and graph your own results." One type of hypoglycaemia is 'reactive', when the blood sugar shoots right up and then falls way down, then goes back up to fasting. Mine didn't go up at all. As soon as I tasted that sweet coke, my sugar level dropped, because my pancreas was pouring out insulin to drive the sugar level down. When it got dangerously low, the adrenal gland kicked in to produce adrenaline, which started bringing the sugar level back up. They stopped my test very early due to my terrible reaction. Doctor Atkins says that this is a pre-diabetic hypoglycaemic curve and if you don't change the way you eat, you're going to end up with diabetes. I was wearing out my pancreas and adrenal glands whenever I ate sugar or white flour.

• Thyroid and Metabolism

The thyroid needs iodine to function well. I grew up in Michigan where many residents suffered goiters. It was a long way from the oceans and the soils were depleted of iodine. Once iodine was added to the boxes of salt, goiters hardly ever occurred. The success of solving the goiter problem in Michigan resulted in our whole country having iodised salt available, but not enough. Doctor Gerson recommends Lugol's Solution as an iodine supplement to help the thyroid better manage metabolism.

I take desiccated porcine as my thyroid supplement and my thyroid stimulating hormone test (TSH) is perfect. It was 3.7 and now it's 0.4. When I started Gerson, my weight went from 170 to 118 pounds. I make my own clothes and wearing them is a lot of fun.

• High Blood Pressure

I had a call from my little brother – he had high blood pressure and other health problems. I had him change his diet, and start taking the yoghurt with Udo's Oil.

The next time he went to the doctor, he said: "They made a mistake taking your blood pressure – I need to take it again". After three days of eating differently, his blood pressure was normal and he had stopped his medication. Three months later, he is still off his blood pressure medicine. I'm so happy about my little brother.

Doctor Gerson says that blood pressure goes down in three days with the right diet change.

Mantle cell lymphoma is an aggressive type of lymphoma that represents about 7% of non-Hodgkin's lymphoma cases. It is a difficult type of lymphoma to treat and often does not respond to chemotherapy. It is found in lymph nodes, the spleen, bone marrow, and gastrointestinal system. Mantle cell lymphoma usually develops in men over age 60.

(University of Maryland Medical Center http://umm.edu/health/medical/reports/articles/nonhodgkins-lymphoma#ixzz35SclsRkf)

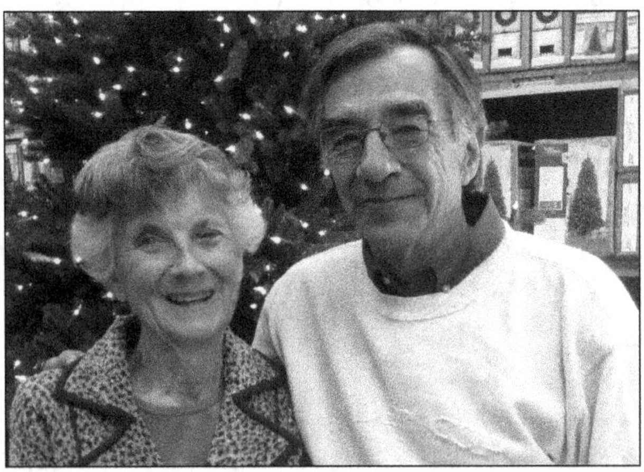

Joyce Forsythe with her husband Pete.

Judith Hansen, 53 years

California, USA

Diagnosed with scleroderma at 40 years

I was still living in New York in 2000 when I started having symptoms. I would have to say that fatigue was the first symptom. It was unexplained fatigue, unrelated to a cold or the flu or anything like that. I felt like I was carrying a lot of weight around.

After fatigue, the next symptom was swelling. I started getting swollen hands when I woke up in the morning, then it spread to my feet and a little bit to my ankles. I kind of had sore joints. All the while, I was preparing to move to New Zealand, so maybe the stress of moving countries was exacerbating my symptoms. The symptoms were mild until a few weeks before I actually got on the plane and moved.

When I got to New Zealand, one of the first things I did after I got a job was find a doctor. I had medical insurance through my work, so I just went to a doctor in my insurance plan. She looked at my hands and could tell right away that I had Raynaud's[1] disease and said that it may be related to an autoimmune disease.

It turned out that I had a positive ANA[2] test. By that time, I had started getting skin-tightening and under my skin was kind of mottled. If I stretched, it would be hard to move. By now I had joint pain, weakness and really crushing fatigue. My doctor sent me to a diagnostician of some kind, who diagnosed me right away as having scleroderma. That was a bit of luck to get a diagnosis when it was early on with my symptoms.

I had never heard of this disease and was quite baffled by it, but the diagnostician was pretty certain that this was what I had. She was not very positive about my prognosis at all, which she said was pretty grim. She didn't use those words, but after she listened to my symptoms, she thought it had spread to my lungs, my thyroid and possibly my kidneys. By that time, I was having shortness of breath, acid reflux and some trouble swallowing.

By the time I was diagnosed, my body was completely tight all over. The skin on my body – I mean from my feet to my face, neck, arms, legs and even my

1 Raynaud's disease is a circulatory disorder that causes discolouration of the fingers and toes, in a characteristic 'glove and stocking' effect. It is usually triggered by stress or cold, when constriction of the blood vessels decrease the blood supply to the extremities.

2 ANA – anti-nuclear antibodies. The presence of ANAs in the blood help to diagnose autoimmune disease.

back – was tight. I couldn't squat to do the garden for a long time, because my knees wouldn't support my body or my ankles, but I can do those things now.

Systemic scleroderma can be a very brutally progressive-acting illness. It was really moving very fast. Every morning I would wake up and there would seem to be something new happening.

My blood work, however, still was normal at that time, except for the positive ANAs. My doctor was surprised at this, but thought that it was only a matter of time before my internal organs would be affected, so she sent me to a rheumatologist. I was scheduled to see the rheumatologist she referred me to in about six weeks. There was a few weeks in between all these visits, because it takes time to get an appointment.

While I was waiting for my appointment with the rheumatologist, I was researching and researching on the internet. I came across this article that told the story of a woman who had systemic scleroderma and had found the *Road Back* website.[3] She took antibiotics, which really turned her life around and she got better. It said on the website that people were using this benign antibiotic that had been around forever. It wasn't harmful and it was reversing symptoms. When I found the *Road Back*, I knew I was on the right track.

Then I read the book, *Arthritis Breakthrough*,[4] which described this theory that arthritis and other connective tissue diseases are caused by bacteria. I got a doctor's name from the *Road Back* list and he worked with me. He had a couple of books on antibiotic therapy for connective tissue diseases in his office. He just asked me what I wanted to do, so I asked, "Can you prescribe this antibiotic for me?" and he said that he would. He prescribed it for me and I started taking it. He was a real find, so I referred other patients to him.

About two weeks after I took the *Minocin*,[5] I started to feel better – some of the fatigue lifted. I don't know if I believe the theory, or if I don't believe it, but it doesn't matter to me really why it works, or how it works, because I know it works.

By the time I went to the rheumatologist, I had already started antibiotic treatment. When I told her what I was taking, she just sneered at me. She said: "You know, that's for acne. People who take that have problems with acne."She suggested methotrexate[6] and I said that I didn't want to take it, so that's kind of the last time we saw each other. She was mad about it – she was angry. She thought that stories of recovery were just "patient anecdotal stories, with no scientific background", but people who say this haven't read the studies! The studies are small and there's no money to be made here really, so no pharmaceutical companies are interested. I think that's why the word isn't getting out.

3 *The Road Back Foundation* http://www.roadback.org

4 *The New Arthritis Breakthrough: The Only Medical Therapy Clinically Proven to Produce Long-term Improvement and Remission of RA, Lupus, Juvenile RS, & Other Inflammatory Forms of Arthritis* by Henry Scammell.

5 *Minocin* is a broad-spectrum tetracycline antibiotic.

6 Methotrexate was originally designed as a chemotherapy drug, but is now used for autoimmune diseases like rheumatoid arthritis and connective tissue disease. It is highly toxic and has a range of serious side effects that include mouth ulcers, immunosuppression leading to various infections, hair loss, nervous system disorders and bone marrow suppression.

The rheumatologist was just not informed and it went against her training. Why would an autoimmune disease be helped with antibiotics? It didn't make sense to her medical brain, but it was a very rigid way of thinking. She had very rigid ideas about how you treat scleroderma, and that was with steroids and methotrexate. To contradict what she went to school for kind of upset her identity in a way.

Just for anti-inflammatory purposes, an antibiotic is going to be helpful. Some rheumatologists look at it and say: "Oh, it's helping the inflammation – this is why they're getting better." But there's another aspect to *Minocin* that helps people with scleroderma. It somehow helps loosen the skin, so there's an anti-collagen effect too.

I felt confident about using antibiotic therapy, because I had found a doctor who believed in this treatment and I had the *Road Back* organisation. There were people on its bulletin-board who had had success. Not only were the people there knowledgable, but they were also kind and compassionate. When I talk about the *Road Back*, I'm still moved by their combination of compassion and knowledge. I can search on the website for any kind of trouble I have and somebody's going to know about it. Patient support and advocacy is so powerful, because then you can empower yourself and build the confidence to then go to your doctor and say: "This is the treatment I would like and if you don't want to treat me this way then I will go somewhere else."

It was a long process to get better. The weeks and months that were the hardest were in the beginning when I was so sick. It was quite a dark time. But with the return of my energy, then I felt like I had my life back. I can deal with pain, I can deal with financial trouble, I can deal with work issues, but when you lose your energy, that is the greatest physical loss I can think of. When my energy came back, I started feeling like myself again – that was just such a blessing.

As I said, my recovery was so gradual. But suddenly last year, I found myself wanting to finish a marathon. Now, why did this happen, when I was 53 years old and had never wanted to do one before? I always admired those people who could finish a marathon. It wasn't the people who were winning, but of course I admired them too!

In New York, I lived between First and Second on 75th Street on the East Side. The last ten miles of the marathon would go right by the apartment where I lived. I would go out there and stand on First Avenue and watch it. Eight hours after the marathon had started is when you see the guys in the wheelchairs, on crutches and the girls who are blind – all these people, eight hours after they had started, still on their journey to complete a marathon. I remember being in tears, I was so moved by these people with this toughness to be able to do this with such incredible determination. Probably the memory of that had something to do with my wanting to finish a marathon.

When I first started training, I didn't know what I was doing, or really why, but

I happened to get into the New York marathon. There's a one-in-four chance to get in by the lottery, and I got in, so I thought: "I'm supposed to do this New York marathon." I was very, very slow, but I'd done the 26 miles in training and I knew I could do it. It has taken me about seven hours, which is about a 15-minute mile. My rheumatologist thinks it's remarkable. As it turned out, Hurricane Sandy cancelled the New York marathon, so I didn't get to run it. Now I've decided to run the Oklahoma City marathon, which is where my mother lives, is where I grew up, and I have two sisters there. I'm running that at the end of April.

Even my current rheumatologist, who knows that my antibiotic protocol helps me and helps people, is not one hundred per cent sold on it. He acknowledges that my antibiotic treatment has helped me, but he also thinks part of it is simply luck, or that it's "spontaneous remission". I hear that a lot – that it's spontaneous remission.

Maybe there is luck involved. We all have luck and we all have bad luck, good fortune and bad fortune. It's pretty balanced out. I think I was very fortunate, but I also did a lot of research. I found that the *Road Back* shows a medical background for the reason why antibiotic therapy works – there are scientific reasons. I try not to argue, because arguing doesn't get anywhere, but my recovery wasn't spontaneous. It wasn't like 'all of a sudden' I got better. It was hard-won. I started recovering a couple of weeks after I started taking the antibiotic, but my whole recovery was gradual, over time. This is hard to explain to doctors – they don't want to think that the antibiotic is what did it, because that is threatening. They get very angry and defensive.

It's puzzling; you know, methotrexate shuts down your immune system, and that scares the hell out of me. Shutting down the immune system? That's crazy to me. The rheumatologist said: "Well, this has been helpful for people in the past for scleroderma." I believe that, but at some point it stops working and starts hurting the person. That drug really scared me and I did not want anything to do with it. I never took a steroid, which I'm very grateful for as well. If your lungs are affected by the fibrosis, methotrexate isn't going to help that. You have to start treating the lungs with another drug, and then are you using methotrexate to stop the skin involvement? It's one drug on top of the other, becoming more and more destructive. I don't see how a body is supposed to live with those kinds of drugs and have the illness as well. That's very disturbing to me.

This disease can be devastating. With scleroderma you have a 50 per cent chance of living over five years. I met a couple of people with scleroderma at a support group in New Zealand. They were very thin and stooped and disfigured with shrunken mouths and unable to eat solid food because they couldn't swallow, so were on a liquid diet. One lady's hands were completely contracted. When I met them, it so scared me, I never went back.

You know, it's hard. I have a very good doctor, but before I go to see him, I have to build up this confidence. I have to be organised and I have to be able to say: "Why?" or: "What does that mean?" or: "I don't want that." It's much less so now, but in my mother's generation, you didn't question the doctor, you just did what he or she told you. Doctors were people who could help you and heal you and make you or your loved ones better.

Now, we have this wonderful thing called the internet and patient advocacy is growing. It's so empowering to be able to learn about this stuff and take it into your doctor. The people from the *Road Back* have such a great knowledge base – much more so than the doctors I've spoken to.

The antibiotic treatment isn't a cure. The improvement happens over time and it takes a lot of patience. I think I got back to normal by about 2005. Gradually, the tightening loosened. I get tests done every six months to a year, just to keep an eye on things, and I do still have positive ANAs.

I'm not completely back to normal, although I feel pretty normal. I still have Raynaud's and skin tightening in my fingers. It doesn't limit me, but there are things I wouldn't do, like snow-skiing, scuba-diving, or any winter sport involving severe cold, but I can practice yoga.

I'm working full-time as an executive legal assistant at an education company. It's a very busy and demanding role. I'm also a poet, I have two little dogs, I'm married and have a step-daughter who lives in New Zealand. I have a very busy, very normal life.

I don't consider myself cured, but I don't think of myself as a sick person either. My hands are swollen and I get little sores on them. This is really the worst of my disease, so I think I'm pretty lucky.

Scleroderma, or 'hard skin' is a chronic, autoimmune connective tissue disorder that has no known cause or cure. If the disease is the 'limited' form, the outlook is more positive than the 'diffused' or 'systemic' form, which affects the rest of the body, including internal organs. The 5-year survival rate is about 85%, the 10 year survival rate is less than 70%.

(Merck Manual of Diagnosis and Therapy, 1999, 17th Edition, Centennial Edition)

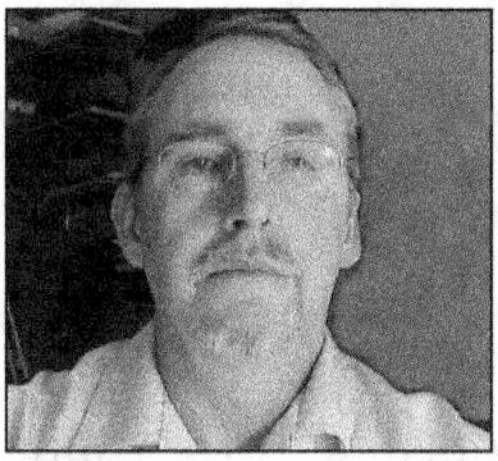

John Hobbs, 55 years

Ozark, Missouri, USA

Diagnosed with rheumatoid arthritis at 40 years

From the time that I was 30 until about 40 years of age, I struggled back and forth with increasing pain and becoming increasingly depressed, because I was unable to really function effectively. When I first started to feel ill, I spent a great deal of time and effort going to various general practitioners, attempting to get to some kind of an explanation of why I was feeling this way. I was 30 years old. I was told that this was old age, and everybody feels this way when they get approximately to my age: "Everybody has aches and pains and goes through something," and that this was my little problem to deal with.

The first symptom that I had was tremendous pain located in the arches of my feet. One day I was fine then the next morning when I woke up, it felt like someone had taken a knife and sliced the tendons in the bottom of my feet. I was unable to walk very well – it was passed from a general practitioner to a podiatrist. I was told that it was because I had flat feet, that I had this sudden onset of terrible pain. I was given arch supports for my shoes and ibuprofen[1] for the inflammation and sent on my way. That was probably the first rejection that I had from the medical community. I never really felt like that explained it, but I did gradually get better. Whether it was my own body fighting back, or the anti-inflammatories, I did improve.

From that point, I would get what I describe as a floating or wandering pain. It was typically one of the major joints of my body, either a hip, a shoulder, or my back. It would be very intense and require a lot of pain relief. Ibuprofen was the only thing that I ever took to essentially manage it. After a period of two or three weeks of intense, continuous pain, overnight it would disappear. Then maybe two or three months would go by and a similar thing would occur in another large joint.

It literally went on like this for years. It wasn't just something where you have trouble using your hands, or something like that. It was a whole body experience. Every time, I was told by a general practitioner if it was my shoulder: "Well, obviously you've strained your shoulder," or if it was the hip: "Well, you did something, or maybe the heels of your shoes are worn," or something like that. There was always some easy explanation.

1 Ibuprofen is a Non Steroidal Anti Inflammatory (NSAID) drug used for musculoskeletal and other pain.

Eventually it came to the point where I asked to be tested for rheumatoid arthritis, just based on the symptoms, but the only thing that showed up was a slightly elevated sedimentation rate.[2] I was told: "Lots of people have this level of inflammation, so it doesn't really mean much. You're a little bit high." That's why I ended up with this ten-year period of time where I was suffering a great deal.

The biggest thing that I remember is that it had an impact not only emotionally in the form of depression, but also on my self-confidence. I think it damaged my self-esteem to the point that I really didn't really care about much of anything. I was doing what I had to do, to get by and stay employed, but I really didn't care much for any of it. Because my blood tests were negative, the doctors that I went to suggested that I had psychological problems. My doctor was willing to refer me, but there was no point in sending me to a rheumatologist, because the tests were coming back negative. So he would refer me to a psychiatrist or somebody that could help me mentally, but that was all.

I was insulted by the suggestion that I had something mentally wrong that was causing these very obvious physical symptoms. I was a bit annoyed by that, because maybe the general practitioner is lacking in their background or training if they cannot tell a person who's weak mentally from a person that has a true medical problem. That was really the point at which I started to question the system that I was trying to work within. Here, healthcare has grown into these big business entities where you are limited in your choices of what you can do.

Mostly, I had an overall weakness. I was getting to a point where I had to ask for help to lift things. With the type of work that I do, I should have been able to lift. My own family had to help me lift things into the car. To go down a set of stairs I had to more or less go down sideways, one step at a time, because the forward motion was just excruciating to me. I had a lot of difficulty with my hands and my grip, which are essential to my work. I mostly tried to hide all that, because I was scared – I really was. I would get up very early and take really hot showers to try to loosen my joints, and I would take as much ibuprofen as I could to try to feel normal by the time that work was required to be done. It was mostly the depression though, that really got to me.

My wife had to pick up the slack for the fact that I wasn't able to be active, or have enough energy to play and have fun, or go on trips and things like that. It did have an overall impact. Mostly, it was frustrating from the point that I didn't really want a lot of sympathy and people feeling sorry for me – I just wanted to be better. But when you have no diagnosis and none of the tests are coming back as an indication of what you have, it probably looks to them the same way it looks to the doctors, that maybe it's all in your head.

I had to drive a lot with my job. By the time I was 40, I had reached a point where the pain in my shoulders and my neck was excruciating. I was literally

2 ESR – Erythrocyte (red blood cell) Sedimentation Rate is the rate that red blood cells sediment over one hour. It is a non-specific measure of inflammation.

driving the car with my legs, because I had to put my arms behind my back, to straighten out enough to ease some of that pain.

Out of desperation, I ended up going to a chiropractor and he was a very decent guy. He did some simple tests on my strength and asked me what hurt and what didn't. He told me: "We'll try this for a while, but if it doesn't work, I'm going to send you to a neurologist, because it's not normal for a person of your age to be the way you are." Here's a person who supposedly has less training than a general practitioner and less education, yet he could see that there was something that was wrong. So really, that was what got things rolling in terms of getting treatment, because he's the one that warned me away from the doctor that I'd been going to.

When I went back to this different lady doctor, I told her about the pain and what I had to do to be out of pain, she did some X-rays. Mostly, she just listened. By then I think I was a little bit better at convincing somebody that there was something going on. She did some basic strength tests, but a lot of that stuff is kind of subjective, you know – how strong your hands or arms are may be a lot different than mine, so I don't think that proved anything.

When the tests for sedimentation and rheumatoid factor were redone, that's when it flip-flopped. The rheumatoid factor[3] came back positive and the sedimentation rate was even higher. That's when I went to the first rheumatologist. He was arrogant, not very well educated and essentially he told me that I needed to start on diclofenac.[4] He didn't give me any hope that if I took the diclofenac that it was going to make me any better. He explained to me that what we were doing was "climbing the ladder". There was never any indication or any hope that I didn't have to go to the next rung of the ladder. It was: "This is the accepted way that we do it and we're going to have to do this over a certain period of time," and: "You're going to end up on one of these newer biologics and that's the best way to treat you for what you have."

He was good about explaining it all. He spent quite a bit of time telling me about the chemistry that was involved and which drugs were successful, but at this point, through my own reading and research, I already knew that people were taking antibiotics for this condition. So I waded through many appointments – *many* appointments – to see if he was going to mention that, or to see if that was an option, but it was never suggested. I had to actually bring it up in order to see whether he would or he would not. When I did, he reacted badly. I could tell that I had caught him off-guard. He got flustered, he stuttered, he got a little bit angry and he chided me for having used the internet as a research tool, that it was all misinformation and it wasn't really going to help. At the end of his speech, he gave me the antibiotic prescription anyway. He was insulted, but he did prescribe it. He told me that the effect would be only temporary, that I was buying a little

3 Rheumatoid factor (RF) is the autoantibody first found in rheumatoid arthritis.

4 Diclofenac is a Non-Steroidal-Antiinflammatory Drug (NSAID) used to reduce inflammation and pain.

bit of time, that it may help a little bit with the inflammation, but I was still going to have to take one of the other drugs and move on "up the ladder".

His preferred course would have been to start me on the stronger anti-inflammatories and the next step would have been methotrexate.[5] Because I admitted to alcohol use, he suggested sulfasalazine.[6] I can't remember the names of all the rest of them – I don't want to remember them, but it goes up from there. There wasn't a lot of emphasis about side effects of the standard medication – mainly how effective it is. The impression that I had at that time was that because people like myself are so desperate by the time they get there, most of them will just go ahead and do whatever he suggests. I think that's what made him mad. I made him mad because I wanted to do what I wanted.

At the time that I went to see him, I was having terrible problems with my shoulders, so I let him give me a cortisone injection in one shoulder. Other than that, I haven't taken any of those drugs and I don't believe I should have taken that injection. I've had three oral doses of some type of cortisone, and that one shot. Other than that, it's all been the antibiotics.

What things turned into very quickly was this disruptive pattern of me sacrificing my time to appease the doctor's requirements for certain procedures. I would go in for an appointment, he would spend no more than 30 seconds in the room, give me a prescription and ask me if things were going okay. The rest of the time was spent on blood work. I was having to go in there every two weeks, wait for a couple of hours in order to have my blood drawn, so he could tell me I was getting better. I already knew that I was getting better. The way that he explained it was that minocycline[7] was at least, if not more, dangerous than methotrexate and I had to be monitored closely while I was doing this.

From the very first time I laid eyes on him, the way that he came up to me was as if to say, "Don't get your hopes up." He really was saying to me: "You're going to be sick, you're going to always be sick, you're going to have to take all this stuff and you're going to have to come in here all the time." I reached a point where I felt like my time was being wasted. From what I already knew from my own reading, I didn't feel like it was necessary. He had told me that the minocycline was at best a temporary treatment and that I was still going to have to go back and "climb the ladder" and take the other drugs. That's when I bailed. I completely dropped out, called and told them I wasn't coming back.

My doctor had been told, "This is the way you treat people." There didn't seem to be any big commitment to me on his part. He did make the statement to me when I first went to him that I was going to get very, very sick and that I

5 Methotrexate, originally a chemotherapy drug, is now used for autoimmune diseases like rheumatoid and connective tissue disease. It is highly toxic and has a range of serious side effects that include mouth ulcers, immunosuppression leading to various infections, hair loss, nervous system disorders and bone marrow suppression.

6 Sulfasalazine is a sulpha-based drug that was developed in the 1950s specifically for rheumatoid arthritis, when it was believed the cause was bacterial in origin.

7 Minocycline is a broad spectrum tetracycline antibiotic.

should prepare my life around that fact. I still to this day think that's a terrible statement for anyone in healthcare to have made to anyone – even a terminal patient.

Within one week of taking the minocycline, I felt so much better. Everything that had been bothering me started to subside in the very slightest way. A big part of it was sleep, because when you're in pain and all your joints are hurting you, you can't sleep well. Immediately upon taking that drug, I started to sleep better.

Gradually, just the sleep alone started to allow me to feel better, combined with everything that I'd read on the internet and all the people I had contacted. I literally found email addresses from people that had given testimony and I asked them: "I know this is crazy and I know that you don't know me, but is what you're saying true? Are you a real person? Is this real; does this really work?" I got enough responses to convince me that there were all these people out there who were using antibiotic treatment and doing well – they were healthy. It was difficult for me to believe what I was reading, which was essentially that people were taking this very simple, cost-effective treatment and improving. It's great to know about people who have been successful in using other treatments.

When I was first trying to find some help, the success stories were what helped me. The medical profession was saying: "Anecdotal evidence doesn't count – the only thing that matters is proven studies," when the fact is: most of the studies done are manipulated in one form or another anyway.

I read the book[8] early on. I don't recall a lot of passages from it, but I was very impressed by the commitment that was demonstrated in the composition of the book. That had a big effect on *my* commitment to proceed with this.

When I went to see a *Road Back*[9] doctor for the first time, I went there pretending to be a person that needed a doctor. We kind of connected and he figured out why I was there. He was, I would say, inspirational, in the sense that he could see that I was already doing better and that there really was no reason to change what I was doing if I continued to improve. The rheumatologist was telling me that even if I improved, I still had to "move up on the ladder."

Within a year and a half of taking the minocycline, I was pain-free. By that, I mean range of motion, pain, sleep patterns – every aspect of it. After two years, I felt normal. The depression cleared very early, because I had hope and my energy started to come back. I simply paid attention to my overall health with more physical activity and the depression subsided very rapidly. I was able to have a more fulfilling life.

---

8 *The New Arthritis Breakthrough: The Only Medical Therapy Clinically Proven to Produce Long-term Improvement and Remission of RA, Lupus, Juvenile RS, & Other Inflammatory Forms of Arthritis* by Henry Scammell.

9 *The Road Back Foundation* www.roadback.org informs the public about research, treatment and practitioners who use the Antibiotic Protocol (AP) for musculoskeletal diseases.

I probably went to the *Road Back* doctor every six months and he continued to prescribe for me. After that I maybe went once a year for the blood tests. It's been a couple of years now since I've had one. It's been up and down. I'm not perfect, but I did get my levels of rheumatoid factor low enough to be considered 'negative'. I'm probably a 'mild weak positive' right now, but it's much, much better than it was.

I still take minocycline. A couple of years ago it seemed to have stopped working, so I stopped taking it and experimented with a number of other antibiotics. It was a slow process, because you can't tell anything on the first dose. Now I've gone back to the minocycline and I can feel that it's working again.

The doctor that I had been going to is close to retirement age. He's been pressured by one of the insurance companies in the healthcare system to stop treating arthritis with antibiotics. You go to these clinics and they're all part of a larger group, so the guy that was helping me all these years won't prescribe for me anymore. Now, he will only refer me to a rheumatologist and I refused that. I asked him directly: "If I allow you to refer me, do you know a rheumatologist who will allow me to continue on this treatment?" His answer was: "No."

So, at this point I have no alternative but to self-treat. The problem is that I have to pay for everything just like a guy that has no insurance, because I'm not doing orthodox treatment. The way the system works is: they want to pass all that cost back onto you. You're paying out of your own pocket, even though you have insurance. What I'm looking at now is the lowest cost way of getting what I need to be healthy. I can go up the street and get methotrexate or the *Enbrel*[10] at $20,000 a year, but if I want to take something that's less harmful, I have to pay for it. They're not getting any trips to Aruba[11] for the prescriptions that they write. It seems ridiculous that you're living in the midst of some huge country paying all of these insurance premiums and you end up not being able to use it.

I'm stable now. I've gotten a handle on being able to tell if I'm getting better or worse. From years of doing treatment, I know what my level of inflammation is. I can't give you a number, but I know when it's high and I know when it's low. I've managed to avoid joint deformity. I have some nodules where you have a bump on a joint that gets larger or smaller. I'm not convinced that it isn't just from taking the antibiotics, because that's one of the side effects – the tendon pops like that. But I have no real deformity. Physically, I'm okay.

My message is that I'm much better now than I was 25 years ago when I first had symptoms. That's the opposite of what the rheumatologists told me would happen. Orthodox medicine is a wonderful thing, but if it's not working, it should be open to other treatments.

10 *Enbrel* is a biopharmaceutical drug used to treat autoimmune diseases, most specifically rheumatoid arthritis.

11 Aruba is an island in the Southern Caribbean Sea.

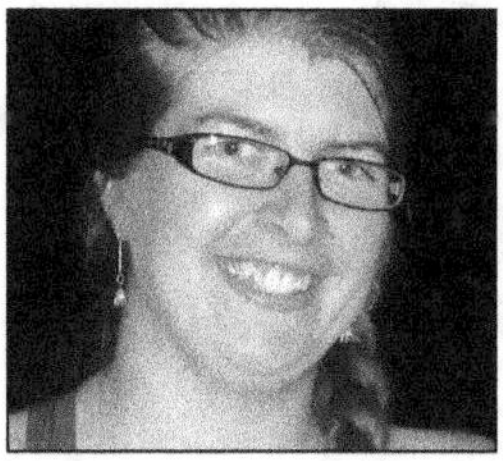

Gabrielle Hogg, 26 years

Napier, New Zealand

Diagnosed with Asperger's syndrome at 15 years

I'm number three of four children. There were developmental delays from the beginning. My behaviour started to deteriorate after I was about one year old. I didn't walk until I was three years old and I started talking at about three and a half. During primary school, my language was limited – I think I only spoke around two or three words at a time. I had speech and language therapy from three and a half until I was about nine years old. I was given a lot of developmental assessments during primary school, but no-one really knew what the truth was.

At ten years old, they thought that maybe I had dyspraxia and dyslexia. Then when I was 12, I visited my dad in Australia and went to an autism specialist there, who diagnosed me with Asperger's syndrome and borderline intellectual impairment. The diagnostic evaluation was sent to my mother in New Zealand, but unfortunately it was all too much for her at the time, so nothing was really done until I was about 15.

I really didn't have a lot of friends – probably none. In high school I was assessed as being eight years behind in my development and I wasn't able to keep up with anything. At 15, they re-evaluated me and that's when I got the diagnosis of Asperger's syndrome. They disregarded the earlier diagnoses of dyslexia and dyspraxia and said that I had more of an overall global developmental delay. My IQ[1] was tested and it came out as 70. Average IQ is about 90.

At around 21, I was diagnosed with an anxiety disorder and they suggested that I had post traumatic stress disorder as well. That was after I spent some time in a psychiatric unit because of self-injury. A little while after that, I started to get some psychological therapy with an autism specialist in New Zealand. Then I was re-evaluated and diagnosed with high-functioning autism instead of Asperger's syndrome, because of the speech, language and general developmental delays that I had.

Then someone got me in touch with a naturopath who works with individuals on the autism spectrum. She immediately put me onto a diet which was

1 IQ – intelligence quotient.

basically gluten-free and casein-free.[2] That really helped me a lot. For once in my entire life, I started to look people directly in the eyes. My anxiety levels started to go down and I was able to concentrate more in examinations, so it was really good.

Everything changed after I went on the diet. Before I started the diet, I would say I was disconnected from my body. I was unable to control my body in the way that I wanted to. The diet gave me the ability to have a clear head and be in control. Once all the symptoms are taken away – like headaches, stomach aches, asthma and eczema – then you're cognitively more there and in a better space to learn. It felt marvellous to be finally connected with my body, to be able to work out what I was feeling and be able to connect the dots. Now, if I eat something that I'm not supposed to eat, I can connect it to the symptoms I get.

As well as gluten and casein, I have to stay away from artificial colours, aspartame[3] and MSG.[4] I have to have as low a sugar intake as possible, so I have limited fruits. I mainly drink water and I don't have juice, except on a special occasion.

My eczema and asthma also disappeared after I went on the diet. As a child, my eczema was really bad in the joints of my arms. The doctors gave me special ointments to use, but I don't think they were really working, because I had eczema all throughout my childhood. It got to the point where my skin was cracked and bleeding. Initially, my mum had all us kids dairy-free, then when I was eight years old we started having dairy again.

My asthma was more mild. I was using asthma inhalers and it went away when I got a bit older, but not completely. It was still there every time I had a cold. With this diet, I don't get so many colds either.

With my naturopathic treatment, there was a stage of having to detoxify my system first, so I was going through detox symptoms before getting any positive effects, which I started to notice within a month. It was quite hard to give up the foods that I had obsessively eaten for ages and ages – that was really difficult.

As a child, I had migraines really badly. During the detox the headaches became intense, but then my brain fog disappeared as well as the headaches. As far back as I can remember, I was constantly in this brain-fog, unable to do much, connect, or process the stuff going on around me. I was more disconnected from the world and it was all a blur to me. It made me feel like I was locked away. [*becomes upset*]

Feeling better made me realise for the first time that I wanted and needed friends. In some ways, that caused a lot of depression to come in, because before then I didn't really care about having friends or not. Suddenly, I started

2 Gluten-free, casein-free diet – excludes all gluten-containing grains like wheat and dairy products.

3 Aspartame – an artificial sweetener, originally marketed as *Nutra-sweet*. Its safety is controversial.

4 MSG – monosodium glutamate is a food additive used to enhance flavour, used in many processed foods. Reaction symptoms include headache, flushing, sweating, facial pressure or tightness, numbness, tingling or burning in the face, neck and other areas.

caring and I wanted to fit in with everyone else. I have more friends today than I had growing up and a lot of them happen to be neurotypical[5] friends.

After my stay in the psychiatric ward, they redid my IQ test and it was 87 instead of below 70. The only thing I can put that down to is diet and supplements.

In 2008, I went to university, studying psychology. I wasn't doing so well in the examinations, so they tried me on different anxiety medications, which weren't working and I was reacting to them. University is good now, although I have decided to discontinue with psychology and do naturopathy, because with naturopathy, it's about fixing the underlying causes, rather than saying: "We can't do anything to help you, you've got your condition for life."

The gluten-free and dairy-free diet has made a huge difference to my life. With being able to focus more, it has meant that I can put more ability into studying and sit longer during the exams. Before the diet, I was unable to sit in an exam, I would walk out after five minutes. Now I have slowly increased the time I'm able to sit during an examination, which is really helpful.

I do officially have ADHD,[6] which was diagnosed last year, alongside a bipolar diagnosis and possibly a Tourette's[7] syndrome diagnosis as well. After doing the basic gluten and casein-free diet, I started to realise that I had symptoms of ADHD. I think that was because the autism was coming under control. As you start to progress along the autism spectrum, you kind of move towards ADHD. I probably did have ADHD as a child, but the autism wasn't managed well enough to separate it all out.

I try and do everything naturally as much as I can. They did put me on quetiapine[8] for the bipolar, but I found that I was getting more suicidal on it – I've only just figured that out. I've got a marvellous GP[9] at the moment, who's into all the wholistic stuff, so he's started to wean me off the quetiapine and haloperidol.[10] They put me on haloperidol for the Tourette's syndrome, which does seem to be working, but as much as possible I do everything else naturally. I'm not on any medication for ADHD or autism at all and I'm definitely not taking any more anti-anxiety medications either.

Interestingly enough, after I researched Tourette's syndrome and what the possible causes could be, I came across 'PANDAS', which is Paediatric Autoimmune Neuropsychiatric Disorder Associated with Streptococcal infection. I went to my psychiatrist and got a streptococcal blood test and the blood titres came back positive. It possibly did start in childhood, but I can't say I've got PANDAS today, because supposedly it's a childhood disorder and I haven't had a course of antibiotics for it. The way I try and treat it is by going

5 Neurotypical – people with a normal mental and emotional development.
6 ADHD – Attention Deficit and Hyperactivity Disorder.
7 Tourette's syndrome is a neurological disorder with involuntary body tics.
8 Quetiapine is an antipsychotic medication used to treat schizophrenia, bipolar disorder, autism and depression.
9 GP – general practitioner.
10 Haloperidol is used to treat Tourette's syndrome, along with nervous and psychiatric disorders.

sugar-free, which is very difficult, and by using probiotics. My psychiatrist didn't recommend any treatment for me, because he was unaware of what PANDAS actually is. New Zealand is quite behind other countries in this area. If you go to America, it's more studied over there than it is in Australia and New Zealand. That was a recent revelation to me.

My Tourette's symptoms are upper body and head tics, although it's controlled at the moment. I have some local tics of snorting, but apart from that I don't have any other symptoms. Magnesium Taurine is marvellous for treating Tourette's syndrome, because it relaxes the muscles. When you're stressed you use up more magnesium, so you're more likely to have tics. Magnesium took away a lot of my upper body tics and I started to sleep better as well. Before that I was getting only four hours sleep a night – no-one can function properly on that. It took me forever to find the right formulation of magnesium and taurine, but once I found the right one and the right dosage, it worked really quickly and really well. Then I slept for eight to twelve hours a night. I'm on melatonin as well, although that has to be prescribed by a doctor in New Zealand. Now I take magnesium in a form with a lot of B vitamins.

I'm always deficient in iron, so I'm on iron supplements. I take cod liver oil as well and my doctor has prescribed me vitamin D. I do Epsom Salts[11] foot soaks and that really helps me to calm down – I do them whenever I feel an anxiety attack coming on.

I was trying to get my supplements, which are specifically to treat my disability, included in my disability allowance. I had to get a lawyer involved because they didn't believe in any of it. At the time I went on the allowance, my doctor had ticked the 'mental retardation' box rather than 'autism', so they were confused about why I was asking for stuff for autism. We finally got the supplements included in the disability allowance – or at least half of them. It was the first case in New Zealand to get that to happen. The punchline was: "Do you want her to be in the workforce or not?"

I'm not studying at the moment. I've had a year off to try and get my bipolar under control. Hopefully I'll be starting a naturopathy course next year. When I get my naturopathy degree I can start to work more on the nutrition side of things.

I'm working now with special needs individuals on a holiday programme, which I love. I've been working there for a couple of years now. It's like any other holiday programme, except we have more staff available, more understanding and we're trained in the area. I see the kids with autism coming to the holiday programme and they're all coming in with chips and fizzy drinks – the whole disaster. One individual only ate chips, chocolate chip cookies and chocolate milk. I wish I could just go in and change it all, but I can't. They're actually

11 Epsom Salts – magnesium sulphate ($MgSO_4$) is an organic salt traditionally used as a component of bath salts. Medically, the salts are used for aches and pains, to remove splinters and internally as a saline laxative. In biomedical treatment, Epsom Salts are used as a detoxifying agent.

addicted to the food. Sometimes changing the diet has a psychological impact. If parents are in doubt about this, they can change their child's food for three months and if it doesn't work then they can move on. There's no *harm* in changing their diet from the limited diet they're already on, because they're not getting enough nutrients in the first place. A behavioural or ABA[12] therapist can come in and work with the child to help with food issues. Even if dietary treatment doesn't become standard in my lifetime, it might happen in the next generation.

I do a lot of work in the area of talking to parents about autism. I'm an advocate for disability in general, but mainly for autism. I currently sit on the Consumer Council with the Hawkes Bay District Health Board. I'm on the Ministry of Health Disability Support Services Consumer Consortium as a representative for those on the autism spectrum for Autism New Zealand. Previously, I was on the Autism Expert Advisory Group with the Ministry of Health. Currently, I'm on *Kaituitui*, which is basically where you get the communities together for a disabled person assembly. It's really good for my self-confidence to get out there and do that sort of stuff and it helps other people as well. I advise them on policies to do with disability and we've lined up with the Convention on the Rights of Persons with Disabilities.[13]

I earn an income from some of the advocacy groups, but not all of them. I'm not completely financially independent, but I'm much more financially independent than I used to be. I don't think I would be able to do all the stuff I do now if I hadn't done the diet.

A group of professionals and individuals in the biomedical[14] community run quite a lot of biomedical seminars in Auckland where I go and talk about my journey with autism. We get parents and practitioners talking about it, which is really helpful for parents. Basically, I tell them if they get a diagnosis early on, like when their child is two years old, it's best to go onto the biomedical pathway straight away, before they become teenagers, when it's a lot harder to get them onto the right diet. Once children are on the diet, there's more of a chance to learn and they can start school with only a six-month speech delay and not a longer one. Unless they're on a proper diet, autistic children have got all this gluten and casein floating around in their heads causing inflammation and they're unable to learn. It's hard going to school when you don't have a lot of speech because you're unable to communicate your needs.

When you get autism as a diagnosis, it doesn't have to be a disaster – there is hope. You can learn things and do something about it and hopefully move along the spectrum or recover completely. Then children can go to school with less teacher-aid hours required. It does depend on the individual child. There

12 ABA – Applied Behavioural Analysis is an evidence-based, intensive education therapy for children with an Autism Spectrum Disorder.

13 *Convention on the Rights of Persons with Disabilities* http://www.un.org/disabilities/convention/conventionfull.shtml

14 Biomedical – type of treatment for Autistic Spectrum Disorders by correcting metabolic errors using nutritional and other therapies.

can be genetic factors involved – some might have Fragile X Syndrome.[15]

I would say that I am more mildly autistic now. Not fully recovered, but definitely not moderately autistic anymore. If you think about the fact that I was diagnosed with borderline intellectual impairment, global developmental delay, or whatever they called it, I no longer fit that category anymore.

The Global Autism Collaboration *website http://www.globalautismcollaboration.com provides information on the biomedical treatment of autism.*

15 Fragile X Syndrome is an inherited condition characterised by an X chromosome that is abnormally susceptible to damage, especially from folic acid deficiency. Affected individuals tend to be mentally handicapped.

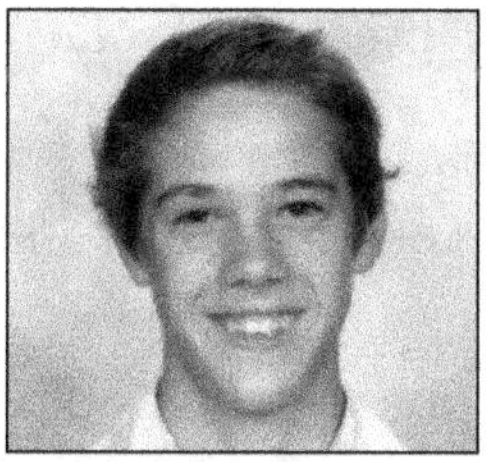

Joel Hooker, 13 years

New South Wales, Australia

Diagnosed with Attention Deficit Hyperactivity Disorder at 7 years

Interview with Sonja Hooker, Joel's mother

Joel was a really easy baby. He slept well, he ate well and got a lot of attention because he was four years after our last child. He reached all his milestones, he was happy and I didn't think there was anything unusual about him at all.

By the time he was about 18 months old, we noticed that he was doing things that were a little bit odd, like having a glazed look on his face when you spoke to him. He did silly things that didn't seem normal and he was very hyperactive. He would never hurt people, but he would do damage to things from jumping around – always by accident and he had no idea how it happened. It could be damaging peoples cars, or getting into house paint – really bizarre things. Because I home-schooled him, I didn't notice it being so unusual, but people around me did and they would say: "He's very hyperactive, he doesn't sit still."

Joel talked well, but he didn't learn his colours, or the alphabet, even though we did it with him every day. By the time we tried to teach him to read, he really struggled – that's when we really started noticing that things were a bit odd. He got that glazed look on his face and had no idea. Each day it was like he had never been taught anything before in his life and he was still hyperactive with destructive behaviour.

He would get frustrated with other people really easily, because they noticed what he was doing and would say something to him. That would make him really upset, then he would lash out at them – mostly with my children or people that he knew. He would be really irritating to other children and they didn't like playing with him. When he talked to them he would get right up close to them, then they would throw sand at him. He didn't know that the other children were being nasty to him and would say to me: "They're my friends." Even if I explained to him that they were being mean to him, he didn't understand or believe me. He thought *I* was being mean to *him*. I was worried about his welfare and scared that he was going to get hurt by somebody, so I was trying to make him aware. Joel could deal with people, but he didn't understand the signals he got from them, or their body language.

I ended up sending him to school in Year Two. When Joel was seven going on eight, we went to see a paediatrician and he was diagnosed with ADHD.[1] He didn't think that there was any autism, although there were signs of it, especially socially, which is what I was really concerned about. He prescribed *Ritalin*,[2] which concerned me, even though it did help. It reduced his hyperactivity and gave him the capacity to actually sit and learn something. It helped with all the bad behaviours you could possibly think of that he had no control over. He calmed down and started learning.

Even though the *Ritalin* did make a huge difference, as soon as he was off it, he was back to the fairies. I gave it to him for his schooling, but the next day I still had to go over the same work again and he wasn't learning as quickly as a normal child would. I know the *Ritalin* was only a cover for his behaviour. It wasn't going to help any of his issues, because as soon as he was off it, he was back to being hyperactive and unable to concentrate or socially cope with life.

Then I had a new baby and I was at my wits end, so I went to see a naturopath. All I wanted out of it was to see him be socially accepted and be able to learn. If he couldn't learn properly, I didn't know how he was going to go into adolescence and high school without upsetting his peers. I was concerned that if he couldn't learn properly, he wouldn't be able to get a decent job. I really wanted to find something that would help him to recover from his ADHD and be cured. I didn't like the drugs, because they were just a mask. I would do anything to try to help this child.

The naturopath ordered a hair mineral analysis which found that Joel had very high levels of copper. There was also a bit of mercury, arsenic and other things in there as well. Once the naturopath gave me the diagnosis of the high copper levels, she gave him some vitamins, minerals and homeopathic remedies that were suited to him. He was given high doses of B vitamins, vitamin C, fish oils and zinc.

After a while, his behaviour started to settle and he could sit for longer periods of time. After three months, I was able to take him off the *Ritalin* and he would stay calm. The glazed look in his eyes wasn't there anymore. When we spoke to him, he understood. Before, you just knew he wasn't understanding what you were saying to him. It was a remarkable difference.

He was also having psychological treatment, because he had been socially backward for a very long time. Through the naturopathic treatment, he was able to understand what the psychologist was asking him to do. He started to understand other people's body language. Gradually the fog lifted from him, his hyperactivity went down to about ten per cent and he became a normal boy that you could talk to. He started learning and managing his schoolwork. It took about 18 months, but by the time he was nine or ten, he was a normal boy.

1 ADHD – Attention Deficit and Hyperactivity Disorder.

2 *Ritalin* is the trade name for methylphenidate, a central nervous system stimulant, which affects the chemicals in the brain that contribute to hyperactivity and impulse control.

It wasn't an overnight thing, but after three to six months, he had responded amazingly well. You could tell that the treatment was working and that gives you the momentum to keep going with it, to make sure that he gets the best out of it. Bringing the copper levels down was a huge thing for him.

Joel is 13 now and he is an awesome child. He's a very generous and kind person. He has always been caring and emotionally aware of what's going on in the household. He can sense if I'm upset before anyone else does. If he's given a gift he is overly grateful. His empathy is very high and he gets upset if he doesn't do the right thing. He doesn't like to upset other people – he comes to me now and says, "I'm sorry, I didn't mean to do that."

He's also very smart. When any machine or device goes wrong, he can figure it out when no-one else can. Joel would say to people who have had an oven in their house for ten years: "Did you realise that your oven can do these things?" We don't know why, but he enjoys doing that! If I have an issue with anything computer-wise, television or phones, I will ask Joel if he can fix it and it's done. I never have to call anybody for anything.

Now he's at high school and he just learns. He settled in well and there's been no trouble. He's not in the top grade, he's in the second or third grade. He works really hard at everything to the best of his ability and is kind of a perfectionist. In his monitoring report he got five As and three Bs – and that's in the second highest class in his school. He struggles a little bit in English, but generally does well in his exams. He's just done an essay on geography by himself at home and all he asked me to do was check it. He sat down and researched it by himself. He's mature and capable. He has many friends and they all love him. He fights with his brothers and sisters, as all kids do. He helps me out at home.

I got a letter from his teacher congratulating Joel on his outstanding performance. His report card says that he contributes well in class. That makes me happy.

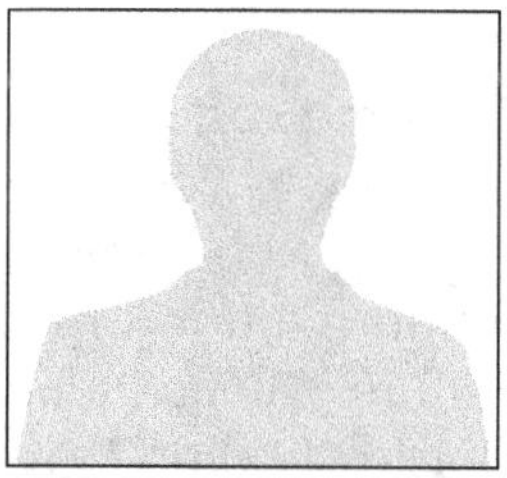

Glenn Hopkins, 59 years

New Mexico, USA

Diagnosed with diabetes at 49 years, heart disease at 54 years

About ten years or so ago, I was having some issues associated with sugar diabetes, when my sugar levels started elevating. I had frequent urination and did have to go a number of times during the night, and my eyesight wasn't real good.

I finally went to a medical doctor and she prescribed me some metformin.[1] She didn't seem to think that it was too big of an issue – that's the impression that I got from her, so I really didn't pay a lot of attention to it. I just continued what I was doing and took the metformin for a little while, then I quit taking it. I thought: "Well, she didn't seem all that concerned about it," so I just figured I didn't need to be.

Seven years ago, my wife was diagnosed with breast cancer and underwent surgery. They convinced us that she needed to have chemotherapy. She wound up getting acute myeloid leukaemia from the chemotherapy treatments, so she had to undergo a bone marrow transplant for that. It was just one thing right after another. We spent probably a thousand days and nights over a three-and-a-half to four-year period in the hospital, so I had a lot of stress during that time period. My sugar levels continued to rise, and about the time she was getting the bone marrow transplant, they got up over 900. The doctor wanted to put me into hospital, but I told her, "I can't do that at this time." We had to go to Phoenix for my wife to undergo this bone marrow transplant – I had to be able to take care of her and I couldn't do that in hospital. So the doctor gave me another prescription for metformin, told me to monitor my sugar levels every day and gave me a prescription for glycoside[2] as well. I was monitoring my sugar, but I didn't change any of my eating habits especially. They said to use these artificial sweeteners and just kind of: "Watch your sugar intake," and that was basically it. That's what I did, but my sugar levels were still two and three hundred.

A few years later, I was hurting real bad and I was short of breath. I couldn't do anything and I couldn't walk anywhere. I'd take ten or 15 steps, I'm short of breath and I've got to stop and rest. You have to go to the doctor every so often

1 Metformin is an anti-diabetic drug for people with normal kidney function.

2 Glycoside is a type of anti-diabetic drug.

to be able to get medication for your diabetes, so I went down to my primary care physician and I was telling her about that. It was a very good check-up. She said: "You need to see a heart doctor."

I made an appointment with the heart doctor. He did some tests and a sonogram[3] on me. He patted me on the legs and said that this was very, very bad. He actually told me that he didn't think that I was going to be able to make it past the next few months. He told me the ejection fraction of my heart was at 18 per cent and that I had congestive heart failure. My heart had really swelled up, I was retaining a lot of fluids and he basically didn't give me a lot of hope.

Looking back, he did a lot of good things, in my opinion. He prescribed a number of different heart medications. I think I was taking about eight in total. He told me to go get CoQ10,[4] to take this slow-release niacin,[5] and drink pomegranate juice. I did everything he told me to do. I had an external defibrillator put on. He said he needed to go ahead and put this pacemaker and cardioverter defibrillator in and they did that.

After I had those procedures done, I developed a blood clot – a deep vein thrombosis in my left arm. I think it was related to the surgery with that cardioverter. I was in hospital for 11 days. After I got out of hospital and I was able to talk to my heart doctor, he said that he wanted to have a surgeon remove where that blood clot was. So they did that and they put a stent in. I'd had this angioplasty[6] done a couple of times in that time frame also.

Of course, my sugar levels are still high, but now I've got congestive heart failure as well. At one time, I went into cardiac arrest four times in one week.

I developed a condition on my arm. There were big rings and small rings and they were raised up and looked like ringworm. My wife's oncologist in the hospital in Albuquerque wanted me to go get that checked out. She didn't know if what I had was contagious and if I should be in the room with my wife.

So I went to a dermatologist who did a culture on it and it wasn't ringworm. He didn't know what it was, so they did a biopsy on it and it turned out to be 'granuloma annulare'.[7] That's associated with diabetes and SLE.[8] I didn't do anything else about it and I just kept going along until my wife passed. Just prior to her passing, I found out that my daughter knew a girl that worked at the Integrative Medical Centre in Las Cruces. I made an appointment and we both went over there.

---

3 Sonogram is another term for echocardiogram using ultrasound.

4 Co Enzyme Q10 was discovered by Professor Fredrick L Crane in 1957. Peter Mitchell received a Nobel Prize for his work on CoQ10 in 1978. In 1972, Littarru and Folkers also demonstrated a deficiency of CoQ10 in heart disease.

5 Niacin – vitamin B3.

6 Angioplasty is a technique of mechanically widening narrowed or obstructed arteries, usually resulting from atherosclerosis.

7 Granuloma annulare is a rare, chronic autoimmune skin condition where reddish bumps on the skin are arranged in a circle or ring.

8 Systemic Lupus Erythematosus ('Lupus', SLE) is an autoimmune disease that attacks healthy tissue, causing inflammation, swelling and damage to joints and organs. Symptoms can be vague, making diagnosis difficult. Two thirds of patients with Lupus suffer from sun sensitivity.

I saw Doctor Berkson at the Integrative Medical Centre and he did a big blood work up on me. I took all my records from my heart doctor and my primary care physician. He'd looked everything over prior to me talking with him. He knew what the rings on my arm were as soon as he saw them. He's the only practitioner I'd been to who knew what that was and what it was associated with. He told me that I just wasn't getting the things that I needed in my diet and to take a number of different supplements – CoQ10, ALA,[9] B complex, Omega 3 fish oils, along with some selenium and vitamin D. My vitamin D levels were low and my Epstein-Barr[10] levels were high. He put me on quite a regimen of supplements.

I did get some dietary recommendations, but I didn't follow the diet real good. I used to have a pretty good weight problem as well. I'd do a diet for a little while, then I'd get off of it. Doctor Berkson told me about the dangers of sugar and carbohydrates and how important it is to eat all these coloured foods, like green leafy vegetables and to have plenty of cabbages, broccoli, cauliflower and all that kind of stuff.

I didn't have any problem giving up the grains and the bread, but I would fall off a few times. Maybe over Christmas, you have a few sweets and whatnot. Now I know they're bad. You just eat things and you don't really know what the dangers are. I was told what we eat is probably more important than anything else we do.

Doctor Berkson also told me that I needed to take some intravenous (IV) treatments of Alpha Lipoic Acid. I went and took a two-week course of the IV treatments. He also prescribed me some oral LDN (Low Dose Naltrexone).[11] I take three milligrams of that, every night, along with my supplements. After I received 12 treatments of the ALA, I told my daughter: "You know, I think I'll just go over there and get one treatment a month and that way it will keep my ALA maybe where it's supposed to be," and that's basically what I've done.

I was still seeing the heart doctor every single week. I didn't tell him all the things I was doing. I thought: "I'm feeling better, I can get around better," and I had been having trouble taking ten steps at one time. Now I can walk ten miles and not get short of breath.

I also had pins and needles in my feet and excruciating pain in my legs. I went to a diabetic shoe doctor in El Paso, a couple of hours away. He told me: "You need to have somebody check your feet every day – you have no feeling. I had some feeling because they were killing me – that's why I went down there to get some shoes. My feet were always killing me. It wasn't something that was hurting periodically, this neuropathy – it was in both feet and it was constant.

Four or five months after I started treatment from Doctor Berkson, my daughter

9 ALA – Alpha Lipoic Acid is a nutritional supplement.

10 Epstein-Barr Virus (EBV) is a human herpes virus which causes Infectious Mononucleosis, or Glandular Fever.

11 Low Dose Naltrexone is the off-label prescription of the FDA approved drug *Naltrexone*.

asked me: "Dad, how're your feet doing?" I hadn't even thought about it – if you're not in pain, you don't even think about these things, but I told her: "I don't have that pain anymore. I don't have any neuropathy."

I have a very dear friend who is 68 years old. Six weeks ago she was diagnosed with a Stage IV breast cancer. She knew she'd had the cancer. A doctor told her that eight years ago and she just didn't want to go back. It got to bleeding real bad so they took her by ambulance to the hospital. They did a CT scan[12] and told her she had cancer in her lymph nodes and some spots on her liver.

We went to see a surgeon and of course, the surgeon told her: "We're not able to operate on it, it's just too large." I went with her to the oncologist and he told her: "Well, you've got six months to a year, if that." He said if they could give her chemotherapy, he really needed to start it that week and that it would give her a couple of extra months. She told them she wasn't interested in that.

We have a very large group of friends – we all get together pretty regular and she's part of that group. She's on a very limited income, so I told her: "If you'll go to see my doctor, I'll just pay for it."

I gave her all the supplements that I thought she needed and I made an appointment over at the Integrative Medical Centre with Doctor Berkson. Now she's receiving vitamin C and ALA intravenously and she told me today she thought that thing was getting smaller. It's healing up and I'm just grateful for that. She says she's never felt better and she's got a great outlook. I have a lot of confidence in her being able to get through this ordeal, even though she's been given no hope whatsoever. She's just doing great.

It was the death of my wife that led me to seek other treatment for myself. I watched my wife, I watched my dad and I watched my mother die from cancer. Neither one of my parents died from the cancer – both of them died from the treatments. Then I watched my wife suffer the most horrible death of anyone I've ever witnessed. We did everything just like they said, but I knew they didn't have the answer. I wish they had been honest and up front with us about that in the beginning. Even though they told her she needed this chemotherapy, she was hesitant in taking it – I'll just put it that way. We both discussed it and said: "Well, whatever we do, let's don't look back and regret," but I regret it every minute. About three months after she finished the chemotherapy, she got acute myeloid leukaemia.

My wife was a healthy woman. A relief oncologist came in and asked me about the health of my wife; I told her my wife was healthy all her life. Even when she was diagnosed with the breast cancer, she was healthy. She was healthy after her mastectomy – all she had was a small tumour. She didn't have to have the mastectomy, but they scare you so bad. I told the oncologist my wife was healthy up until the day she took the first chemotherapy treatment

12 CT scan, also known as a CAT scan, or Computed Axial Tomography is a diagnostic medical imaging procedure that examines cross sections of the body allowing a three dimensional view of specific areas.

and she's been sick ever since – deathly sick. That oncologist got in my face and she pointed her finger at me and she told me: "This chemotherapy didn't cause this leukaemia and I'll prove it to you." I didn't say nothing – I really thought that she was going to attack me, but when we went to Phoenix, to the City of Hope[13] for the bone marrow transplant, the doctor there said: "I guess they told you in Albuquerque that you got this leukaemia as a result of that chemotherapy that you received." We told him: "No, actually they told us that that *didn't* cause it." I've read a lot since then. Everybody should have been able to know that.

By watching the death of my wife and what she went through, how the medications that she took basically killed her, I lost a lot of confidence in the medical establishment. I investigated a lot of these medications that I was on, because I was feeling bad. I had sore muscles and I couldn't control my diabetes. I was taking a statin drug.[14] You read about how dangerous that drug is and I've got all these symptoms. Then I also read that statins even cause congestive heart failure. There was no question that I had congestive heart failure, but I'm here taking a medication that causes that. I've got sugar diabetes and I'm taking a medication that decreases your insulin resistance. It just makes a guy start investigating these things that he's taking for himself.

I don't take that statin any longer – I threw that in the trash. It wasn't very long after that, that I started feeling good. I do take two heart medications now – I was taking about eight. That's a fourth of what I was taking at one time.

After I went to Doctor Berkson, I just got more and more interested in finding out about all of the stuff that I was taking. Even with the supplements, I want to know exactly what they're going to be able to do for me as well as the medications. I want to know if it's something I need, or if it's something I'm being prescribed just because I went to the doctor.

I'm glad we've got medical doctors, but I've lost confidence. You almost get to feeling that these doctors feel compelled to prescribe something that you may or may not need. I know now that they're trained in medicine – they're not trained in health. There's a lot of work going into being a doctor, and there's a lot of studying and a lot of effort and perseverance, but they're trained in pharmaceuticals and they don't know anything else. I wish they did, but they don't.

I've had a lot of blood work done from a lot of doctors, but I've never seen anybody do a blood work up like Doctor Berkson. It's not based upon whatever he wants to sell – it's based upon exactly what your blood work shows, what your cells need.

Anytime anybody tells me of a health issue, I do everything I can to try to

13 The City of Hope, founded in 1913, is one of 41 comprehensive cancer centres in the USA. For the past ten years, it has been rated by US News as one of the '10 best' cancer hospitals in America.

14 Statins are a class of drugs used to lower cholesterol levels by inhibiting the enzyme that helps produce cholesterol in the liver.

convince them: "Hey, you need to take an active part in this, and you need to study your body, instead of putting your confidence in somebody else." They're not with you 24 hours a day, but you are. You know all of your aches and pains, what makes you feel good, what you need, or what you're lacking. You may not know that specifically, but with the right guidance, which is what I got, and with good investigations, you'll get what you need.

I cut my sugar medication way back three years ago and I take hardly any now. My blood work came back good – my A1C[15] was a little high at 6.2, but that's not too bad for someone that has been diagnosed with diabetes.

I feel like I still need to go Las Cruces – I go get a treatment every two weeks right now. Even if the doctor tells me I don't need it anymore for a while, I'm still going to go and have one at least once a month, because it's done so much for me.

Some of my close friends know the kind of shape I was in and how bad I was doing and now they're amazed. I took my daughter and my youngest granddaughter on a two-week cruise to Alaska last summer. There was nine of us altogether. Everywhere we went in Alaska, I'd just run off and leave everybody, carrying my one-year-old granddaughter. They still talk about that today – they just can't believe how full of energy and how full of life that I was.

For the last two years, I've seen the heart doctor once a year and he tells me there's nothing wrong with my heart. Doctor Berkson says the same thing. He says he wishes that he could have got to me before they put this pacemaker and cardioverter defibrillator in. I don't really think I need it, but it's there. I feel great, I'm doing great, and I'm going to continue doing exactly like I'm doing.

I would like to say this: I would encourage every single person that's having any kind of health issues, to do some investigation. Investigate the things that you're taking, try to figure out what your problems are. I would encourage everyone to see an integrative doctor – someone that knows and recognises that there are some good pharmaceuticals, and there are some bad ones. There are also some things that our bodies need as we age. Find someone that can help advise you as to what exactly your body needs, through the blood work.

There was a time when I felt like maybe life isn't worth living. I don't think I'm that old – I'll be 59 in July. I feel good now. Life's worth living. I'm fit. I can do anything and go anywhere.

15 The A1C blood test is the primary test used for diabetes management. It provides information on average levels of blood glucose over the past 3 months.

Kirsten Horner, 45 years

Queensland, Australia

Diagnosed with enthesitis at 43 years

I had been fairly active, training at the gym three times a week. I was also doing boot camp training. At first I thought I had been overdoing it, because my hamstrings[1] and adductors[2] were sore – and a week later, they were still getting worse. It was a gradual progression of increased pain and I started to have trouble lifting my legs. Then everything started hurting and I lost the proper function of my legs. If I was sitting in a chair, I could not physically lift a leg up, as much as I tried. I just had no muscle strength.

I had all-over body pain for nearly a year and a half. I couldn't do anything without it hurting. As well as not being able to lift my legs, I couldn't roll over in bed, bend over, or put my arms over my head. The pain was deep in the muscles – it felt like they were pulled. I had trouble getting dressed, washing my hair and I couldn't pick anything up off the floor. Because I had no strength, I didn't do much. I could only walk slowly with a limp, so I couldn't walk the dog anymore – I just walked her up the path, but walking up the incline on our driveway was really painful. I had to do everything so slowly. My doctor carried out MRIs[3] to identify where the inflammation was.

Because I became less active, I put on weight, so this condition changed everything. I got depressed, because I was told by my rheumatologist that I was going to have it for the rest of my life, so I'd have another blueberry pie with ice cream and put on more weight!

It was a struggle, because it was such a drastic change to my lifestyle. I could still work, because my working day pretty much consisted of working at a computer and driving. I'd have to lift my legs into the car, but I still could drive around.

It took six months to have this condition formally diagnosed. I was told I had an autoimmune condition called 'enthesitis'[4] – which is an inflammation of the entheses, where the muscles join the bone. Apparently, it was a complication of a bacterial infection, which hadn't been identified.

1 The hamstrings consist of six tendons that are connected to the three main muscles in the back of the thigh.

2 The adductor muscles of the hip are a group of muscles in the thigh.

3 MRI (magnetic resonance imaging) – used in radiology for a more detailed image than standard X-rays, used in hospitals for diagnosis, without exposure to radiation.

4 Enthesitis means an inflammation of the entheses, which are the areas where tendons and ligaments attach to the bone. Recurring stress or inflammatory autoimmune disease can cause enthesitis.

First of all, they gave me prednisone.[5] That was fantastic, because I had no pain and it made me very energetic. But when I got fine capillary damage and swelling of my face, neck and body, I realised that steroids weren't so good. But when we went away with friends or went camping and I'd have to go walking, I'd take small doses of prednisone for two or three days, just so that I could get around with everybody and not be hurting. I'd still puff up, flush red really easily and get rosy red cheeks when I took it though, so that wasn't good. Then, as soon as I came off the prednisone, the pain was unchanged. You can't live like that.

I spent the next year trying different drugs like sulfasalazine.[6] I was taking one drug for two months and then another one for the next two months. When one drug didn't relieve any pain, I'd progress to the next drug. A third drug didn't do anything either. The rheumatologist advised me that I needed to get a blood test every month to check my kidney function, and if my vision went blurry, to stop taking it. So I wasn't very keen on these different drugs as a long-term solution.

I was always looking for something else. I just couldn't believe that one minute I could be perfectly healthy and the next minute I had a chronic inflammatory condition for the rest of my life. I thought: "No, I can reverse this." I said to my specialist: "I need a reset button for my immune system, because it's gone a bit haywire." She said, "Well, we don't have one of those."

I saw the DVD, *Fat, Sick and Nearly Dead*,[7] where this guy had an autoimmune disease and was on similar medications to what I was on. He did 60 days of fruit and vegetable juicing and got better. After watching it that night, I got the juicer out of the cupboard and said to my partner: "Do you think I could do this for 15 days?" He said: "Yeah, of course you could." I ended up having only juices for 30 days and I never went hungry. I was consuming fruit and vegetable juice whenever I wanted it, day and night – and getting through the odd craving for blueberry pie and ice cream. [*laughs*] Then I started incorporating dinner and snacks during the day into my diet. I pretty much lost one kilo a week, so over three months, I lost 12 kilos. I felt better – I had no headaches, no period cramps, no constipation and definitely had a better sleep pattern.

At least my body was in as good a condition as it could have been, but even though I'd lost the weight and felt better in myself, I still had the pain. I told the specialist that I was juicing and asked her if there was any nutritional thing I should be doing. She didn't have anything to add, except that the weight loss and less muscle may mean less pain.

5 Prednisone is a synthetic corticosteroid that is effective as an immunosuppressant drug. It is used to treat inflammatory diseases.

6 Sulfasalazine is a sulpha-based drug that was developed in the 1950s to treat rheumatoid arthritis, in the belief that it was caused by a bacterial infection.

7 *Fat, Sick and Nearly Dead* http://www.fatsickandnearlydead.com

After about 18 months, I found a practitioner who did ENAR[8] therapy. She told me: "We just need to reset your system," which was exactly what I had in mind. I had one-and-a-half hour sessions, a week to ten days apart. She began by treating my spine, did quite a bit of work on my hips, then worked on my front, back and feet. She also treated my vagus nerve. I saw her for four treatments over five or six weeks.

What was interesting is that I only had a vague improvement after the first three sessions. In fact, after the second session I was worse. My symptoms were all the same, then I got a lot of tingling and twitching in my calves and legs, which I'd had about five years earlier. I had that treated with acupuncture at the time. I tried acupuncture three times to fix this condition, but with no effect. I said to the ENAR therapist: "I'm not happy. I've got all the usual symptoms plus these ones that I haven't had for five years." She said to me: "Perhaps it's stirring up the underlying cause of this. All I can suggest is to try another couple of sessions to work through it and see if there is any change from your initial reaction." I was still fairly uncomfortable in my legs, then after the third treatment there was a slight improvement, but nothing dramatic.

I remember driving to the fourth session thinking: "Is this doing anything? Shall I keep this up?" Then, the day after the fourth session, I came good. I could bend over, lift my legs up and walk without my hips hurting. It was an 80 per cent improvement and I was just so excited and overjoyed. I haven't been back to a doctor since.

I still had some pain in my hip and my left shoulder, which had restricted movement. That day I rang my practitioner and said: "Order me one of those devices straight away!" She told me it would arrive in three days. She gave me a couple of training sessions and I had some more treatment sessions with her and learned a little bit about using it, so I could start treating myself.

I had stiffness remaining in my neck, my shoulder and some lower-leg issues. I worked out that my hip pain was actually coming from my lower back, so I put the treatment pads on those areas. After that I probably had another three or four sessions with the practitioner, quite spread out. Now she's gone off travelling, so I haven't been able to see her anymore. It would be nice to have a brush-up, but I really feel very good.

The last thing I got rid of was what turned out to be a frozen shoulder. Now, my shoulder has full movement again and my hips are totally better. My lower leg issues have completely gone. Everything else is *totally better*.

I've started treating some people at home myself. I see two or three patients a week who have painful hips, knees, elbows, necks, bursitis and all those sorts of things. It's been really enjoyable and they've had really good responses. One guy had really bad knees. He'd been in a lot of pain for a long time and

8 ENAR – Electro Neuro Adaptive Regulator is a hand-held biofeedback medical device for home use.

couldn't play bowls anymore. He couldn't move well or sleep properly and was very depressed. I treated him only once for about an hour and a half – and the next thing he went bowling! He came back to me and said: "I overdid it," so I treated him a second time and he hasn't come back since. He rang me up recently and said: "Look, I just want to let you know that I've got the flu at the moment. I'll probably come up for another treatment next month, but I'm feeling fantastic." This was an older guy, who was overweight. When I first saw him I thought: "Oh gee, I don't know what I'm going to be able to do to help – this condition might take a while to respond." [*laughs*] He was overjoyed and has told everyone at his bowling club.

I'm so lucky to have found this treatment. I have yet to go back to my specialist and tell her about my recovery. If I rang her office and said: "I've cancelled my January appointment because what the doctor told me I'll have for life, I don't have anymore. If she wants to know more, she can ring me," I suspect I'd never get a call. But I'll follow through and call her office anyway.

SCENAR – Self Controlled Energy Neuro Adaptive Regulator, is a battery-powered, professional-use device about the size of a mobile phone, used for the medical treatment of a range of disease processes – most notably for pain relief. It was developed as a part of a Soviet space program in the 1970s. The goal was to create a portable, effective, non-invasive device to maintain the health of astronauts while in space.

In 1973, Russian doctor Alexander Karasev[9] developed the first TENS (Transcutaneous Electrical Nerve Stimulation) device to block pain, which is now used by pain sufferers all over the world. Following this, Karasev and Alexander Revenko[10] released another device designed to assist the body's healing properties – not just to block pain signals.

SCENAR devices and treatment protocols were produced by the 'Special Design Bureau' in Russia (ZAO OKB[11] RITM). In 1986, the first SCENAR device, having passed technical and clinical trials, was permitted by the USSR Medical Council for application in clinical institutions and homes.

SCENAR became available to the broad medical community after the dissolution of the Soviet Union. Since then, the device has gained popularity throughout the world. ENAR is the home-use version of SCENAR.

Further research in Russia has developed more than 20 modifications of the SCENAR, from simple hand-held devices to complex computer applications. The latest generation of SCENAR devices was patented by RITM with joint authorship: Y Gorfinkel, J Grinberg, M Zenkin, A Murancev, A Nadtochii, A Revenko, M Unakafov, S Uvarov.

SCENAR technology is based on the principles of traditional Chinese medicine and acupuncture, resulting in this form of modern electrotherapy. It interprets biological feedback between the device and the body, then modulates the form and the power

9 http://www.rexresearch.com/scenar/kasarev.htm

10 http://www.scenar-revenko.ru/en/

11 OKB Opytnoye Konstruktorskoye Buro – Experimental Design Bureau.

of its signals. The main goal of SCENAR therapy is to induce the secretion of a sufficient amount of neuropeptides to relieve pain and initiate a healing sequence. The effect of action remains after the treatment has been applied.

'SCENAR' is a trademark registered by RITM in the state list of trademarks in USSR in 1989. Classed as a 'biofeedback-controlled electro-stimulator', SCENAR is regulated by the United States Food and Drug Administration (FDA) under 21 CFR 882.5050.[12] Similar certification was acquired in Europe in 2006.

This 15 minute video outlines the use of SCENAR therapy in acute care in the Russian medical system. https://www.youtube.com/watch?v=np89Y9dGqCQ&list=UU-33VauZpGHbEsRJ_KhGiD7w

SCENAR therapy is available worldwide through individual therapists. To find a therapist, search on the internet: SCENAR therapy + your country. For example: 'SCENAR therapy London, England'.

12 US Food and Drug Administration approval http://www.accessdata.fda.gov/scripts/cdrh/cfdocs/cfcfr/cfrsearch.cfm?fr=882.5050

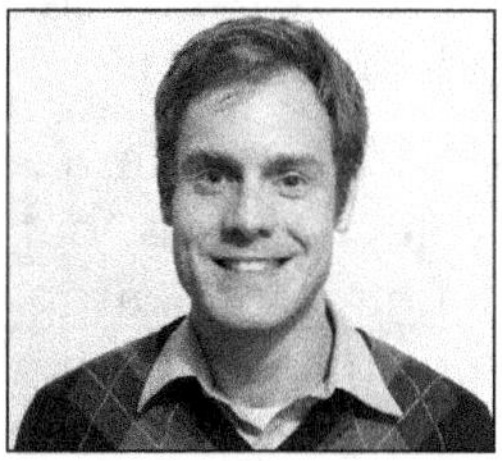

Michael Hurst, 35 years

Washington DC, USA

Diagnosed with ulcerative colitis at 21 years

While travelling with my family in South Africa, I increasingly had irritable bowel type symptoms. I wondered if the sudden shift in daylight from summer to winter triggered it. Quite suddenly it turned into worse diarrhoea, gas and then significant amounts of bright red blood. I held myself together as best I could, with a stiff upper lip, but by that time I had to tell my parents. I also had redness in my eyes that looked like pink-eye, which I later learned was a secondary symptom of ulcerative colitis.

My bowel function has never really been normal. As a baby I frequently spat up and had bad stomach aches. Since infancy, I have been restless, hyperactive and had frequent ear infections that required consistent treatment with antibiotics. After one course of antibiotics when I was two-and-a-half years old, I had a grand mal[1] seizure, which scared my mother greatly. After that, I was raised on the all-natural Feingold Diet[2] for the rest of my childhood, which my paediatrician recommended to my mom. The goal of the diet was to help control hyperactivity and eczema, not specifically for my gastrointestinal symptoms.

My parents are well educated – my father is a law professor and my mother is a school psychologist. In addition to taking me to specialists, they did a lot of their own research, so I was given pretty much the best opportunity to be healthy.

I was always very active and played a lot of sports, including being in the swim team in high school and then college, but I always had frequent diarrhoea, especially after I ate high fibre foods like fruits and vegetables. This increased over the years and became more apparent at college, especially in the winter. Even then, I think that seasonal depression was an issue.

After returning to the US from South Africa, I had stool tests and a colonoscopy. They couldn't find any known pathogens, so the GI[3] doctor diagnosed me with ulcerative colitis instead of infectious colitis or *Clostridium difficile (C. diff)*.[4] I can't recall if they tested for *Clostridium difficile* or not. Even

1 Grand mal seizure – a loss of consciousness and violent muscle contractions, caused by abnormal electrical activity in the brain.

2 The Feingold diet is a diagnostic tool to determine if certain foods or additives are triggering symptoms. The diet eliminates artificial colours, flavours and preservatives as well as foods that contain salicylates. It can be used with medical treatments.

3 GI – gastrointestinal.

4 *Clostridium difficile*, or *C. diff*, is an antibiotic induced colitis, causing diarrhoea which can be severe and life-threatening.

60mgs of prednisone[5] did not bring this into remission. Finally, they added the antibiotic ciprofloxacin that is sometimes prescribed to treat travelers' diarrhoea and that finally enabled me to get the illness under control.

I had been struggling academically in my sophomore[6] year at college. I managed to pass the exams, ending up with some pretty good grades, but I was under massive psychological stress. I was dealing with untreated Seasonal Affective Disorder (SAD), depression, working on election campaigns, as well as having frequent diarrhoea. I was continuing to teach tennis and swimming at summer camp, even though I had been constantly losing significant amounts of blood. Having had good nutrition throughout my life, my energy allowed me to largely carry on. Of course, I was determined not to let something as minor as a physical illness, that's causing me to bleed out, to stop me from doing what I wanted to do!

I tried the Specific Carbohydrate Diet (SCD).[7] That helped me to lose weight which I didn't really need to lose. I had already been avoiding problem foods, but suddenly I was eating no bread. It was like a more restricted version of a gluten-free diet. Having more fibre is not what you need when you have diarrhoea. Eventually I was living on juice, broth, hamburgers, chicken and turkey. While that diet seems to be helpful for some people, I think my case was too severe for it to have made a difference.

I do think that high doses of VSL#3, the pharmaceutical-grade probiotic which contains 450 billion colony-forming units per packet, helped. I was taking as many as eight packets per day – four trillion high-quality probiotic bacteria. It was hard to sustain that though, because it was costing me over $700 per month, in addition to other costs that I had.

My doctor treated me with intravenous *Remicade*[8] for about eight months. This was billed to my insurance company at $10,000 a dose, but it didn't really help. It seemed to cause a secondary respiratory infection and a staphylococcal infection on my skin, which really was terrible to deal with. Then it caused a leg infection – I accidentally scraped my leg and it became necrotic.[9] There was a huge open sore there, causing me to limp my way to the hospital at four o'clock one morning. I'd never had something of this magnitude before. *Remicade* is known to be an immunosuppressant drug used for things like psoriasis and rheumatoid arthritis, but it has some potentially very dangerous side effects, including secondary infections and in rare cases, an aggressive and often deadly form of cancer.

At the hospital I was treated with IV[10] vancomycin[11] for two days and my colitis

5 Prednisone is a synthetic corticosteroid drug, used to treat certain inflammatory diseases. It has an immunosuppressive action.

6 In the USA, a Sophomore is a student in the second year of high school or university.

7 The Specific Carbohydrate Diet (SCD) was created by Doctor Sidney Valentine Haas (1870-1964) to heal digestive disorders.

8 *Remicade* is the trade name for infliximab, an artificial antibody administered intravenously, used to treat autoimmune diseases.

9 Necrotic – death of body tissue.

10 IV – intravenous.

11 Vancomycin is an antibiotic used to treat serious infections that are unresponsive to other antibiotics.

symptoms improved dramatically. It was like night and day, from a bad colitis bowel movement to one that was almost well formed, which was just amazing. This suggested to me that there was some sort of infectious bacteria there, or even *C. diff*.

After that I said, "Okay, I'm *done* with *Remicade*," and sought out a doctor once again, to treat me with antibiotics. The vancomycin treatment did not continue at the hospital. The doctor told me it's because they don't like to use vancomycin any more than is necessary, since it is considered to be a drug of last resort. It's a very expensive drug too. I asked the infectious disease specialist to refer me to a GI doctor who would treat me using antibiotics. I was given a stool test, which once again was negative for any known pathogens. However, since antibiotics had been effective in the past, the doctor was willing to prescribe *Flagyl*, which is used to treat *C. diff*.

I had colonoscopies pretty much every year. Fortunately, I had good health insurance during the first few years – first under my parents' plan, which helped during my college years. Then I worked as an intern for the US House of Representatives, so I was able to afford my own care, but I had some major gaps in my health insurance. During those times I was basically self-medicating, using the same drugs that doctors had prescribed for me. Sometimes after the prescriptions ran out, I ordered the prescribed drugs from overseas pharmacies that were willing to send them to me for just an email 'consultation'. I said to myself: "Why should I go to the doctor and pay if he's going to do exactly the same thing as he did the last five times?"

Then I saw an article on the use of faecal transplants to treat *C. diff*. '*The Enema of Your Enemy is Your Friend. Faecal transplants could be a cheap and effective treatment for gastrointestinal disorders*'. I thought: "Wait a second – even though my condition is not supposed to be infectious, it has often behaved like an infectious condition, rather than an autoimmune illness. It has clearly responded to antibiotics and probiotics on numerous occasions, so there's got to be something to this." So I thought: "Let's have another crack at this, go back to the doctors and see if they can do something other than just the same prednisone when I have a flare, or otherwise take *Asacol*,[12] which didn't really do anything." I was also starting to waste away a little bit, and had lost almost 20 pounds in three months, so I was getting a little discouraged. My doctor said: "It's time to consider surgery. That's really the last thing that we can do for you. We can't get this thing into remission without prednisone, which is not a sustainable drug. Even moderate doses don't seem to be getting it under control." So I was referred for the surgical removal of my whole colon and rectum, then to have the restorative ileal/anal reservoir done – the 'J-pouch.' It was going to be a two-step procedure. I was going to do it at the Mayo Clinic in Jacksonville, Florida, which is a very good hospital.

12 *Asacol* is a commonly prescribed form of mesalamine.

It was near my parents too, because I was not going to be able to take care of myself after the surgery.

I looked at the research and saw that no faecal transplants were available for ulcerative colitis. So, at my doctor's recommendation, I went along in the whole surgery direction. The surgeon recommended that I take protein shakes, because my blood albumin levels were so low that I may not have an optimal recovery from surgery. I took the protein shakes and started mesalamine[13] again. Then I was able to taper off prednisone, so that one month before surgery, I was suddenly prednisone-free for the first time in over six months and I wasn't losing blood. If I wasn't losing blood, I considered that not to be a flare. Usually, normal bowel movements just didn't happen.

I found out about faecal transplantation for ulcerative colitis three days before my surgery date to have my colon removed. My mom handed me a print-out of the Wikipedia entry for ulcerative colitis, which referred to *Treatment of Ulcerative Colitis using Faecal Bacteriotherapy*, an article published by Doctor Borody in the *Journal of Gastroenterology*. It documented six patients who were, in the doctor's words, "cured" – which blew my mind. I thought: "This is too obvious. How could my doctors not know about this? Why are they not trying it? These case studies look very valid. Why is there no other research out there?" It just didn't quite make sense. My doctors had never diagnosed a known pathogen, even though I had clearly gotten better before when given antibiotics and taking probiotics. I really had nothing to lose at that point, other than my colon.

I feverishly dug into the research and stayed up all night until the sun came up, reading and constantly looking things up if I didn't understand them. Even if surgery was successful, the risk of complications was very significant and my quality of life would certainly be worse than it currently was for at least the next year. Eventually I realised that it was elegantly simple. The imbalanced bacteria likely triggered the dysfunction in the immune system and there were pathogens that it was trying to fight against. Straightening that out would probably help things, so I decided to cancel surgery.

After cancelling my surgery in March 2011, I looked for doctors who did faecal transplants. It was very difficult, because it is not employed in widespread practice by conventional doctors. I called doctors Lawrence Brandt in New York, Colleen Kelly in Rhode Island and Thomas Borody in Australia. I was then scheduled to have a faecal transplant in New York, first with Doctor Brandt, and then with Doctor Colleen Kelly in Rhode Island.

About a week before I was scheduled to have my faecal transplant, I cancelled it and found my own healthy donor here in Washington DC. Doing the faecal transplant with a doctor, using my brother as a donor, would have entailed both of us travelling up to Rhode Island and staying up there for a week or more. The doctor's plan was that the first transplant would be done as part of

13 Mesalamine is an aspirin-based anti-inflammatory.

a colonoscopy. After the first transplant, I was going to have to do follow-up enemas at home anyway, using my own donor *and I* was going to have to find that donor. I wondered how much benefit I would get from having one done with a colonoscope, other than the legitimacy of a doctor being involved. That also assumed that I only needed to do the transplants for a week or so.

Then I spoke to Sky Curtis in Toronto, who Doctor Kelly referred me to. She had recently been featured in the *Toronto Star* about how she had helped 'cure' her son's Crohn's-colitis using at-home faecal transplant enemas. Sky had also been in regular contact with Doctor Borody during the treatment process with her son. Since then, she has published a guide book on doing faecal transplants at home. After speaking to Sky, I decided that really I could just do this myself. Her story seemed authentic. The distinction of being cured, over just fighting for remission, gave me a lot of hope and motivated me even more. She told me it was not a quick battle and I was going to have to do the enemas for a lot longer than a week. My brother said: "Well, you want to make sure you get your health back in order as fast as possible and you will have to do most of it yourself anyway."

I found a donor who was a friend of mine and asked him to complete the medical questionnaire which checked his social and medical history, that there was no history of antibiotics and that he had had a lifetime of healthy stools. I couldn't get a lab to test his stool without a doctor's request – by now I was getting frustrated at how long this had dragged out. I had cancelled surgery in March and it was now June.

I read through all the research and knew I wasn't crazy. I was confident that I had a healthy donor and I did everything that a doctor would have done. I wanted give it a good solid try, if for no other reason to simply put my mind at ease, knowing that I had tried everything.

So I took the plunge and did enemas on a daily basis. There were a few mishaps. [*laughs*] I started to get better initially and then I ran out of mesalamine. I thought I would stop taking it, because it cost me $600 a month and I wasn't convinced it did anything. I'd been off prednisone for months too. Then my symptoms started to slowly come back. I found out that this was normal, due to the bloom cycles of some bacteria, which explains the flares that you get with this disease.

I did my faecal transplants for about five weeks. One week after I stopped them, I had an almost spontaneous remission. Even after the new bacteria is established, there is going to be continued healing with some ups and downs. In my case, pharmaceuticals still played a powerful role. I was taking high doses of prednisone, mesalamine and an antidepressant, so the drugs on top of the faecal transplant really tipped things.

I was already labeled as 'non-compliant' by the GI doctor who had referred me to surgery, so when I went back to him, hat in hand for a prescription for more prednisone, he said to me: "You're doing what?" As if he had a rogue patient on his hands. That was fair, I guess. I got some more prednisone from him, agreed to stop doing the faecal transplants and have another colonoscopy. By this time my poop was basically mirroring my donor's – even without the enemas. The colour and smell was different, implying that the new bacteria had established itself.

About a week after stopping the faecal transplant enemas, I sought out more ways to treat my colitis. After uncovering some case studies on the internet, I went back on mesalamine suppositories and got prescriptions for a low dose of doxepin[14] and for bupropion.[15] I had a complete remission of symptoms within 24 hours and then was able to quickly taper off the prednisone. The illness and the symptoms just vanished and I was astonished.

About eight weeks later, after stopping the faecal transplants, I had a colonoscopy which showed significant mucosal healing. There were actually healthy patches separating inflamed patches. Every colonoscopy I had in the past had shown continuous inflammation that was typical of ulcerative colitis. The doctor was surprised and did not have an explanation other than 'remission'. I didn't say it, but I smugly thought: "It worked, and you're not going to admit it." As I saw it, here was evidence that I am better in a way that has not happened ever, in the history of my illness, in spite of any drugs that I have taken. I've rapidly improved my symptoms.

Faecal transplants to treat infectious colitis caused by *C. diff* are growing in acceptance in the mainstream medical community, but back in June 2013, the FDA[16] imposed a rule that required an Investigational New Drug (IND) permit for any doctor wanting to do this procedure. When it came right down to it, this would have effectively prevented most doctors from doing it. Since faecal transplants are in many cases the only effective treatment option for *C. diff*, which kills an estimated 14,000 people a year in the US, there was significant protest from doctors and patients. One patient, who testified at an FDA hearing, started a group called the Fecal Transplant Foundation[17] that is working to raise awareness of this simple treatment.

While doctors have immense amounts of training, a doctor is not a magical person. All the doctors I went to have been to the top ten medical schools in the US. They were very well qualified, but sometimes they missed things and they were not privy to other information.

None of the doctors I met knew about faecal transplantation, even though an article had been published in their own *Journal of Gastroenterology*. That's what really motivated me to do my own research on everything. It would have been one thing for them to tell me: "Here's an off-the-wall option. We don't

---

14 Doxepin is a medication for insomnia.

15 Bupropion (brand names: *Wellbutrin, Zyban*) is a quit-smoking aid and a psychiatric drug for depression. Studies indicate it may lower the inflammatory mediator TNF-alpha, similar to *Remicade* and *Humira* that are used for Crohn's disease and ulcerative colitis.

16 FDA – US Food and Drug Administration is an agency of the United States Department of Health and Human Services, responsible for protecting and promoting public health.

17 *The Fecal Transplant Foundation* http://thefecaltransplantfoundation.org

personally think that it has much validity, nor will we even do it, but it's out there." But they didn't seem to be aware of it. In fairness, doctors face many constraints from using pioneering new treatments, like long working hours, a practice to maintain, huge student loan debts and many demands from a complicated health insurance billing system. They have to keep detailed patient records and defend their reputations against attack from other doctors, regulatory authorities, insurance companies and the legal system. Their hands really are tied when it comes to pushing the limits, unless they're at the end of their career and they don't care if anyone hurts their reputation. For young ambitious doctors, over-stepping the box they're put in is a sure way to jeopardise all the time and money they spent getting there.

While I truly think that doctors believe they are helping people, the business reality is that gastroenterologists make most of their money by treating people with chronic illness who never ever get better. If self-administering faecal transplants proved to be effective for large numbers of patients, it could severely undermine business for doctors and pharmaceutical companies.

The faecal transplants definitely helped me. So did the protein shakes; some of the diets I tried didn't provide me with enough protein. The antidepressant drugs, including bupropion, made a significant difference. These drugs were very cheap in comparison with the existing, expensive drug treatments for ulcerative colitis. I went through all of them. I really couldn't afford them, and they didn't work. They also had secondary side effects, like causing nasty infections or making me manic, in the case of high doses of prednisone.

Surgery has major effects and does not cure this illness. You can't have an inflamed large intestine if you don't have one. Surgery changes the nature of the problems, but doesn't eliminate them. Oftentimes the J-pouch becomes infected with *C. diff*, or you can get 'pouchitis', which has to be treated with antibiotics. That happens within the first two years to almost half the patients who have this procedure. There are also side effects to prescribed medications.

Having faecal transplantation as a first line of treatment can be very effective. There haven't been any large, controlled studies on faecal transplants for ulcerative colitis or Crohn's disease yet, but there was a small study at the university of Michigan which appeared to be beneficial, but not totally curative.[18] Studies at Baylor University and the University of Pittsburgh are scheduled to start soon.[19]

Once I discovered that faecal transplantation could help me heal and avoid surgery, I realised: "Wait a second – they were going to do surgery, even though they aren't aware of all of the medical literature out there." This other information wasn't worthy of even being considered by them.

18 *Safety, tolerability, & clinical response after faecal transplantation in children and young adults with ulcerative colitis* J Pediatr Gastroenterol Nutr 2013 Jun;56(6):597-601.doi:10.1097/MPG.0b013e318292fa0d. Kunde et al, http://www.ncbi.nlm.nih.gov/pubmed/23542823

19 http://clinicaltrials.gov/show/NCT01947101 and http://clinicaltrials.gov/ct2/show/NCT02108821

Finally, in pushing to do it without doctors, I felt almost like I was in that movie *The Truman Show* with Jim Carey, who in trying to get off the island, he suddenly realised that everything was this huge illusion and they had been messing with him the whole time, like a laboratory animal.

At a certain point I thought: "I don't care if this kills me, I am going to do this." It took me a while to really completely make that decision. I was like: "Okay, I'm going to make myself better," but was still holding back just that little bit. I was still afraid of what would happen, even though all the facts told me this was safe. Once I made that decision to fix this quickly or bust, everything became easy.

The message that I try to communicate is that you are ultimately responsible for your own health and wellbeing. You have to do your own research and be your own best advocate. There's still a lot that is unknown and it's hard for any one healthcare professional to be aware of all of the information that exists in their field.

It is documented that there is a gut-brain connection.[20,21] Therefore, clinicians should look for certain disorders in patients with inflammatory bowel disease. My GI doctors told me that patients often appeared to have a flare of the illness during stressful times, or in the fall as the days get shorter and darker, suggesting that Seasonal Affective Disorder could play a role. I believe that psychological stress can trigger diarrhoea and muscle spasms, which upsets the balance of bacteria in the intestines and leads to an overgrowth of bacteria that then causes inflammation. It's a self-perpetuating cycle of diarrhoea and inflammation.

My bowels are better now than they've been in my whole life. I don't need medications to treat colitis, although I do still take antidepressants if I need them. After 12 years of having doctors tell me that this was an incurable condition, it's hard to believe that I have been in remission since December 2011 without any medications for my bowels.

I now consider myself cured – and I still have my colon. I am grateful for all of the support I received from my parents, from Doctor Kelly, Sky Curtis and of course my faecal transplant donor. I hope that I can help others be done with this disease too.

Michael Hurst has written about his experience in an e-book called Poop Power, *which shows you how to do faecal transplants yourself or with a doctor. It lists a range of studies and research. His e-book and videos are available on his website http://fecaltransplant.org/*

---

20 *Impact of depressive mood on relapse in patients with inflammatory bowel disease: a prospective 18-month follow-up study* http://www.ncbi.nlm.nih.gov/pubmed/14747641 "Psychological factors such as a depressive mood associated with anxiety and impaired 'Health Related Quality of Life' may exert a negative influence on the course of IBD. Therefore, assessment and management of psychological distress should be included in clinical treatment of patients with IBD."

21 *Emotional disorders and inflammatory bowel disease* http://www.ncbi.nlm.nih.gov/pubmed/22811232 "The comorbidity of emotional disorders and IBD seems to be frequent.

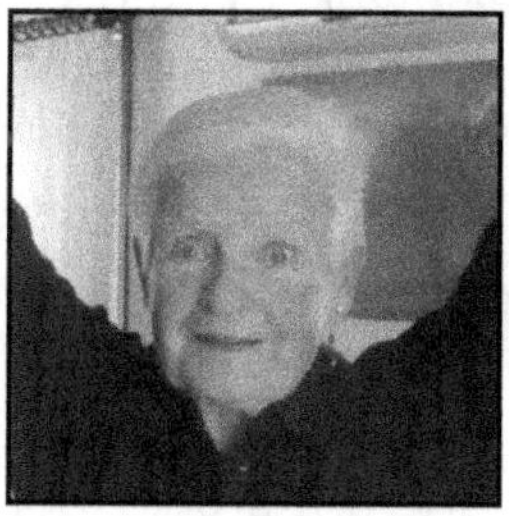

Tina Jackson, 67 years

New South Wales, Australia

Crushed cervical vertebrae with chronic arm pain for 19 years

I woke up one morning and I thought I'd had a stroke or something, because my arm was painful and I couldn't move it. Frank, my husband, had gone to golf down in Bowral and was going to be away for the day. I put up with the pain all day. When he came home that night, he realised something was wrong. By two o'clock in the morning, he just flatly said, "We're going to the hospital," so I went to the hospital. I was in there for a week, with my neck in traction and everything. It wasn't until they gave me a myelogram,[1] where they turned me upside down and put this substance in my back that I got some sort of relief from the pain.

I was told that I had a crushed vertebrae in my neck *and* that it was inoperable – that was a double whammy. They said that all the years of working in a delicatessen, setting up and using the slicer caused it, because I was doing the same movement all the time. Years ago the slicers weren't on automatic slicing as they are now, so that was where the wear-and-tear came into it.

My doctor said that he couldn't guarantee he could fix my neck with surgery, so I said to myself: "Well I'm not having an operation unless he can guarantee that he can fix it." He didn't say anything about me deciding against the surgery. Also, because I had had a heart attack at 45, they didn't want to touch me.

I couldn't lift my arm up any further than my shoulder, so I couldn't stand in the shower and wash my hair or do the housework – my arm just wouldn't work. Frank and my granddaughter, who I was minding at the time, had to help me with everything. She used to peel the potatoes and I would stand there watching her, crying. I couldn't drive the car, and I'm not a walker, so I didn't go for walks. When I was in the car as a passenger I had to rest my arm on a pillow to help with the pain.

I tried acupuncture three times a week for about a year, which semi-relieved the pain for about an hour or two after each treatment, but not a lot. Physiotherapy was more like torture. I saw a chiropractor, but when my doctor found out he said: "Don't even go back," so I didn't.

1 A myelogram is used to help find the cause of pain not found by an MRI or CT scan. It involves injecting a contrast medium into the cervical or lumbar spine, followed by several X-rays. It is used to locate spinal cord injury, cysts or tumours.

The pain was acute and sharp, all the time, down my whole arm to the palm of my hand, which was stone cold and it was worse at night. I could use my fingers, but I couldn't write. I could do virtually nothing with my hand, because if I did, it would trigger the pain. I got through the day by eating painkillers all the time – I had six every day.

I was working at the time it happened, so my life stopped overnight. I didn't drive the car for the next 19 years. I just read books, and lived by the clock, waiting for the next time to take the painkillers. I didn't get depressed – I could have been worse off. I could have had little children. I turned it around sort of, to put up with the pain. You've got to stop and think sometimes, don't you?

The painkillers only kicked in every now and then, but after 15 years, they weren't helping like they used to. Then I got hooked on them, so I weaned myself off them and put up with the pain. The pain wasn't worse without the painkillers – it was just the same! [*laughs*] I tried *Valium*[2] once and lost a day on them sleeping, so I went back to the doctor and told him not to ever prescribe them again for me.

Then I came across a SCENAR[3] therapist. I'm not sure how I came across her, Frank might have heard about her down at the club. Like I said, I'd try anything to get rid of the pain.

The therapist worked with the machine down my back, then down my arm, right to my fingertips and then she treated the other arm. Not that much happened after the first treatment. It was the second and third treatments that helped me. After those treatments, I couldn't believe how I felt, and my hand wasn't cold.

I could move my arm a lot higher and *there was no pain*. I couldn't get over that, because I'd lived with it for so long. Then I got frightened and thought: "Well, if I start using my arm, the pain's going to come back," so I shied away from doing anything. Then gradually, I got back into doing things like driving, but precious little housework, because Frank wouldn't let me do it, which was alright by me!

After six or seven treatments once a week, the pain was all gone. My arm movement is normal now with no pain when I move it. When people ring me up and ask me about this treatment, I tell them: "Well, it's worked for me and that's all I'm going to say." It was worth it, so much so that we went and bought the home-treatment machine.[4] Frank treated me about five times all up, but then I said to him, "I'm not going to do it every couple of days anymore. I want to have it as a back-up in case anything ever happens again." It's a wonderful feeling to have the machine there.

---

2 *Valium*, or diazepam, is a drug that has a relaxant effect. It is used for a range of mental anxiety disorders, muscle spasms and alcohol withdrawal.

3 SCENAR – Self Controlled Electro Neuro Adaptive Regulator is a hand-held biofeedback medical device http://en.wikichiro.org/index.php?title=Scenar_Therapy

4 ENAR – Electro Neuro Adaptive Regulator is a hand-held biofeedback medical device for home use.

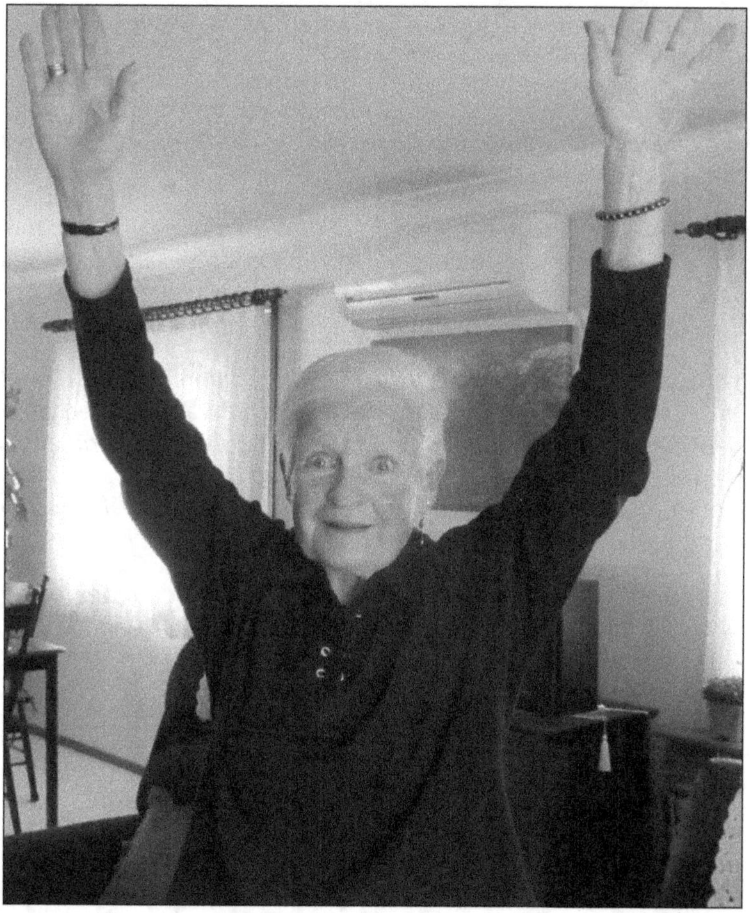

Tina Jackson celebrating having no arm pain after 19 years.

SCENAR – Self Controlled Energy Neuro Adaptive Regulator, is a battery-powered, professional-use device about the size of a mobile phone, used for the medical treatment of a range of disease processes – most notably for pain relief. It was developed as a part of a Soviet space program in the 1970s. The goal was to create a portable, effective, non-invasive device to maintain the health of astronauts while in space.

In 1973, Russian doctor Alexander Karasev[5] developed the first TENS (Transcutaneous Electrical Nerve Stimulation) device to block pain, which is now used by pain sufferers all over the world. Following this, Karasev and Alexander Revenko[6] released another device designed to assist the body's healing properties – not just to block pain signals.

SCENAR devices and treatment protocols were produced by the 'Special Design Bureau' in Russia (ZAO OKB[7] RITM). In 1986, the first SCENAR device, having

5 http://www.rexresearch.com/scenar/kasarev.htm

6 http://www.scenar-revenko.ru/en/

7 OKB Opytnoye Konstruktorskoye Buro – Experimental Design Bureau.

passed technical and clinical trials, was permitted by the USSR Medical Council for application in clinical institutions and homes.

SCENAR became available to the broad medical community after the dissolution of the Soviet Union. Since then, the device has gained popularity throughout the world. ENAR is the home-use version of SCENAR.

Further research in Russia has developed more than 20 modifications of the SCENAR, from simple hand-held devices to complex computer applications. The latest generation of SCENAR devices was patented by RITM with joint authorship: Y Gorfinkel, J Grinberg, M Zenkin, A Murancev, A Nadtochii, A Revenko, M Unakafov, S Uvarov.

SCENAR technology is based on the principles of traditional Chinese medicine and acupuncture, resulting in this form of modern electrotherapy. It interprets biological feedback between the device and the body, then modulates the form and the power of its signals. The main goal of SCENAR therapy is to induce the secretion of a sufficient amount of neuropeptides to relieve pain and initiate a healing sequence. The effect of action remains after the treatment has been applied.

'SCENAR' is a trademark registered by RITM in the state list of trademarks in USSR in 1989. Classed as a 'biofeedback-controlled electro-stimulator', SCENAR is regulated by the United States Food and Drug Administration (FDA) under 21 CFR 882.5050.[8] *Similar certification was acquired in Europe in 2006.*

This 15 minute video outlines the use of SCENAR therapy in acute care in the Russian medical system. https://www.youtube.com/watch?v=np89Y9dGqCQ&list=UU-33VauZpGHbEsRJ_KhGiD7w

SCENAR therapy is available worldwide through individual therapists. To find a therapist, search on the internet: SCENAR therapy + your country. For example: 'SCENAR therapy London, England'.

8 US Food and Drug Administration approval http://www.accessdata.fda.gov/scripts/cdrh/cfdocs/cfcfr/cfrsearch.cfm?fr=882.5050

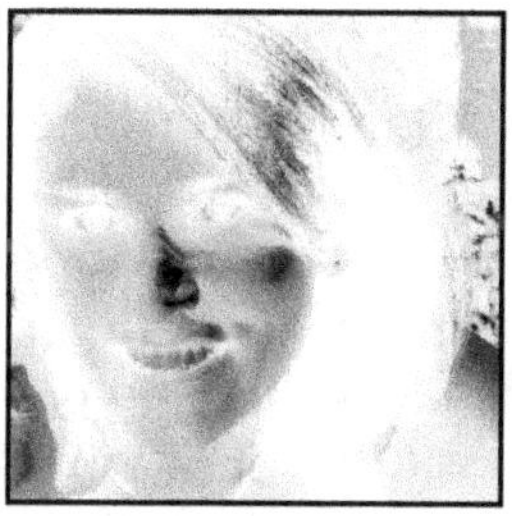

Genevieve, 32 years

Colorado, USA

Diagnosed with Crohn's disease at 25 years

I probably had Crohn's disease for at least seven years before I was diagnosed. After I graduated from high school in 2000 and went to college, I noticed a change in my digestion during my freshman year, when I started having frequent diarrhoea. I would go for a run and couldn't make it very far without needing a bathroom.

I was diagnosed in January 2007, only because I took a job in Denver and so had health insurance for the first time since college. Up until that point, I just kind of lived with my symptoms. During college I thought: "Well, I'm eating crappy food and drinking a bunch of beer and my stomach hurts, so go figure!" When I finally got health insurance, I decided it was time to go to the doctor and ask why I had to go to the bathroom so often. They did a colonoscopy and diagnosed me with Crohn's disease on the spot. The doctor prescribed some medication and sent me on my way.

I didn't really know what Crohn's disease was. My Crohn's is in my large intestine – mainly in the descending colon and the rectum. Most people develop Crohn's near the terminal ileum in the small intestine, which is the area that can cause severe pain and blockages. Since mine is lower in my intestine, I haven't experienced much pain.

I've come up with some of my own little theories as to what caused it. I think emotions have a lot to do with the overall health of your body. If you don't deal with traumatic events in your life, and truly process and acknowledge your emotions, you can store the hurt and pain in the cells of your body. With that theory in mind, one reason for my Crohn's could have been the emotional trauma of my dad going to jail when I was 14. I don't think I ever fully processed that event – I just pushed down the hurt into my body.

When I was in high school, from 1996 to 2000, I would get upset stomachs at sporting events for track or cross-country and that's when the diarrhoea started. I thought: "Oh, I'm just nervous." Maybe it wasn't really nerves, but the beginning of my Crohn's.

Other contributing factors could be toxins in our environment and food supply, and the introduction of genetically modified food in the US in the early to mid-nineties. We weren't educated about the dangers of processed and non-organic food when I was growing up. I assume that these factors had an effect without me knowing it.

When I was diagnosed, they immediately put me on *Asacol*[1] and prednisone.[2] *Asacol* didn't do much, so soon afterwards they switched me to 20 pills of *Pentasa*[3] a day! That didn't have much effect either, so then I was put on a drug called *Imuran*,[4] which landed me in the ER.[5] After ten days on *Imuran*, I developed severe abdominal pain, a high fever and started puking my guts out. My white blood cell count was through the roof, so they admitted me to hospital for the night and gave me some pain meds. They couldn't figure out what was wrong with me and discharged me in the morning. They said: "That's just your Crohn's disease. This drug is fine and you should keep taking it." I told them: "My Crohn's disease has never acted like this before – it's weird and I feel like it's this medicine that I'm on." So I went home and did a test. I took the *Imuran* and the same thing happened again. I got a high fever, puked my guts out and had terrible abdominal pain, so I was like: "Well, obviously, it's the *Imuran* and I don't need to try it again – that was terrible!"

That was the first time I realised that doctors don't always have all the answers. The next drug they put me on was *Remicade*,[6] starting on a fairly low dose. I was on that for a few months, but didn't really notice much improvement from that drug.

During the fall of 2007, about nine months after my diagnosis, I got some food testing done and found out I was sensitive to gluten. I thought: "I'm going to cure my Crohn's disease by giving up gluten – screw *Remicade*," so I went off it.

Around the same time, I moved from Denver to Colorado, which is where I live now. It was a stressful time, due to the move and a new job. It was then that I experienced my first serious flare. I lost about 12 pounds, had no energy, lost a bunch of hair, had weird pain and gas, and I just felt terrible. It turns out just going 'gluten-free' wasn't the answer to my problems! I went back onto *Remicade* – they doubled the dose and it worked. Within 48 hours, I started feeling better.

Remicade got me out of my first flare, and it continued to work for the next one and a half to two years, from 2008-2010. It's an IV[7] medication and the infusion takes three hours. The benefit is supposed to last for eight weeks. When I first took it, I could go for ten weeks, then it was nine weeks, eight, then seven. After a while, I would barely make it for four weeks. All of a sudden, my 'well-controlled' Crohn's disease was not so well-controlled

1 *Asacol* is a commonly prescribed form of mesalamine, an aspirin-based anti-inflammatory.

2 Prednisone is a synthetic corticosteroid drug, used to treat certain inflammatory diseases. It has an immunosuppressive action.

3 *Pentasa* is a trade name for mesalazine, an anti-inflammatory drug used to treat inflammatory bowel disease.

4 *Imuran* is a trade name for azathioprine, an immunosuppressant drug used for autoimmune diseases and organ transplantation.

5 ER – emergency room.

6 *Remicade* – (infliximab) is an artificial antibody used for autoimmune diseases, administered intraveneously.

7 IV – intravenous.

anymore. My doctor switched me to *Humira,*[8] which is another injectable, but you can do this one at home with a spring-loaded pen – it feels like a bee sting. I had to have my husband give me the injections – it was just too scary for me to push the trigger!

In the fall of 2010, when I switched from *Remicade* to *Humira,* I also happened to tear the ACL[9] in my left knee, which needed reconstruction. As with any surgery, they pump you full of antibiotics before you leave the hospital. I think the combination of the high doses of antibiotics, trauma of surgery, and an already compromised gut, was too much for my body to handle. It was a downhill slide for all of 2011 and I couldn't regain control of my Crohn's.

I tried *Humira* for a couple more months, then another drug called *Cimzia,*[10] which didn't work either. The next drug I took was injectable methotrexate,[11] plus combinations of prednisone and *Flagyl.*[12] Methotrexate is a hard-core cancer drug. I took it about three times, but I was just so afraid of it that I said: "Forget this – I'm not going to do it."

In the Spring of 2012, my doctor said to me: "Well, you've failed all your meds so I think we should cut your colon out." I said: "That's a terrible idea – let's not do that." He was super-closed to any alternative and said: "I treat Crohn's disease with drugs and surgery. You've failed all the drugs so now we have to try surgery." He even went so far as to schedule an appointment for me with a local surgeon. I was disgusted – I couldn't believe that he was just throwing up his hands. I thought: "I'm too young to have my colon removed!" That's when I started seeking alternative therapies.

My first stop was to meet with a nutritionist down in Boulder. He recommended several dietary changes – organic unprocessed food, raw milk and fermented foods. He was the first practitioner to key me into the concept of 'gut dysbiosis', which is an imbalance between good and bad bacteria in the gut. I'm pretty sure the massive dose of antibiotics during my ACL surgery contributed to this. He gave me a CD that discussed Doctor Thomas Borody in Australia using faecal transplants to cure gut dysbiosis. I thought: "Hmm, maybe I should try that."

Then I had my second significant flare. I lost about 15 pounds, became severely anaemic, had constant fevers, terrible digestion and I was very weak. I had to have iron infusions in order to cure the anaemia. I was barely able go to work and couldn't really function. My body just wasn't absorbing any nutrients. I had unexplained swelling in my ankles and joints and developed Erythema

8 *Humira* (adalimumab) is a tumour necrosis factor (TNF) drug.

9 ACL – Anterior Cruciate Ligament of the knee.

10 *Cimzia* is a trade name for certolizumab pegol, and is a tumour necrosis factor (TNF) drug.

11 Methotrexate, originally a chemotherapy drug, is now used for autoimmune diseases like rheumatoid and connective tissue disease. It is highly toxic and has a range of serious side effects that include mouth ulcers, immunosuppression leading to various infections, hair loss, nervous system disorders, bone marrow suppression and loss of consciousness.

12 *Flagyl* is a trade name for metronidazole, an antibiotic medication used for anaerobic bacteria and protozoa.

Nodosum[13] on my legs. I had so much inflammation everywhere in my body and I was just a mess. My CRP[14] was off-the-chart high. By now, no drugs were working, so I stopped them all.

Out of desperation, I decided I should try faecal transplants – what did I have to lose? I decided to use my husband as my donor. You're supposed to have your donor tested for a slew of diseases, but I opted not to, because he is so healthy. He's a professional mountain bike racer and super fit. I thought: "I don't think you have anything that I don't want, so... [*laughs*]

I did the faecal transplant at home with a blender and an enema bag, for four consecutive days at first. My doctor freaked out when I told him I did a faecal transplant: "You did what? You did a faecal transplant? There's no research on that!" So I stopped doing them, basically because he scared the crap out of me. Then I thought: "He doesn't really know anything – never once has he mentioned gut dysbiosis, so I'm going to do it again." I did another five in a row. The two transplants that I did were within two and a half weeks of each other.

Within two weeks of the last transplant, I was on the road to recovery. Suddenly, everything was turning around. My digestion got better and I started feeling better. I started gaining weight and my stool was more formed. It was still a long process to heal my body through that whole summer of 2012. I had to work hard to regain my strength and weight, get the inflammation down and my anaemia under control, but the faecal transplants were the turning point.

The transplants got me mostly normal. My 'normal' is being able to mountain bike in the summer. I was able get back on my bike, go hiking and be active again. My digestion was never perfect, but it was much better. I had much more formed stools than I'd ever had before. At that point I thought: "I'm cured! I did a faecal transplant and I'm all good!"

In November of 2012, I started to regress again. Turns out that faecal transplants are not a magic-bullet fix – there are other factors at play. I had another flare in January of 2013. I tried some faecal transplants with my husband as my donor again, but they didn't do anything. At that point I tried an elemental diet from Jini Patel Thompson's book called *Listen To Your Gut*. She 'cured' her own Crohn's with these special shakes she developed, called 'Absorb Plus'. I tried her diet for about six weeks, but I got worse and lost more and more weight.

In March of 2013, I met with an acupuncturist here in town, who encouraged me to try the GAPS[15] diet. Within a few weeks of following that diet, I finally felt that I was coming out of the flare and starting to heal. GAPS emphasises no grains, homemade bone broths (probably the most healing aspect of the diet), increased consumption of fermented foods, no dairy and no sugar (honey only). Even so, I had to do 15 iron infusions to get my iron back up. I was

13 Erythema Nodosum is an inflammatory condition where fat cells under the skin cause tender red nodules or lumps, often on both shins.

14 CRP – C-reactive protein, a blood test that measures general levels of inflammation in the body.

15 GAPS – *Gut and Psychology Syndrome*, written by Doctor Natasha Campbell-McBride, promotes a Specific Carbohydrate Diet (SCD) based on the work of Doctor Sidney Haas (1870-1964), who pioneered a low-carbohydrate diet to treat coeliac disease.

down from 120 pounds to 100 pounds.

I found out that I was super-low in vitamin D. No-one had ever tested that before, which really surprised me. I discovered that vitamin D was important when we went on a trip to Florida last April. Within a week of being in Florida, I gained back five pounds just from lying in the sun. I thought: "Oh my God, it's the vitamin D." My body just didn't have enough, so I started vitamin D supplementation and saw a huge improvement. I take 20,000 IU a day in winter and reduce it to 5,000 IU a day in summer. It's a lot, but it's important for my body. I followed the GAPS diet strictly until about February of this year, 2014.

Then I had some stool testing done. I had no overgrowth of pathogenic bacteria in my gut and no candida, but there was still a dysbiosis. There was just nothing good or bad in there, but I had super-low levels of good bacteria. The GAPS diet had worked by not feeding my body any grains or sugar so all the pathogenic bacteria had died off, but so did all the good bacteria. To feed the good bacteria, I started reintroducing starches, gluten-free grains and rice into my diet. I also started a prescription strength probiotic called VSL#3[16] and I'm taking three of those every day. Actually, I have seen the most improvement with my digestion than I've ever seen since I started the VSL, so I'm very encouraged with taking probiotics.

I'm still not taking any medications. *Remicade* was the only medication that noticeably worked for me – but it wasn't a long-term cure, as it stopped working after two years.

I guess I am really disillusioned with western medicine; they are so consumed with treating the symptoms of your disease that they forget to treat, or even consider, the cause. My western doctors always told me that, "Diet doesn't matter in Crohn's disease." They couldn't be more wrong! Now that I've learned how powerful acupuncture, diet and other natural ways of healing can be, I'll never turn back.

When I first did a Google search on faecal transplants, I barely came up with anything. Now it's everywhere – it's completely exploding, which I think is really exciting. At some point I think society will finally understand that the reason we have so much sickness is because our gut health is so poor. The gut microbiome[17] is not very well understood, but it's so important to our overall health.

The *Power of Poop* website[18] has been a great resource for me. The FMT[19] Facebook page is where I get a lot of useful information from people who are posting and sharing their experiences. When it was started a little over a year ago, I think I was member number 40. Now there are a couple of thousand

16 VSL#3® is a high-potency probiotic medical food for patients with ulcerative colitis, an ileal pouch and irritable bowel syndrome.

17 Gut microbiome – community of symbiotic and pathogenic organisms found in the gut.

18 *Power of Poop* http://thepowerofpoop.com

19 FMT – faecal microbiota transplantation.

people – I've learned so much about the gut through that page!

I've sought out several doctors. The doctor who prescribed me the probiotic was not a gastroenterologist, she was just a family doctor. The reason I went to her was that she was a registered clinician who did stool tests with one of the companies. I thought: "Well, she's half-way there, so I'll go contact her and see if she can sign off on this test and order these other tests for me." I got her involved that way. When I came back for the test results, I was the one who led the discussion and determined my own treatment plan. I just needed her signature on the prescription for the probiotics. That was about all she helped me with. It might be that I'm in a small mountain town in Colorado, but doctors never know what I'm talking about. They've never heard of faecal transplants, the GAPS diet, or gut dysbiosis.

I've realised that I'm my own doctor now, and that's fine. I go to a doctor to get a blood test ordered, or a stool test form signed, and that's all I really need them for.

I've been feeling super-healthy lately. My digestion is not normal, but it's much better. I have my energy back and I can exercise again. Besides the fact that I still have to be near a bathroom, there's much less diarrhoea now and I'm doing pretty damned well!

In 2012, when my doctor told me I had "failed all my meds" and had no options left other than having my colon removed, I felt completely hopeless. Now I feel like: "Oh my gosh, there are so many options out there in terms of supplements and diet and faecal transplants." I'm almost overwhelmed by: "What do I do next? There are so many things to try!"

There has to be a three-pronged attack – heal the gut lining, deal with the dysbiosis and calm the inflammation, which are all so interconnected. If you deal with just one, like the dysbiosis through FMT, but not work to heal the gut lining or calm the inflammation, your body will continue to flare.

I think I will do FMT again in the future if needed. There is such an ick-factor with the whole process, but when you're really desperate, you'll do anything to feel better, including putting someone else's poop up your butt! Once you're feeling better, you're like, "Oh, I don't know if I want to make a poop smoothie today!" They're pretty disgusting.

The way I view it is that it's little puzzle pieces. I haven't gotten my whole puzzle figured out yet, but I've got a lot more pieces now than I had when I was first diagnosed. Figuring out the vitamin D was huge, also staying away from gluten, processed grains, sugars, going organic, eating fermented foods, drinking raw milk, and consuming homemade bone broths are big pieces. I keep finding pieces to my puzzle that work. I'm not quite there yet, but one day, it's going to be cured. I can't fail, doing this myself.

Now I can function well and enjoy my life. Energy-wise, I'm 85 to 90 per cent back to normal. My digestion is around 75 per cent normal – for me that's great! There are times when I feel hindered by my Crohn's, but for the most part it doesn't bother me too much. It feels good to control it through good foods and natural methods. I know the things I am doing are only helping my body heal. I'm an accountant for my real job, but if I could go back and redo it, I think I would study the gut.

It's now June of 2014 and I've been flare-free for over one year now – that's the longest I've gone in three years. I feel great. I'm healthy, strong and still finding puzzle pieces. The newest addition to my diet is raw goat's milk, which seems to be helping immensely. I can't wait to find out what my next puzzle piece will be.

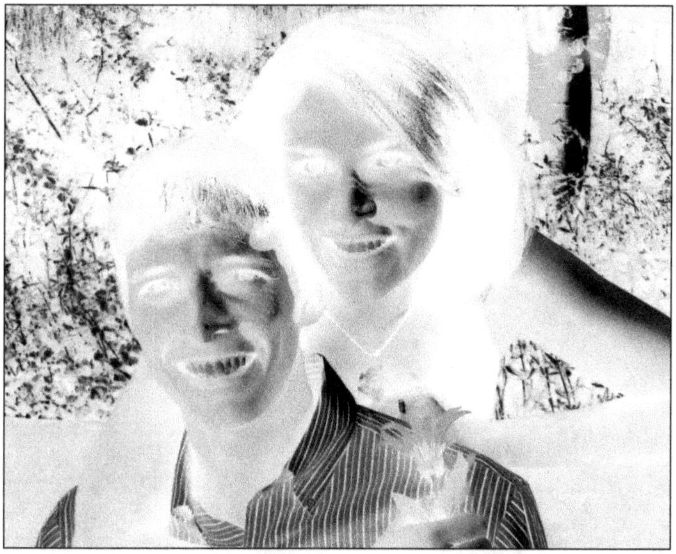

Genevieve with her husband.

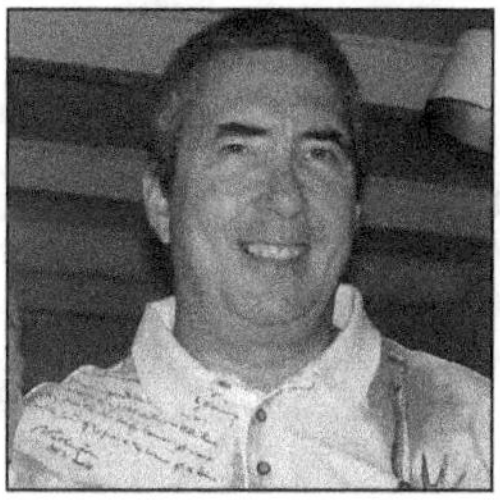

Bud Lindley, 63 years

Powell, Ohio, USA

Diagnosed with lymphoma at 59 years

Bud:

I was diagnosed with lymphoma in March of 2009. Actually, my wife found a lump that I had on my back. It was a benign lump that was changing a little bit. It was getting more of a purplish colour and she got to be concerned about it. Twenty years ago, we were told it was a benign lump, but it had changed in appearance, so that's what got our interest piqued. I went to my skin doctor and they did a biopsy on it. Initially, the skin doctor thought it could have been skin lymphoma that's called 'follicular lymphoma' and it's not as serious as full-blown lymphoma because they can usually treat it with radiation locally. He found out that it had systemic lymphoma cells in it, and told me that I might have lymphoma in another part of my body, so he removed as much of that lump as he could.

I went to Ohio State University, the James Cancer Center, and they did a bone marrow biopsy there. From the bone marrow biopsy they found B-cell lymphoma. My cancer doctor gave me a percentage: 30-40 per cent involvement in my bone marrow. I had two lymph nodes in my abdomen that were sightly swollen. They were so deep down in my abdomen, they said that until there was something closer to the surface that they could get to easier, it wouldn't be worth the risk digging all the way down in there just to see exactly what kind of lymphoma I had, so they could 'stage' it – you know: one, two, three or four.

My lymphoma is what they call 'non-Hodgkin's' and it's 'B-cell'. It's a low-grade, slow growing type, but this kind of lymphoma can transform into a faster growing one at any time. That's kind of what they've been watching for, for the last four years – whether or not my lymphoma was going to transform into a more aggressive type, which would require chemotherapy and/or radiation.

My wife, Connie, and I (we've been married 43 years) were kind of startled at the diagnosis and it didn't sit real well with either of us, so we asked if there were any nutritional things we could do. The oncologist said that there was nothing that we could do – no vitamins, no supplements, nothing.

When we first got the news, we were shocked, because my health has always been pretty good. When I was 25 years old (I'm 63 now) my company doctor told me I needed to get more exercise, because I was having a lot of stress and tension headaches and he put me on an exercise programme. About the only thing I really stuck with was the walking and jogging part of it. I've been doing that since I was 25 years old – almost 40 years now. I ran a marathon and a half marathon and that seemed to help my blood pressure. I'm not as young as I used to be, but I'm still in pretty good shape, I think. The only thing that had changed was that lump on my back.

We came down to Florida in our Spring break in 2009. Connie had talked to her sister, who has a daughter who's an attorney in Miami. She recommended a naturopathic doctor around Sunnyside Beach. His name is Doctor Martin Dayton. He was a great doctor and he must have spent about two hours with Connie and I talking about lymphoma and things that I could do. One of the things he mentioned was LDN – Low Dose Naltrexone[1] – and he prescribed it for me. We found a compounding pharmacy close by there to Miami and they gave us powder in these little packets and told us: "Mix these with distilled water and drink it before bedtime." So that's how I got started on it.

Doctor Dayton gave me the name of a naturopathic doctor, Doctor Richard Mason, for when we came back to Ohio. Actually, he lives about five minutes from us, so it really worked out good. He prescribed LDN, but when I went to the compounding pharmacy here in Columbus, they gave it to me in capsules, so I take it in capsule form now. I buy 90 days supply and when I run out of my prescription, I go for another appointment with my doctor and talk to him and he gives me some more. That's how I get my LDN.

We had an interesting experience at the Cancer Center in Columbus Ohio. The lady oncologist I had stated: "Well, we think we've found this in the early stages," but they couldn't 'stage' it, because that would involve going way deep into my abdomen and getting samples from the couple of swollen lymph nodes that I had. So she said: "Just go home, and if you develop any further symptoms like night sweats, anaemia, stuff like that, get back with us and then we can start your treatment." They were waiting for lymph nodes to pop out on my neck so it would be easier to biopsy that way. She [the oncologist] said that eventually I would get very tired, and I would have swollen lymph nodes, probably within six months. "When you develop those symptoms, come back and we will further evaluate you and then we'll be able to treat you."

About a month or so after that, I found the Cancer Treatment Centers of America[2] online, and I started talking to them. One of the centres is in a little town north of Chicago called Zion, Illinois. That's where we go. The Cancer Treatment Centers are private hospitals and there's five of them in the United States. They propose a full body outlook as far as your disease goes – mind,

1 Low Dose Naltrexone is the off-label prescription of the FDA approved drug *Naltrexone*.

2 Cancer Treatment Centers of America: http://www.cancercenter.com

body and spirit. They also put a lot of emphasis on the nutritional aspect of fighting cancer. For me, basically it was keeping my immune system as strong as possible. I take lots of supplements as well as the LDN. I take green tea extract, curcumin, fish oil, vitamin C, vitamin D3 and a baby aspirin every day. Something they recommended, because I guess it's good for other things, is to take 5mg of melatonin at bedtime. That's the same time that I take my LDN. I take them pretty religiously every day.

At the Cancer Treatment Centers, I have my oncologist, a naturopathic doctor, and I also have a nutritionist, so you have three doctors there to compare notes about your case and then they recommend things to do. They also have a mind and body therapist. With my diet and nutrition, they told me to have less sugar (I'm a sugaraholic!) and more fresh fruit and vegetables. They said I was slightly low on my protein level at one time, so they encouraged me to eat a little more lean protein every day. That's about it as far as my diet and stuff. They don't want me to lose weight. I'm six feet and five inches and weigh 230 pounds. I could probably lose a little bit of weight, but they just don't like you to lose weight over there, because that's a sign something could be going on, you know.

It's very inspiring for us to go to the Cancer Centers of America, because we see and meet people in all different stages of cancer and they're all fighting so hard. They have a pretty good success rate there, too. One of the things they're doing more of now is personalising the chemotherapy, based on what kind of cancer cells you have. You can go on their website, and they'll give you their success rates on the different kinds of cancer. They even have folks that recover completely from Stage 4 pancreatic cancer – it's remarkable! It's quite a humbling experience when we go over there.

I've had absolutely no side effects from the LDN that I'm aware of. I hope it is working in keeping my tumours and things at bay. I'm definitely not going to stop taking it, unless my doctor tells me to. People take it for all kinds of different things, like lupus and autoimmune system problems. My naturopathic doctor over there at the Cancer Treatment Center will not prescribe it for me, but they have told me not to stop taking it – I do not believe it is approved by the FDA.[3] I take 4.5mg at bedtime. If you're a drug junkie, you can get 50mg real easy, but for cancer patients it's like pulling teeth unless you know a DO,[4] or a naturopathic doctor.

Every nine months or so, at the Cancer Treatment Centers, I get full blood work and either one of a CAT[5] scan or a PET[6] scan. Then the same day I go meet with

3 FDA – US Food and Drug Administration is an agency of the United States Department of Health and Human Services, responsible for protecting and promoting public health.

4 DO – osteopathic doctor.

5 CAT scan, also known as a CT scan, or Computed Axial Tomography, is a diagnostic medical imaging procedure that examines cross sections of the body allowing a three dimensional view of specific areas.

6 PET (Positron Emission Tomography) – a nuclear medical imaging technique that produces a three-dimensional image of the body to assess the metabolic activity of tissues. It is used to identify cancer cells and their possible spread through the body.

a cancer doctor and he goes over it all and sees if there are any changes or anything. I can report that I've been stable for four and a half years. No changes, no need for anything. The lesion on my back has gone. As much of it as could be was removed surgically after my biopsy. I also had some lesions here on my chest, which I had my skin doctor biopsy and she said: "Oh yeah, that's lymphoma." So we contacted my oncologist in Chicago and he said: "Don't have her take those off, because whenever they pop up there, it's probably going to show up as lymphoma." They have disappeared – they're gone. My lymphoma continues to be completely stable on the scans. There's been no changes that he's told me of, as far as my internal organs or lymph nodes or anything like that. My doctor says the internal lesions haven't disappeared, but everything is stable, and my blood work is excellent. For people who have lymphoma, 'stable' is a very good word. I'm very thankful for that.

At one time, I had a slightly enlarged spleen, but they said that was insignificant. They're shocked that they don't see the normal progression of lymphoma and changes in the blood. My white blood cell count always comes back excellent. Everything always comes back excellent.

My family is very supportive and we're just all thrilled that I'm doing as well as I'm doing. To be perfectly honest with you, it's like I don't even have a disease, because I have no symptoms. I just hope and pray it stays that way. I had a cancer doctor telling me he wished he had the blood that I had. [*laughs*] I feel healthy, I stay active and feel very blessed that I can do everything I can do.

I have not been back to my original cancer doctor at all. Once we got feeling like we needed to be a little bit more proactive, we just left. We wanted to see what we could do with this kind of diagnosis.

Connie:

When we go into the Cancer Treatment Center, there's all these people who are really sick and they're doing treatments in rooms all along the area that we go to.

It's kind of interesting to watch the doctors' reaction to him. Every time that he goes for a check-up there, they seem amazed that he's still in this good of condition, because they felt like it would have transformed by now. You can tell that they know there's something that he's doing right. It's almost like the doctor's afraid to say: "Well, you're cured." They can't tell him that there's a thing wrong with him. They act like his blood is as good as theirs, or as good as mine or anybody that's free of any type of blood disease or blood cancer. It's really kind of amazing to go and hear their reactions. They're not willing to let go of the fact that once you've got lymphoma, it's always there. They will never say that you're cured – they'll only say that you're in remission. We thank God every day for that. We feel like that is a gift to us from God.

I want to say to them: "Why did you tell us it would have transformed by now and nothing's happened? If something miraculous is happening here with something he's doing, if there's something that you know that he's doing right, why don't you now find out what that is? If it is LDN, then let's push to get that drug on the market in this country to fight cancer."

There are too many people dying of cancer. Every single day you hear of another person who has died, or another one who's been diagnosed. You just get sick of hearing the word. There just has to be a way. You feel that it's too big of a money-maker for the doctors and the medical companies. All the stuff that they give people that supposedly kills the cancer in their body, but the chemo[7] also destroys their body's ability to fight disease. That's always the amazing thing to me – you go in there and you see the looks on their faces and the report that comes back from the testing. They will just not concede to the fact that we're seeing something here that we didn't expect to see. I want to say that maybe we need to search deeper into what it is that you are doing that the rest of the people that come in here who are so sick are not doing. We don't know what else it can be. We really think that it needs to be researched more.

We know other people have had the results with LDN that we have had. That's why I think that it needs to be out there more. It's just not being given the credit where it's due. It's all money that seems to matter here in the United States. Nobody wants to open up that drug and do all the research on it, because they're not going to make the money. With the FDA in this country, all it is, is dollars. When they release drugs, they make so much money off of them. When they become generic, they don't make any more and there's too little. That's the same thing with LDN – they can't make the money on it, and that's very tragic in my heart. They let people die that might be saved.

Bud:

In conclusion, I just want to say: Don't take the first thing that somebody says to you about your cancer or any kind of illness as gospel – *dig deeper!* In our case, we had this feeling that there's got to be something else that we can do, instead of sitting, waiting for the lymphoma to get worse. Never, ever, ever give up – there is always hope! We hear stories all the time of people who are given up for dead, and they're still alive. I tell my story, every chance I get. I tell them that I don't have any symptoms and I'm taking this stuff called LDN. It's like a God-send to us. As of right now, we're sitting four and a half years out from my diagnosis and I'm feeling pretty good and very blessed.

Lymphomas are the most common form of blood cancer. Most diagnosed are non-Hodgkin's lymphoma (NHL). The incidence of lymphomas has more than doubled over the past 20 years and is continuing to rise, for no known reason. The causes of lymphoma are not yet known. Exposure to radiation and certain chemicals puts some people at higher risk. Exposure to viruses such as the Epstein-Barr

7 Chemo – chemotherapy.

virus or HIV increases the risk of developing lymphoma. Treatment options include chemotherapy, radiotherapy, monoclonal antibodies, or a stem cell transplant if the prognosis is poor.

(Cancer Council Australia http://www.cancer.org.au/)

The overall five-year relative survival rate for people with NHL is 68%, and the ten-year relative survival rate is 57%.

(American Cancer Society 2013 http://www.cancer.org)

Harvard educated Bernard Bihari, MD (1931-2010), discovered the clinical effects of FDA-approved Naltrexone using low doses (Low Dose Naltrexone or LDN). In 1985-86, he conducted a groundbreaking clinical trial on patients with HIV/AIDS. Doctor Bihari says that the immune system normalising effect of the drug application he discovered applies to a wide range of autoimmune diseases.

Research trials can be found at http://www.lowdosenaltrexone.org/ldn_trials.htm

79-minute interview with Doctor Bihari: http://www.youtube.com/watch?v=x54Jc-cr8GT879

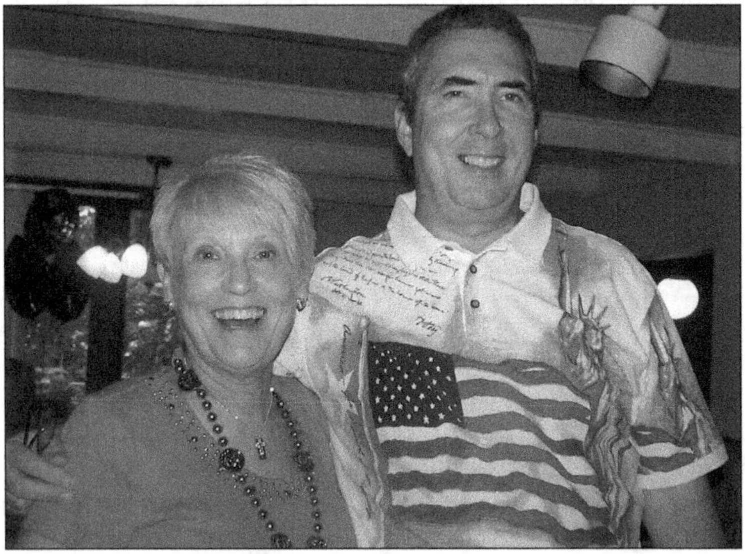

Bud Lindley with his wife Connie.

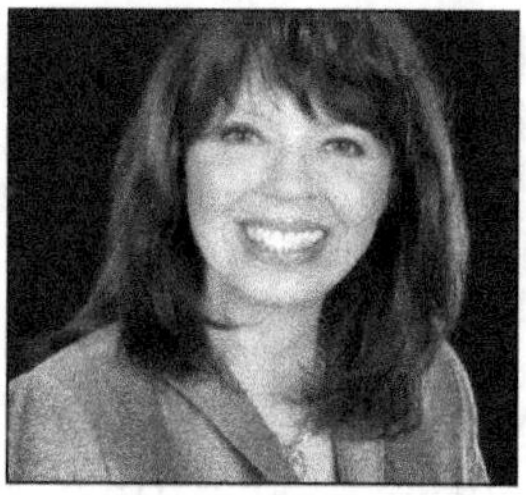

Lexie Lindstrom, 66 years

Seattle, USA

Diagnosed with Parkinson's disease at 60 years

I was diagnosed with Parkinson's disease (PD) in 2008, when my motor symptoms surfaced. However, my non-motor symptoms developed 25 years before that, shortly after my divorce when I was 40. I had symptoms, but I didn't know what they were at first. I started having terrible problems with anxiety. I thought: "Well of course, I'm getting divorced and I'm anxious," but it was really severe anxiety. At 41, I started having terrible insomnia and chronic constipation, which I'd never had before.

The strangest thing that happened way back then was that I totally lost my sense of smell. Firstly though, I would smell some kind of pungent odour, like cardamom, and the smell wouldn't go away. Once, when I went into a bakery to get some cookies, I started panicking, because the smell was so overwhelming. After I left the bakery, that smell stayed with me for several weeks – I couldn't get it out of my nose. Then, if I got a strong whiff of something else very strong, another smell would take its place and *that* would stay in my nose for the longest time. I worked in the cosmetic business, so I thought I must have overdosed on perfumes. Now, they call it 'olfactory hallucinations'.

About six months after that, I totally *lost* my sense of smell. It was really embarrassing, because I was going into department stores training staff about fragrances – I just had to remember what they smelled like.

Two years later, I started having urinary incontinence. I've never had children, so I thought: "Why in the world am I having this?" It was severe enough that I went to a urologist and had some extensive testing done. He told me that I had 'neurogenic bladder spasm' and it was 'idiopathic'.[1] I really don't believe that there is such a thing as idiopathic – something has to cause it, especially when the symptoms are so severe. He did say that neurogenic bladder spasms could mean either Parkinson's disease or MS.[2] I started panicking and thought: "Oh my goodness, maybe I have MS." He said: "Well you don't have Parkinson's, because you don't have any symptoms," and I said: "Oh no, no, it wouldn't be Parkinson's."

1 Idiopathic – a condition that has no known cause.

2 MS – multiple sclerosis.

The urologist sent me to a neurologist who did an MRI[3] and ruled out MS. So I said: "Okay, I'll go with it being idiopathic," but I knew in my mind that it had to be caused by something. My symptoms kept getting worse and worse over the years, to the point where I couldn't even make it to the bathroom. I had to wear protection and it was a really embarrassing and serious issue. Years later, I was diagnosed with Parkinson's.

The insomnia was really problematic. I thought that it was another symptom caused by my divorce. I went for one period of almost three weeks where I was unable to sleep. I was getting up each morning and teaching eight-hour seminars to 40 or 45 people, totally running on adrenaline. Every night I kept thinking: "I'm tired now, I am going to sleep," but I just didn't sleep. Finally, my doctor said that he would have to put me on sleep medication, which worked beautifully.

For the anxiety, I was given *Paxil*,[4] which my doctor told me would fix my anxiety. I think I'll probably be on it for the rest of my life. I had a question mark on all of these things – was the anxiety from the stress of my divorce? The loss of smell was a real clincher, but I just decided not to worry about it.

I went to different doctors for different things. I saw a psychiatrist for my anxiety, my primary care practitioner for insomnia, the urologist for my bladder spasms – three different symptoms and none of them connected the dots. Now, they know that losing one's sense of smell is a really common precursor to Parkinson's disease.

I'd been in my job with the cosmetics company as a Regional Training Executive for 14 years, but because the travel was really just too much for me with my anxiety, bladder spasms, insomnia and constipation, I reluctantly left that job. I took a year off and then trained as a medical aesthetician.[5] I wanted to do something that would be a little bit more calming, without all the travel. I got my license, then started working in a plastic surgeon's office. I loved it there. I was doing chemical peels, micro-dermabrasions and other medical treatments like that. I still had all my symptoms and I couldn't smell anything, but I had a bandaid for everything.

After working for the plastic surgeon for six months, I was approached by another cosmetic company to work as a sales representative. I worked for them for the next ten years. I loved working there too, but it was very high pressure.

In 2007, we were remodelling a farmhouse and living in a barn house on the property. My husband and I both worked out of our home, which at that time was the barn. We took the walls of the farmhouse down to the studs, cleared it out and redid *everything*. There were all these huge decisions to

3 MRI (magnetic resonance imaging) – radiology test for a more detailed image than standard X-rays, without exposure to radiation.

4 *Paxil* is the trade name for paroxetine, an SSRI anti-depressant used for a variety of anxiety disorders.

5 Aestheticians are licensed beauty professionals who focus on advanced skincare, makeup, and hair removal. Medical aestheticians work in doctor's offices, hospitals, and surgery centres.

make about the tiles, light fixtures, colours – I drove myself crazy looking through magazines and trying to make the right decisions for our dream home. That took about a year and a half and I was still working full-time.

About two weeks before the farmhouse was finished, I remember walking from the barn to the farmhouse and the thought came into my head: "This is going to be my healing house." A short time after that, I started getting a right foot drag and was tripping on my right foot. Then I knew something was seriously wrong. My brain wasn't telling my foot to lift high enough. I'd walk up a flight of stairs and I kept missing a step with my right foot. I would fall on the stairs unless I consciously used my brain to lift my foot. I knew that was abnormal and it really frightened me.

I went in to my primary care physician and told him about my right foot drag. He said that it sounded like I had Parkinson's disease and recommended that I go to a neurologist. That was the first time I'd really heard it where it stuck. He said: "I hope you don't have Parkinson's disease, but if you do, there are some good medications for it." I thought: "Oh, *great* – just what I need is more medication." The thought of having Parkinson's disease terrified me.

That's when I started my quest. I was also starting to have a really severe symptom of bradykinesia,[6] which is when it feels like you're walking through quicksand or against the current of a river all the time – your body feels so slow. I also started getting debilitating fatigue along with pain, stiffness and problems with balance. I went to three different neurologists. For my third opinion, I flew down to the Mayo Clinic[7] in Arizona and went to one of the top neurologists there. All three of them gave me the same diagnosis of Parkinson's disease. I was completely devastated.

My voice started getting soft and crackly, which was really embarrassing when I was on the phone to clients. All of a sudden my handwriting was tiny and cramped. I used to have really loopy, big handwriting and now I could hardly even read my own handwriting. My Parkinson's disease was right-sided and I had no right arm swing. I was still able enough to keep working and make good money, so I thought: "I'm just going to push through this," not wanting my clients or the company to know.

I also started having cognitive issues and found that I was losing my ability to handle stress. Usually I thrived on a whirlwind of high-stress jobs that I loved. It was glamorous and fun, but stressful. I remember coming down to my desk in the morning and my brain would just short-circuit. Things that used to be second nature to me, I just couldn't do anymore and I would become paralysed by everything I had to accomplish. That's when my husband and I

6 Bradykinesia – slowness of movement, which is the most characteristic clinical feature of Parkinson's disease.

7 The Mayo Clinic is a not-for-profit medical practice and medical research group based in Rochester, Minnesota. In 1864, Doctor William Worrall Mayo settled with his family in Rochester, Minnesota and opened a medical practice that evolved under his sons into the Mayo Clinic. It is the largest integrated medical practice in the world, employing more than 3,800 physicians and scientists and 50,900 allied health staff. Noted for its integrative approach to healthcare, it is considered to be one of the best 20 hospitals in the world.

started getting worried. I stayed with the company until 2010 and finally had to tell them that I had Parkinson's disease. They offered for me to just do what I could manage, but I couldn't even do that anymore. Stress relating to work just sent me over the edge.

All this time, my mom had Alzheimer's disease and we had her in a facility close to where we live. I'm her only living child and I was visiting her all the time when I wasn't working.

My neurologist put me on a medication called *Requip*,[8] which was one of the new Parkinson's drugs at the time, but I had terrible side effects from it. I spontaneously fell asleep at the wheel four times while I was driving to work. By the grace of God, I didn't kill myself or anybody else, because I was always in traffic when it happened. I would wake up in another lane or on a line – some place I shouldn't be. I also developed a shopping compulsion. I've never had any kind of addictive issue in my life, but I became addicted to thrift stores, goodwill stores and consignment stores – I just couldn't pass them up. I would go there after work and rummage through things for hours [*laughs*] then bring them home and say to my husband: "Look what I've found!" I'd never done that before. I said to myself, "What is wrong with me?"

It was definitely the medication. Many people who take *Requip* get gambling, sexual, or shopping addictions. Fortunately, my addiction wasn't with the high-end shops where I would normally shop! Even so, I spent quite a lot of money. It was putting a lot of pressure on my marriage, because my husband couldn't believe that what I had was an addiction.

My neurologist changed me to *Sinemet*,[9] which I was very fearful of, because when I was first diagnosed, the doctor at the Mayo Clinic said: "Whatever you do, don't let anyone put you on *Sinemet*, because you can only be on it for about five years, then you have to take more and more and the side effects that you get can be worse than your original symptoms." So then I was on the dreaded *Sinemet* that I didn't want to go on.

Finally, I said to my neurologist that I could no longer function on my job and she agreed to write a letter to my employer. I was accepted for disability, because my cognition was so bad, along with my other now debilitating symptoms. To qualify for disability, I took a test with a psychologist for almost four hours. I was drawing and trying to remember things. I felt like a different person and I failed miserably. I started crying, saying, "What's happened to my mind?" That was pretty tough.

I was able to continue with my insurance plan for a while, which was great. I then took Medicare at age 62 instead of 65, because I was not doing well.

---

8 *Requip* is the trade name for levodopa (also called L-dopa). It is the most commonly prescribed and effective drug for controlling the symptoms of Parkinson's disease, particularly tremors and rigidity.

9 *Sinemet* is carbidopa and levodopa combined, a commonly prescribed medication for Parkinson's disease. Its side effects include involuntary movement disorders ranging from a slight hand tremor to uncontrollable movements of the upper body or lower extremities.

After I quit work, I started researching everything I could. I got online, looking for all sorts of alternative ways to treat my disease with supplements and so on. Then one day I stumbled upon Low Dose Naltrexone (LDN).[10] After three visits to my neurologist, I was finally able to get a prescription from her. She didn't want to give it to me, because it was an off-label[11] drug she'd never heard of. She said: "I've heard that it helps some people with MS, but you don't have MS." So she did a little research then came back to me and said: "Well, at least I know that it won't harm you. Maybe you'll get some kind of a placebo effect out of it."

I began taking LDN along with my *Sinemet* in 2009 and started getting better. What I noticed first of all was a feeling of wellbeing. The feeling of anxiety just melted away, due to the increased endorphins in my body from taking the LDN. My symptoms were still there, but they weren't as bad. I kind of did my own experiment at the time, because not a lot of people were taking LDN for Parkinson's disease. I very slowly started titrating off the three *Sinemet* tablets I was taking each day. Over the next six months to a year, I titrated off all of the *Sinemet* and the *Azilect*[12] that I had been taking along with it.

Today, I'm not on any Parkinson's medication except for an occasional dose of controlled-release *Sinemet* that I take as a bandaid. When we had friends from out of town here and were away for four days walking all over and were really busy with a lot of activities, I took a *Sinemet* then, and do at times like that, to keep my energy up. It's a shot of energy, like a cup of coffee is. I need that about twice a month. Other than that, it's just the LDN that I take.

My bladder symptoms have improved tremendously – oh my goodness. I still have bladder issues, but I can make it to the bathroom now. It's 85 per cent better.

I have REM sleep disorder[13] now. They put me on *Klonipin*[14] for that, which I take at night and it really helps my sleep. Many people with Parkinson's disease have that sleep disorder and it's a really disturbing symptom, but it can be controlled for the most part with the proper medications.

My sense of smell has come back more than 95 per cent. A few years ago, we were on holiday down on the Oregon Coast and we wanted to get a latté. As soon as we walked into this coffee shop, I could smell the coffee. It was the first time I had smelled anything in years. I looked at my husband and said: "I can smell the coffee!" People looked at us as if we were crazy, saying, "Yeah, you're in a coffee shop." [*laughs*] After that, I could gradually smell a little bit more and a little bit more. I still can't smell a single flower like a lilac or a rose, but if you put a bouquet together, I can smell that – and I can smell and differentiate fragrances again. I've never heard of anybody's sense of smell

10 Low Dose Naltrexone is the off-label prescription of the FDA approved drug *Naltrexone*.

11 Off-label means the use of a pharmaceutical drug in an unapproved indication, age group or dosage.

12 *Azilect* is used alone or with other medications for movement disorders caused by Parkinson's disease.

13 REM sleep behaviour disorder (RBD) – the paralysis that normally occurs during REM sleep is incomplete or absent. RBD is characterised by the acting out of dreams that are vivid, intense, and violent. Dream-enacting behaviours include talking, yelling, punching, kicking, sitting, jumping from bed, arm flailing, and grabbing.

14 *Klonopin* (clonazepam) is a benzodiazepine which has sedative, hypnotic, anticonvulsant, muscle relaxant, and anti-anxiety actions.

coming back with Parkinson's disease and I never thought that my own sense of smell would come back. That's huge.

My mom died two years ago in April – she was my closest friend in the whole world and I took care of her for her last ten years. I had been preparing for her funeral for a long time – I put together a videotape of her life and really put a lot of thought and energy into it. On the day of her funeral, everything went perfectly, but when the funeral service started, my body started shaking like a blender. The right side of my body shook like it had never shaken. It was just during the hour of the funeral. Afterwards at the reception I was fine, but ever since then, I've had problems with tremors. That was a new symptom. Before then I just had tiny tremors. My disease had accelerated because of another trauma. Everything else remained the same, but I got that new symptom. I take a prescription medication for it and I don't tremor all the time – I only tremor when I'm stressed, or when I'm cold.

The last time I went to see my neurologist, about six months ago, I had zero symptoms of Parkinson's disease. She took me through all the tests and all the mental examinations and I didn't have one tremor or any indication of Parkinson's. She knew that I was off the *Sinemet* and that I was only taking it about twice a month. She couldn't believe I was taking that little and looked astounded. She just didn't think it was possible. I said to her: "Doctor, it's the LDN." At first she thought I was having a placebo effect, because I got all of her notes when I went to get Social Security Disability. I had a chuckle when I read the notes she had written about how I was obsessed with LDN and how she finally relented and gave me a prescription because she found out that it wouldn't do me any harm and maybe I'd get some placebo benefits from it. For about a year, she said: "You're just having a tremendous placebo effect." After that year, as she watched me get better and better and better, she realised it was more than that. I didn't have one shake. It was almost comical – she looked at my knee and said: "I think I saw a tremor," and went right up to my knee and said, "Oh, I guess not." Then she was talking to herself, saying: "This isn't possible – it just isn't possible." That was the last time I saw her and she wrote me a one-year's prescription for LDN.

My husband suggested that I change neurologists, because she was about an hour's drive from our home, but she's a very well-known doctor in Seattle and I wanted to show her that LDN would work for me. If it worked for me, it could work for other patients.

Recently, I was at a very sad funeral of a young mother who had left behind a young child and I was very upset. We were standing up praying and a man behind me said: "You have Parkinson's disease, don't you?" I thought: "Darn it," because I knew I was shaking. I don't usually tell people I have Parkinson's disease. Some people treat you differently – they think you might be mentally disabled or something, which I'm not at all now.

I lead a fairly normal life. I'm 66 now and I don't really want to go back to work, nor do I feel I could handle the constant stress of it. My anxiety is so much better, although I still take the *Paxil*. My bladder spasms are still gradually getting better. The debilitating fatigue was a horrible, horrible symptom and I have zero fatigue now. I sleep well all night – when I wake up in the morning I've got as much energy as my husband does. I used to not be able to make it through the day without a nap, or a few naps. My soft and crackly voice has gone away. I have an arm swing now and I haven't had a right foot drag for years. I still have a little bit of bradykinesia on my right side. I can get out of the driver's side of a car really easily, but when I get out of the passenger side I'm a little bit slower.

My cognitive issues are really good, but I have started worrying about that, because I had the "23 & Me" test done at the Michael J Fox Foundation[1] and found that I have the APOE gene,[2] which is the gene for Alzheimer's disease. So now I'm doing everything I can to prevent that and to keep my brain sharp. Up to 70 per cent of people with Parkinson's disease go into Parkinson's dementia. I don't want to go in the direction of my mom, so I take coconut oil every day and I cook with it too, hoping that it will work as a preventative for Alzheimer's. Now, my brain is as sharp as it always was, but it wasn't that way before I took LDN.

I improve all the time, but I always tell people that it's not a quick-fix. I speak to many people every day who have started taking LDN and they'll call me up after taking it for a month and say: "I'm not cured yet." "Well, no, LDN is not a cure for PD – it 'cures' the symptoms of PD while you are taking it." I say, "You have to take it for years." I will probably take it for the rest of my life, or until there's a cure for Parkinson's disease, which I don't expect to see.

I have a folder for people with PD who are on LDN and who I am currently coaching. Some didn't get it from the right compounding pharmacy, so it didn't work for them. You do need to get Low Dose Naltrexone from a pharmacy that knows how to compound it. Whenever I find someone who is not being helped by LDN, my first question is: "Where did you get it from?" There's a list of nine pharmacies on the LDN website[3] that compound it properly.

The only thing that I can relate my getting Parkinson's to is being faced with a devastating divorce. I've read that you can get it from pesticides and herbicides and exposures like that, but I'm a city girl and have never really been exposed to those types of things. I am a person who always sees the glass half full, but I've had a lot of trauma in my life – my father was an alcoholic, my younger brothers, who I loved dearly, both had problematic issues, and I took care of my mom for the last ten years of her life. In addition, I've always kind of thrived on really high-stress jobs. I do think all that stress finally got to me. It feels like it was traumatic, chronic stress over a lifetime that triggered and maybe even caused it.

1 *Michael J Fox Foundation* https://www.michaeljfox.org

2 APOE – apolipoprotein E www.nia.nih.gov/alzheimers/publication/alzheimers-disease-genetics-fact-sheet

3 http://www.lowdosenaltrexone.org

Practically everyone I chat to online in various online forums say they have had really traumatic stresses in their lives prior to getting Parkinson's. I have come to the conclusion that Parkinson's can be a by-product of that.

In 2011, I did a Blog Talk Radio interview with Robert Rodgers, PhD, who is the founder of *Parkinson's Recovery*.[4] He turned it into a 30-page book called: *LDN for Parkinson's Disease*.[5] It tells you a little bit more about my journey in the first couple of years when I first started taking it.

Harvard educated Bernard Bihari, MD, (1931-2010) discovered the clinical effects of FDA-approved Naltrexone using low doses (Low Dose Naltrexone or LDN). In 1985-86, he conducted a groundbreaking clinical trial on patients with HIV/AIDS. Doctor Bihari says that the immune system normalising effect of the drug application he discovered applies to a wide range of autoimmune diseases.

Research trials can be found at http://www.lowdosenaltrexone.org/ldn_trials.htm

79-minute interview with Doctor Bihari: http://www.youtube.com/watch?v=x54Jc-cr8GT879

4 *Parkinson's Recovery* www.parkinsonsrecovery.com

5 *LDN for Parkinson's Disease* by Lexie Lindstrom is available on Amazon.

Butch M, 65 years

Mexico

Diagnosed with ALS (Amyotrophic Lateral Sclerosis) at 59 years

Before, I think I was kind of normal. [*laughs*] When I first started getting symptoms, I didn't realise what was happening. I remember one incident early in 2007, where I went to step over something and fell down because I caught my right foot. I didn't think anything about it – I had bad knees from my past, so I thought that's what it was. All of those times I had accidents the doctors always told me: "When you get older you're going to have lots of pain and lots of difficulty."

In December of 2007, I said to my wife that I thought I had ALS.[1] Her comment was: "If you think you're going to get it, you get it, so don't think about it." [*laughs*] But she noticed I seemed to be getting worse. I was having difficulty walking and going up and down steps. I felt like I had a whole army of pacmen in my leg, and they were all chewing on something, which is common with the disease. So in March 2008, we went to the doctor to get a diagnosis.

The ALS started in my right foot and moved up my leg. I had difficulty standing for very long, like standing in line. I was putting more pressure on my left leg and had problems with my back and both knees. By the time I got through the diagnosis process, my leg was almost asleep, but not quite numb. I could touch it and feel my hand, but didn't have any real sensation. I started noticing the muscles, especially in my thigh, were starting to get smaller.

I got one of the common symptoms of ALS, when your saliva gets real thick, especially at night, making you almost choke. I was also having troubles when I tried to roll over in bed, because one leg didn't move like it used to. It's surprising how much you need your legs. [*laughs*] I was losing a little bit of weight and having troubles getting dressed. It was kind of aggravating, but that's the way it goes with ALS.

Getting diagnosed required a whole series of tests. They measured both legs every time I went in. I had two MRIs[2] and two spinal taps.[3] I don't know how many EMGs[4] I had. That's always fun, because what they do is hook you up to

1 ALS (Amyotrophic Lateral Sclerosis) is also known as Lou Gehrig's Disease, or Motor Neurone Disease.

2 MRI (magnetic resonance imaging) – radiology test for a more detailed image than standard X-rays, without exposure to radiation.

3 Spinal Tap, or lumbar puncture, is a diagnostic procedure performed on the lower spine to collect a sample of cerebro-spinal fluid.

4 EMG – electromyography, where electrical activity of muscles is performed on an electromyograph.

a computer, stick a needle in you and run electricity through it to measure how long it takes to get from point A to point B. They put the needles in – fortunately only one at a time [*laughs*] – but they put them in all different parts; your arms, your hands, your legs and more! The worst one is when they push a needle up through the underside of your chin and into your tongue. Then they tell you to stiffen your tongue muscles, relax, then they wiggle the needle around and they don't give you anything for the pain. It's one of those things that causes you to start moving away when you see the needle.

By the middle of September 2008, they finally decided I had ALS. It's a very difficult disease to find, so a lot of times the doctors say: "It's not this, and it's not that, so it must be this." Kind of like car mechanics. By that time, I was having more difficulty walking and needed to use elevators instead of stairs.

After I was diagnosed, I flew back to see my family to tell them, "Hey, I'm temporary." That's when my sister bought me a cane, because she said, "You need this," and it was true.

I've done a lot of things in my life – I should have died numerous times in all the accidents I've been involved in with motorcycles, cars, hang gliders, skydiving. But for some reason, I'm still here, so for me it wasn't a big deal. My thought was: "We've all gotta die someday. At least I know about when and kind of how." So for me that was okay, and it still is.

I inherited my disease from my mother. She died of ALS after about eight years with it. We didn't know exactly when her disease started, but there was one incident that was an early sign. When our front yard accidentally caught fire, my father told my mother to run in and call the fire department, but she couldn't run. Later on, when I had difficulty and fell down, I started putting things together. I started checking on the net, and found I had seven of the eleven symptoms.

Unlike most people with ALS, I've always had it with me – my symptoms just didn't start until I was 59 and its progression was slow. My mother's started when she was around 60.

All my life, I've had a problem with pain – I've had it since I was a child. It would just hit me – mainly in my chest or my organs. The pain could last anywhere from a few seconds to a couple of minutes and doctors could never figure out what it was. When I was in my early twenties, I had an exploratory operation to find out what the problem was, without success. The last thing my mother ever said to me when she could still talk (she had a tracheostomy) was that I needed to enjoy every day, because I was going to end up just like her. At the time it seemed really weird – it was in late 1986, about three months before she finally died. Then when I got the ALS, I thought: "What did she know that I didn't?" The only thing I can think of is that she had the same kind of pain.I saw my mother for the last time about three months before she died. All she could move was her eyes and she could hardly move her mouth to talk.

The doctors said she finally died because her heart just quit, but it was a slow process.

My father took care of my mother the whole time she had ALS. He was her caretaker 24/7 for all of those years. When she went on a respirator, he promised her she would not die in a hospital and he kept that promise! When she died, they had been married for about four months short of 50 years. Several months afterwards, he told me it was the hardest promise he ever made.

ALS is a rare neuromuscular disease, that less than one per cent of the population in the United States has. After the doctors have diagnosed you, it's kind of like: "Well, why should we waste our time with you, because you're going to die anyway." It's sad, but that's kind of how it works. Fifty per cent of people with ALS die within three years of being diagnosed and 80 per cent of them are normally dead by the fifth year.

There are different types of ALS. 'Sporadic', or 'Classic', is the type most people get when there's no history of ALS in the family. The inherited type is 'Familial', which is what I have. And then these types: Bulbar, Upper Limb Onset and Lower Limb Onset. 'Bulbar' has the fastest progression. It starts by affecting the lower part of the brain and the throat. 'Lower Limb Onset' is what my mother had, and what I have. Eventually, lower onset affects you everywhere. People with the inherited type of ALS tend to live a little bit longer than the average, but the outcome is still the same. Only about ten per cent of all the people with ALS live for eight to ten years after its onset. It's similar to Alzheimer's and Parkinson's disease, but with ALS you end up being the opposite of Alzheimer's disease – you're trapped inside a body that slowly doesn't work. Your brain is still functioning, but your body just quits. There's no good disease.

When the doctor diagnosed me, he said, "It's a terrible disease." I asked: "Is there a good one? That's the one I want." He's like: "Grrrrrr" – they don't have much of a sense of humour. [*laughs*] He just said I had "from three to five years to live".

My mother survived for eight years after her onset. I am now in my seventh year and improving. When I go to see the neurologist, they look at me like I'm one of the walking dead, because for them I should be dead by now, or at least close to it. I should at least be in a wheelchair. Instead, I'm walking with the aid of crutches!

After I was diagnosed, I contacted the ALS organisation in the United States and asked: "Can I help in any way? Is there anything that I can do?" One of the tasks they gave me was to look at webpages, so I started looking at webpages every night. It would take maybe half an hour and I would send them a report at the end of every week. I found coconut oil that way, and one thing led to another. If I can help other people a little with what I've learned, I'm glad! Hopefully it will help their family too.

On the web you find people selling everything. Somebody's got a cure, you eat totally organic, or you think positive all the time. I found one link to something that said: "What if there was a cure?" I thought: "What are they selling?" But it was a video of Doctor Mary Newport and her husband, Steve, and how coconut oil helped him with his Alzheimer's. I thought: "Hmmm, Alzheimer's is a neurological disease." I knew that ALS, Alzheimer's and Parkinson's are all related in some way. In fact, some doctors have said whatever they find to help one, may help the others. So it made me think: "What do I have to lose?"

Before I started taking the coconut oil, somebody sent my wife a link on magnesium chloride, because her family has a history of diabetes. We found it also helps people with epilepsy, because it helps the brain. By that time, I had a terrible drop foot and I had lost so much muscle mass in my right leg, that I could feel the bone in the underside of my thigh. The pacmen had moved on – they were starting on the other leg by then. [*laughs*] My wife said: "Well, there's nothing else – what's it going to hurt?" So I started taking magnesium crystals in mid-September 2009, one year after my diagnosis. About two weeks later, my leg started to feel funny. I couldn't say what it was, but it was feeling different. Six weeks later, my leg was starting to feel more like it was 'my leg' again.

Before I started taking coconut oil, I did extensive research on what it is. I'm not one of those people who says, "Oh yeah, I'll just go out and do it." I want to know what is it, why does it work, how does it work and what does it do? It was kind of an experiment. The stuff won't kill me, and if it does, maybe I'll die faster and it'll be easier. [*laughs*] I read that one to four tablespoons a day is what most 'normal' people take, so on October 31st, 2009, I started taking three tablespoons a day. For all of November I didn't notice anything different. One person commented: "But coconut oil causes high cholesterol and you could have a heart attack!" I thought, "Yeah, that'd be terrible, wouldn't it, to die quick, instead of slowly." [*laughs*] (I had my cholesterol checked in January 2011 and everything was fine.) Then I thought: "With ALS, I'm not 'normal' and maybe I should take more." Everything I read said that it can't hurt you, so I started taking six tablespoons per day for the month of December. In January, I moved to eight, and took eight for the next year. I now take nine tablespoons per day, and have been for about two years.

There is a risk in taking too much coconut oil too fast, because coconut oil cleans your system out, so if you take too much too soon, you can get an upset stomach. This is because at least 25 per cent of people in the industrialised world have viral infections in their intestinal system and coconut oil is an anti-toxin. You might think you are allergic to the coconut oil, but it's actually all that bad stuff coming out of you.

I didn't tell the doctors about taking it all through 2010, because I wasn't sure if it worked. Several months after I'd been taking eight plus tablespoons of coconut oil daily, my left foot was getting a little bit weaker. I was dropping dishes and breaking glasses. There was a question as to whether we should buy plastic dishes, or I should stop washing the dishes. [*laughs*] But some time after taking the higher amounts of coconut oil, those things improved. My strength came back in my left foot and I could wash dishes without breaking or chipping them, because my hands were stronger. Now I can hold a glass without a problem! These are little things, but important first signs, because people with ALS eventually get to the point where they can't even hold a glass.

I got some physical therapy at one of the local clinics here. They did some additional EMG testing. It hadn't progressed, so they said it couldn't be ALS. I told them it had been in my left foot and hands, but it wasn't there when they did the tests. I was still on nine tablespoons of coconut oil a day and the magnesium chloride.

In March of 2011, I went to my neurologist for my annual EMG. When we told him about the other EMG, he said: "Well those people don't know what they're doing – you still have ALS." Then when I went back in March of 2012, the guy doing the tests compared the 2011 and 2012 results, and said I had had some improvement in my left leg, both hands, and my right leg was stable. He couldn't say why, but he thought the progression had stopped. When I'd tell them about taking coconut oil, they would kind of pat you on the head and say, "If you think it works, then keep using it." [*laughs*]

By the time I had the appointment with my neurologist to formally analyse the test results, I had written about what the coconut oil had done for me. I gave him a copy, but I doubt he ever read it. It's difficult for doctors and most non-medical people to believe, because there's no official proof – there's only me. To my improvements, he doesn't say much and I can tell he doesn't understand. I think I could tell him: "It's magic!"

The good thing is he's not concerned. I'm still improving and it's not his problem as to why. He sees so many other people with so many different problems that he can't be concerned with one who doesn't fit the medical profile. His attitude is: "Well, I'm not here for that, I'm not into research." I've also sent similar information to the two doctors who were responsible for my diagnosis, but never heard anything back. Even though most of the doctors understand what ketones[5] are and what they do, they're focussed on what they see today, and: "Oh, here's some medicine."

When I say that this stuff works on the ALS webpages, some people complain. They say: "I'm not going to take *anything* that's not approved by the doctors." My comment back is: "Well, it's going to be long time before they have something that works, so it looks like you're going to die."

I have 'non-official proof' coconut oil helps, because I've been tracking and

5 Ketones result from the metabolic effects of consuming coconut oil.

recording my symptoms since March 2008. I wanted to be able to compare my symptom progression with my mother's. I try to record my status once a month on an Excel sheet. It's not difficult once you realise how important knowing from month to month what's happening. This way you have a 'mark on the floor'. I track my symptoms, weight, measurements, and more. Originally, I made an approximate timeline of my mother's and my symptoms progression. Then I put the timelines together. Our timelines were almost identical as far as problems with walking and hands, until I started the coconut oil in higher amounts.

Taking higher amounts of coconut oil – that's the key. On the net somebody said: "Coconut oil doesn't work, I took it for six months and it didn't help me." So I asked them: "Did you take it every day at higher dosages? It has to be every day." The answer was, "No," because their doctor didn't tell them and they don't think to do it on their own. It's kind of like being a diabetic. You have to take your insulin every day to avoid a problem. The difference is with diabetes, if you don't take your insulin, the reaction is quick. You're going to know it that day or the next day. But with ALS, the disease is there working 24/7, but the problems are small and slow to appear.

One guy on a webpage said coconut oil was really good for lubricating squeaky doors, but no good for ALS, even though he admitted to never trying it, because his doctor hadn't prescribed it for him. I said: "Well, you can believe what you want. You can go use it on the doors – I'm going to keep using it on me, and I'll probably be here long after you're gone." He died about six months after our conversation. These kind of people say: "It's unofficial. You have documentation, but it's unofficial."

The thing is, there is no regimen for it – there are no rules, so I call it 'unofficial' documentation. [*laughs*] I have it all the way back to almost the beginning of my ALS journey. I've had to figure out what are my rules as I've gone along. I now know it takes eight-plus tablespoons every day. It takes discipline and time, but people want to see and feel a change in the first month. I tell them: "It's not that way." The other thing that I always mention is: "Are you tracking your symptoms?" That's critical. Otherwise, how do you know what's changed? People are looking for the magic bullet, a magic concoction that's going to cure them – and there's no cure. Based on my personal experience, coconut oil is not a cure!

I've been fortunate – I've had a good life. I had a sister who was a little over one year and a month older than me. Just before I was born, she got sick. She was perfectly normal, then she got polio, chicken pox and rheumatic fever all at the same time. It was 1948. They couldn't get her temperature down, so she became physically and mentally disabled. Mentally, she was always the age of a six year old. She had difficulty walking and with her hands. She could talk and think, but on a lower level than normal. Growing up, I always thought it was the worst thing to be related to someone who was this way. As I've gotten older, I've apparently gotten a little smarter and realised how easy my life has been. She died about six years ago. She's one of the reasons why my outlook with my ALS is different from other people's. Most people look at it like: "Geez, I've got this, I'm going to die – it's terrible." It depends on their situation. If they're younger, have a family, have children and things like that, it's different. I'm over 65 and retired, so I'm an old man. [*laughs*] As my father use to say: "If you're over 50, you have more past than future!" So that's me – ALS is okay, because I have to die of something.

Now I'm walking better and I'm not breaking dishes. My mental state is still kind of the same, depending on who you ask. The problem now is, I don't know how long I'm going to live. [*laughs*]

My attitude is still the same; taking coconut oil is an experiment. I'm kind of disappointed, but in a way I'm also really glad. I can prove that my ALS is reversed. I looked up some of my dimensions and I have increased approximately three and a half to four centimetres in my right thigh. My right leg has more muscles now so I can't feel the bones anymore in my leg. I still have a slight drop foot, but it's less.

Even though the neurologist said I was dead, the doctors replaced my knee in my non-ALS leg. The orthopaedic surgeon looked at me and said: "We have to replace the knee in that leg." He took the time to read all the information about my ALS and said: "You're going to live longer." The neurologist now says I'm going to live another ten to 15 years more. Apparently they talked, because after all that, they said: "We can replace your knee." To prepare for the knee replacement, I had to do exercises three times a day. I used this vibrating machine I stand on and it helped enormously.

My knee operation was only supposed to take an hour and a half, but it took three hours. I was half asleep and it sounded like they were building a house. They were drilling, hammering, sawing with a power saw and talking like there was a problem. The doctor told me the next day they had difficulty with my leg because the bone was so hard they kept having to change the blades. I told him it was because of the machine, and he said: "Uh huh." But it is true – those machines are used by astronauts to strengthen their bones.

Because of the exercises I had to do for my new knee, my right leg has improved even more. I thought: "I might as well do the exercises for both legs." My goal was to walk into my next appointment with the neurologist using a cane, instead of crutches. But the advantage of the crutches is, you get more respect. [*laughs*] People drive different here in Mexico.

I am now taking twelve tablespoons of coconut oil per day, starting last November. I take the extra three just before I go to bed. That way I keep the ketones in my system, because they only stay in your system for two to three hours. There is no risk in getting too many ketones in your body, because any excess goes out when you go to the bathroom. It does keep your system clean – you go regularly. [*laughs*] Constipation is one of the problems for people with this disease. I now also take 1000mgs fish oil every day, to get the omega-3.

Every so often I stop taking the coconut oil and the magnesium chloride, just to see what happens. What I always find is, sometime within the next two weeks, I start feeling a little bit different, because the ALS is trying to do its thing.

There's another treatment outside the medical profession called 'Deanna's Protocol.' It was invented by a retired doctor, Vince Tedone, who I met through Doctor Newport. His daughter has ALS that started in 2007 too. He started her on palm oil just after she was diagnosed, but she didn't like it. Being in the medical profession, he thought that pills were the way to go. When I met him, Deanna had just started using a cane and was starting to have weakness in her hands. When we started comparing notes, Vince realised I was getting more ketones each day than Deanna, so he increased her amount. The result was her progression stopped and she improved. She no longer needed a cane, and her hands were stronger. That's when I made the connection between coconut oil and Deanna's Protocol and why both treatments help people with ALS, Alzheimer's, and maybe even other neuromuscular diseases. For this opportunity, I say thank you to the Lord for giving it to me.

I have been in contact with people all over the world – from Europe to Pakistan, to the hills in South Africa, because of what has happened to me. Not all of them, but many of them have improved. If nothing else, they have made small improvements and they have hope. I tell them: "It's not a cure. You have to be disciplined, and you have to work at it. It's not going to happen on its own."

There are lots of places where medication is not available, but where they can get coconuts and coconut oil. People in the US, Canada and Europe can get the supplements in Deanna's Protocol and have more trouble getting coconut oil. Here in Mexico, supplements are too expensive, because Mexico makes a lot of drugs – not just cocaine and marijuana! [*laughs*] They have drug companies here, so there are high tariffs on drugs and medicines coming into the country. I can buy coconut oil and magnesium chloride here for less than a dollar fifty a day, so for me coconut oil is the way to go. Even though I don't have 'official proof' it works, I do have a new knee. That's proof enough for me!

For those who read this and say coconut oil doesn't work, I say: "How many people in the world who have been diagnosed with ALS have also had a new knee put in?" I've improved. That's pretty rare.

Amyotrophic lateral sclerosis (ALS), also known as Lou Gehrig's disease, or Motor Neurone Disease, is a rapidly progressive, invariably fatal neurological disease that attacks the nerve cells (neurons) responsible for controlling voluntary muscles. Motor neurone diseases, are characterised by the gradual degeneration and death of motor neurons. (http://www.ninds.nih.gov/disorders/amyotrophiclateralsclerosis/detail_ALS.htm)

Death is usually caused by failure of the respiratory muscles. Fifty per cent of patients die within three years of onset, 20 per cent live for five years and ten per cent live for more than ten years. (Merck Manual http://www.merckmanuals.com)

Directors Patricia Tamowski and Alan Scott Douglas are currently producing a full-length documentary Healing ALS – Motor Neurone Disease – Lou Gehrig's Disease *on people who have healed from ALS. The link below shows interviews with 11 patients who have survived ALS and the doctors who treated them.*

https://www.indiegogo.com/projects/healing-als-mnd-lou-gehrig-s-disease

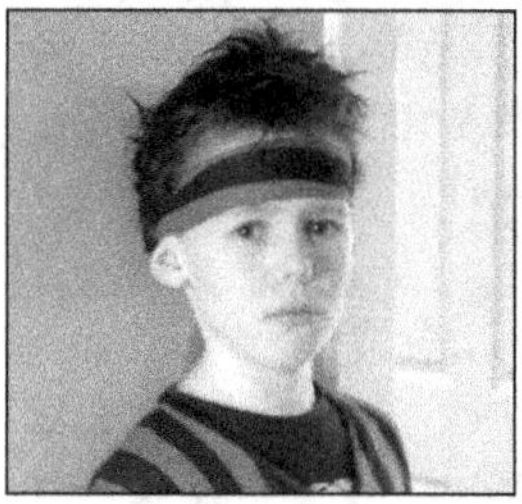

Ryan Middleton, 15 years

Wollongong, New South Wales, Australia

Sleeping problems since birth, violent behaviour, with no diagnosis

Interview with Lorraine Middleton, Ryan's mother

Ryan is the eldest of my four boys. When I was pregnant with him, I was constantly nauseous and I had sciatica. There were also a lot of emotional stresses – I couldn't say it was a pleasant pregnancy.

His birth was fairly traumatic. It was all hands on deck, because he was posterior. His head was hitting my tail-bone and he got stuck. I had a forceps delivery and he ended up with a fairly big haematoma[1] on his head. The doctor said that he could be unsettled for a time, because he would have a fairly big headache. That was the understatement of the century. [*laughs*]

He wasn't at all a settled baby – nobody could settle him. While I was in hospital, the lactation consultant sent me off to have a shower and thought that she would be able to settle him by the time I came back, but she hadn't been able to either. He was so uptight, but the reason why was a mystery.

I breastfed him and he always fed pretty well, but when he was awake he would cry for hours. Every time I put him down to sleep, he'd scream. He'd cry for two and a half hours, feed, doze off for around 20 minutes, then he'd start crying again – 24 hours a day.

I did the controlled crying technique, but that didn't work. He'd just scream for five or six hours until I couldn't stand it anymore and I'd go in and pick him up. He would not sleep – he might doze off for ten minutes from exhaustion, but that's all. Reflux was ruled out. There were many times that I'd have to go up to the backyard so I couldn't hear him screaming. I pretty much had to carry him around all day in a pouch. To get him to sleep, we would walk him up and down the hallway – nothing else would settle him.

Once he'd got out of feeding every three hours, on a good day he would sleep from 9.30 to 11 in the morning. Then he'd be awake until 11 at night. After that he would wake at 3am and again at 5am. The morning sleep wasn't regular though. He always dozed and never had a proper, good sleep.

1 Haematoma is a collection of blood outside the blood vessels. In this case, under the skin of the scalp.

When he was about three months old, I took him to a paediatrician. Thank goodness I had my mum with me as my witness, because he told me that I shouldn't be playing with him and stimulating him late at night and that the problem was more my behaviour than his. I went to baby health clinics and they gave me tips on how to settle him, but they never worked.

From three to five years, he got a lot of night terrors and would wake up screaming. Although he was awake, he'd look right through you. He would be hysterical and I just couldn't settle him down. He still couldn't sleep until about 11pm, then he would wake at 5.30am and that was his sleep for the day. I didn't really take him to see anyone after that, because I had been told it was my fault.

Once he had siblings, he developed behavioural problems. Whenever we went somewhere he would carry on. If I put him in the back of the double pram he would sit and whack his brother. If I put him in the front he wouldn't want to be there. Either way, he couldn't be calm – he had to be doing something and he was having severe tantrums.

He didn't sleep through the night until he was four. We were in survival mode. We had our children close together and we didn't know how to handle it. It did put pressure on our marriage. The whole focus was just on getting through each day, as opposed to anything else. It was: "Okay, we made it through another day." One of the techniques the baby health nurse suggested was to put the child in their room, close the door, let them have their tantrum and get over it. You were supposed to hold the door so they couldn't get out. It isn't an exaggeration to say that it would have been two or three hours with him kicking the door in there. We couldn't control him and get him out of it. He was like a possessed demon, but he never knew the reason why. Then he would exhaust himself so much that he would fall asleep. When he woke up, he would be quiet and almost have a sense of remorse, knowing that he'd done the wrong thing. That continued right up until he was around ten.

As he got older, his behaviour became more and more of a problem. He would have these outbursts and he'd just be like a wild animal. If we were shopping I couldn't hold clothes up to him to see if they were going to fit him. When we took him to get his haircut, he'd go crazy and we'd have to hold him down. Anything he didn't want to do, he'd go really crazy. I'd walk him to calm him down, but we could walk for hours and he would scream the whole time.

He put a couple of holes in the walls. When he was five, I put him in the naughty corner and he stood there and kicked the wall until he put a hole in it. I just got the hole patched last week actually! [*laughs*]

His behaviour wasn't consistent. With other people, he was very introverted. When he went to preschool, he was such a perfect child and so sociable, they thought that he'd been in daycare. When he stayed at friends' places he was perfect, which was very frustrating.

He was fine at school and we never ever had a bad report about him. The reports from school were that he was a polite, quiet and well-behaved child, but he wasn't like this at home. At home, he couldn't sit still without doing something annoying. We couldn't take him anywhere. You could actually see his energy build. He would get hyped up and have this silly laugh, then he would explode, kick and scream.

When Ryan was around seven years old, we took him to a cranial osteopath,[2] who asked if he had had a traumatic birth. I thought he was a mind reader! He said that the bones in his neck may have been misaligned. After a treatment, he was really calm, but it didn't last. The next day he'd be back to his old self.

I took him to a paediatrician in Sydney to have him diagnosed. He sympathised about the sleep, but he was looking more at the behavioural problems. Ryan was always bright at school and he never struggled socially, so he couldn't tell me what was wrong with him.

We also took him to a psychologist to deal with his behaviour at home, but we didn't go through all the sessions, because we didn't really see the benefit. We never got a lot of feedback from these practitioners. We'd sit there and talk to them, but couldn't find out anything concrete. He never received a diagnosis.

Ryan was such a good reader that he'd get through a really thick book in a couple of days. The teachers thought he was faking it, but when they questioned him, he could answer all the questions. He's got a really good memory. If ever you forgot where something was, you'd ask Ryan.

Ryan's sleep was still poor when he was ten years old. Since he was a baby, he couldn't settle himself and found it very hard to get to sleep. We tried different things, like warm milk, music and a bath before bed. He would go to bed okay at around 10pm, but he'd still be awake at midnight. He could never wind himself down. I'd ask him if there was anything on his mind, but he'd always say that he just couldn't go to sleep. When he eventually went to sleep, then you couldn't get him out of it and he'd be like a zombie in the morning. We could make as much noise as we wanted. If I had the vacuum cleaner on, or his brothers jumped on him, he wouldn't wake up. It was like he was drugged, or in a coma, but he never had a refreshing sleep.

The sleep we'd sort of got used to, but his behaviour flare-ups got to the point where we couldn't go out and do anything. If we did try to go out to dinner, we'd have to get out of there really quickly after we'd had our food, because he would always do something so that we would have to leave. It totally affected our family life – we didn't really have one. It also set up some resentment towards him from the other three children, because it was always: "Ryan spoils everything." With games in the backyard, he would always do something to

2 Craniosacral therapy (CST) was developed by osteopath John Upledger in the 1970s based on the work of William Garner Sutherland in the 1930s. It is a body therapy based on regulating the flow of cerebrospinal fluid by manipulating the joints of the cranium, using light touches to the patient's skull, face, spine and pelvis.

ruin the game.

It used to be that he never had the outbursts in front of people outside of the family. They were getting worse though, because there were a few times where he had meltdowns in front of his friends. One day, two of his friends came and told me that Ryan was going crazy. He had slipped over and gotten dirty and just started screaming. If his father tried to stop him when he got upset, that would make him even worse. Once, he kicked his father.

As Ryan got older, I'd talk to him about it and it sounded to me like he just lost control. There were occasions when he didn't remember what he had done. He would go into this state that he couldn't get himself out of and then he wouldn't know why. In the end, the best way was to just walk away and let him wear himself out, but when he was younger, we couldn't leave him, because he might have hurt himself. We took him to the psychology department at the local University, because his focus was inconsistent. If he was faced with a challenging problem, he had perfect concentration, but for day-to-day things, it was harder for him to focus.

I felt a lot of guilt all along the way, because everything that I had tried had failed. I realised that there was more to him than what I was seeing, but it only came out occasionally. It was like his outbursts weren't him. Your own frustration would be so great too, that you turn into a person that you're not as well, because you don't know what to do. When he was with animals, he was a different person – you could see his calm, gentle side.

I talked to other people about his behaviour. One day a friend referred me to a naturopath, because she'd had a son who had similar problems. By the time I went there, I was at the stage where I was feeling desperate, because of the effect it was having on the whole family. This was my last hope for some relief.

Ryan was actually quite open to going to see a naturopath, who asked similar questions to the osteopath. They were spot-on as to how Ryan was behaving. Previously, it was me telling practitioners who didn't really 'get it'. I went home thinking that the naturopath was reading my mind. The main things he did were a hair mineral analysis and a urine test. He also checked his fingernails, looking for white spots. The tests showed that he had extremely high levels of copper in his system – ten times off the chart, the highest levels the naturopath had ever seen. When he explained what the effects of having that much copper were, they fitted Ryan's symptoms exactly. Ryan has always twitched a lot – his fingers, toes jump when he falls asleep and that is a symptom of copper excess. It's a family thing, because his father does the same.

I don't know if it has anything to do with it, but when I was pregnant with Ryan, we were renovating an old house in Sydney. We did a lot of sanding and I was painting walls one week before I had him. Other than that, we don't know where it came from. His father's family were farmers. They used to go out in the wheat paddocks that were being crop-dusted with pesticides and the dust would just fall on them. Apparently it was extreme.

Ryan was placed on some chelating[3] drops to take each day, which changed over time. He was great at taking them and never missed a day. He was given some magnesium and zinc too.

We started to see a change pretty well straight away. Where there used to be 29 awful days and one good one in a month, we were starting to have quite a few days in a row where he would be okay. He would still have flare ups, but they became less and less. His overall demeanour seemed to be much calmer. He still struggled with getting to sleep, but when he turned his light out he would go to sleep and he woke up more refreshed.

When he went for his monthly follow-ups, he would only have had one or two outbursts. The other thing was that when he had the outbursts, rather than them going on for two hours, they would last for maybe 20 minutes and he would calm down a lot faster. He had two follow-ups for his copper levels. The last one was down to almost the normal range. That's the evidence – the fact that the copper levels went down and his behaviour had improved so much, just had to be why he got better. This treatment was the only thing that had a long-term effect on his behaviour. Everything else lasted for a day or so and then he was back to square one again.

Ryan saw the naturopath for three years. In that time, he became an every-day kid. He would have a few outbursts with his siblings, but overall he was calm. He goes to sleep easily now and doesn't wake up during the night. He's 15 now, so it's hard to get out of bed in the morning anyway. [*laughs*]

On the whole, Ryan doesn't have outbursts now. At one point he had a whole lot of awful emotional things happen, and he tends to keep things in. Before his grandfather died of motor neurone disease, he spent the whole weekend sitting with him, so he had some big outbursts around that time, one of which he doesn't remember.

The change we saw in Ryan is nothing short of a miracle. From before he went on to the minerals and chelating drops to now, he's a totally different child. A lot of people don't consider that natural medicines work by themselves. We did go to quite a few different types of practitioners and nothing worked.

It's important to trust your instincts. If you know that something's not right, don't settle for being fobbed off or being told that it's your fault due to your parenting. It always felt like there was something more than that to me.

I did sometimes think I was betraying Ryan. If you're talking about your kid in a negative way, it doesn't sound good. Unless you meet another parent who has a child who is similar, it's something that you don't really talk about, because it's embarrassing. I found that I had to pick who I spoke to, because some

3 Chelating agents enable unwanted minerals to bond with metal ions, resulting in a water soluble complex, allowing the metal to enter the bloodstream and be excreted harmlessly. There are many types of medical and nutritional chelating agents available.

people thought I was exaggerating – even my family members. It wasn't until they came to stay with us that they believed how bad he was.

I think there are thousands of families battling with children like Ryan. They have tried lots of different things and found that nothing's worked and they just have to accept "that's the way it is" and work around it.

Ryan is 15 now and he has a calmness in himself. The agitation that was always there on some level every day is gone. Day to day, there is a calm environment in our house. His last year at high school is the best year he's ever had. He has a lot more self control and he gets more involved with the family now. He plays with his eight-year-old brother and we can go places together. What I'd really love to discover is how this happened to him in the first place.

Mineral imbalances that cause behaviour disorders were researched by physician and biochemist Doctor Carl Pfeiffer (1908-1988), who was involved with the development of orthomolecular psychiatry, which uses nutritional supplements in large doses to treat mental illness. He ran the Pfeiffer Treatment Center in Illinois[4] *and conducted a 12-year study, which led to him classifying behavioural disorders into four categories based on trace mineral patterns. His work includes conditions caused by copper and zinc imbalance, called 'kryptopyrroluria'. Two of Doctor Carl Pfeiffer's publications are:* Nutrition and Mental Illness: An Orthomolecular Approach to Balancing Body Chemistry (1988), *and* Mental and Elemental Nutrients: A Physician's Guide to Nutrition and Health Care (1976)

Practitioners such as nutritionists, naturopaths and integrative doctors, treat childhood learning and behavioural disorders using biomedical treatment and often include orthomolecular medicine in their treatment programmes.

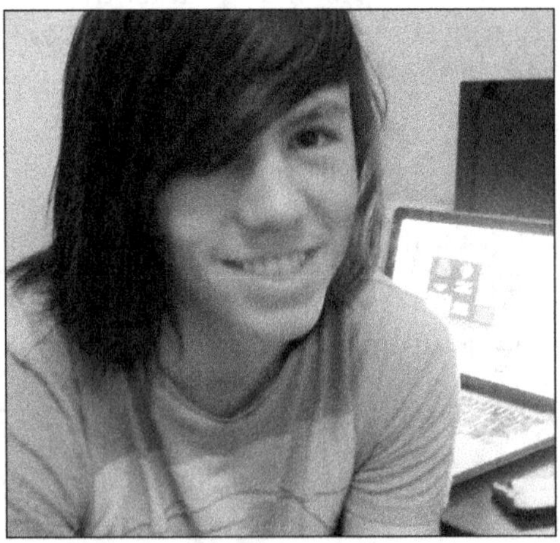

Ryan Middleton at 15 years.

4 Pfeiffer Medical Center Health Research Institute 3S721 West Ave, Suite 300, Warrenville Illinois 60555.

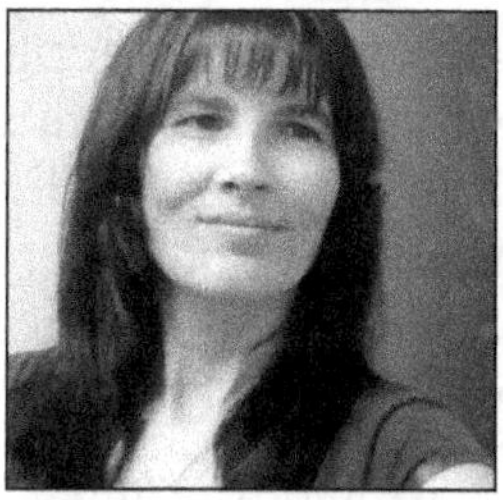

Crystal Nason, 46 years

Philadelphia, Pennsylvania, USA

Diagnosed with secondary progressive multiple sclerosis and transverse myelitis at 38 years

About eight months prior to my diagnosis, I had just married my third husband and I was working full-time for a company in Florida, driving a van around to different places where I would fill in attraction brochure displays. After I had been working with them for almost a year, I would come home with my neck and back hurting and I would need to take a nap to get through the day.

Then I went numb from my chest down, so I went to my regular doctor and he did checks from my lower back down and didn't find anything. He thought maybe it was a pinched nerve, so I went to a chiropractor, who did some MRIs,[1] X-rays and tests. He saw a mass on my spine and said he couldn't touch me until I got into a neurologist. They got me into the neurologist, and did another MRI and a lumbar puncture, which came back positive for multiple sclerosis (MS) and transverse myelitis. I'd never heard of transverse myelitis – it's more or less the same as MS, but where MS affects your brain and your spine, transverse myelitis affects just your spine. A lot of people get transverse myelitis and it will lead to MS, or some people get both, like I did.

A few years before that, I'd had some symptoms, when I lived in Georgia with my kids' father. I would have problems with drop foot and my speech. I was also having a hard time talking and swallowing – all of that. I had back pain, muscle spasms, numbness and tingling in my legs and fatigue. I also had the 'MS hug', where it feels like you've got somebody squeezing you around your ribs. There was also spasticity in my legs, tremors and weakness in my arms.

The symptoms worried me – I wasn't sure what was going on. I wasn't sure if it was some stress, if it was the job I was working at the time, or if I'd pinched a nerve, because I was doing a lot of heavy lifting. But when the chiropractor sent me to a neurologist, it really started making me worry and wonder what was going on. It went from the tiredness, to my neck and back hurting, to the numbness from my chest all the way down to my feet. I was numb in my feet – I couldn't feel anything. I still worked for a week while I was numb.

1 MRI – magnetic resonance imaging is a medical imaging technique used in radiology to investigate the anatomy and function of the body, using magnetic fields and radio waves to form images of the body. MRIs are widely used in hospitals for diagnosis, staging of disease and for follow-up, without exposure to radiation.

After I was diagnosed, there were things that came out. Growing up, there were symptoms of the MS. I'd had viral meningitis after I was born and had seizures up until I was 12 or 13. I was told that things like that could lead to people having MS. I always remember my mother telling me that she would be trying to talk to me and get my attention and I was looking off into space. Finally, I would come out of it and realise she was talking to me. The seizures were caused by the viral meningitis. They had me on phenobarbital until I was 12 or 13, then they just stopped and I never had them again.

I was fine until my mid to late thirties, when I started getting symptoms again. At times I was worried, but then I was accustomed to them too, so it didn't really faze me. When I was in Georgia, I knew something was wrong with my body, but the doctors kept telling me there was nothing wrong and that it was all in my head.

I saw quite a few doctors – regular doctors. I went to emergency a few times and they would do different tests, like CAT[2] scans and blood work, and everything would come back normal. At one point, I had a lot of pressure in my head. It didn't hurt, it just felt like somebody was squeezing my head. I went to one doctor and he was like: "Here, take this medicine, it will take away the pressure in your head." I took it for about two weeks. I woke up one morning and I just didn't feel right, so I called 911. If I hadn't, I would have been dead right now, because he had given me blood pressure pills for the pressure in my head which brought down my heart rate and my blood pressure. The nurses did take my blood pressure when I went to that doctor, but I had nothing wrong with my blood pressure – never have. At that time, I had listened to the doctor, thinking: "Well, he knows what he's talking about," so I took the pills, but they ended up almost killing me. I think the doctors should have looked a little further, a little deeper and done a little more extensive testing, especially with my background, instead of saying nothing was wrong and it was all in my head.

It was very frustrating, because I didn't have the support when I was with the kids' father, before we got divorced. My mother and stepfather were living with us then and we didn't get along very well. It was like I was all by myself and I didn't have anybody. Everybody was saying: "Oh, nothing's wrong, the doctors are saying it's all in your head." It was very discouraging and very stressful, you know, feeling like you're all alone when you know something's wrong. I was in a stressful marriage and I had three kids. My girls were six and seven at the time and my boy was nine or ten. I was working and having to deal with all this. I was down, because I was all alone and everybody didn't believe me. But you know when there's something wrong – especially with your body.

One morning I woke up and my legs were numb from my waist down and I fell down on the floor when I got out of the bed. My ex took me to the hospital. They just laid me on the bed for a couple of hours and then sent me home. The

2 CAT scan, also known as a CT scan, or Computed Axial Tomography is a diagnostic medical imaging procedure that examines cross sections of the body allowing a three dimensional view of specific areas.

numbness lasted for a few hours and then it went away. They didn't do any testing – nothing at all. I recovered from that and got back to a pretty much normal life.

In Georgia, every time I went to doctors, they told me there was nothing wrong, that it was all in my head – panic and anxiety attacks, different stuff like that. I was going through a divorce with the kids' father, and I didn't get a diagnosis until I moved to Florida two or three years after that. Once I divorced him and got my life back together, things were okay for a while. I had been working for this company for almost a year when the symptoms started coming back.

I was in my late thirties when I got diagnosed. I went to the neurologist after a chiropractor sent me there. He did more MRIs, put me into hospital and did a lumbar puncture. Finally, all the results came back positive for secondary progressive multiple sclerosis.

Secondary progressive is the second stage of MS. The first stage is relapsing and remitting, which is what I was going through before, when you would only get symptoms for a certain period of time and then they would stop. So by the time I got diagnosed, in the second stage of MS, it was continuous.

The neurologist put me on steroids in the beginning, and then he put me on one of the injections that they have – *Betaseron*[3] and *Vicodin*[4] tablets for pain. I did those for the first eight months. Within eight months of being on that injection, I went from using a walker, a wheelchair to a power chair – in eight months. Then I got a cellulitis infection in my right upper leg, my thigh – the injection site for the *Betaseron*. I had to give myself the injections every two days. They came all pre-packaged and sterilised, so it shouldn't have given me that, but it did. The doctors didn't catch it soon enough. My neurologist said: "Oh, it's just an infection in your leg, take some antibiotics, walk on it and it will go away." (I could still walk a little with assistance.) It kept getting worse and so I went to the emergency room. The doctor there took one look at it and said: "Do you know what that is? That's a cellulitis infection – you're not supposed to be walking on that." By walking on it or standing up on it, it damages tissue and muscles underneath your skin faster. It got so bad it put me in bed for three months, because of not catching it right away. It's the most painful thing I've ever been through – ever. I was treated at home, then they sent me to a surgeon. By that time, my leg was so blown up it had started to split open by itself. They put a pump in to drain out all the fluid. They taught me how to do all that at home, gave me antibiotics and pain medication. It took a good four months – three of those months in bed, before it finally all healed up.

After that happened, I stopped the injections. While I was in bed for three months, I started doing research online, trying to find something else – something in pill form, that would help MS, because I was not going to do injections anymore. The *Betaseron* made me worse, because it was such a

3 *Betaseron* is an injectable drug from the interferon family, used to treat relapsing multiple sclerosis.

4 *Vicodin* is an analgesic medication derived from codeine, used almost exclusively in the United States.

quick progression. Within eight months of taking the injection, I was in a wheelchair. My doctor didn't really say a whole lot. As far as he knew there was nothing else out there that he could give me.

Online, I kept coming across the Low Dose Naltrexone (LDN).[5] I researched it on the LDN website[6] and followed some other people who were taking it for MS for a good two months before I went to my neurologist about it. The more I read up on it, I realised that there's no bad side effects, which is one of the things that caught me, because all the other medications out there have bad side effects. This medication, the LDN, boosts your immune system, instead of bringing it down like the other medications do. At first, I thought: "It's too good to be true – it's too good to be true."

I went to my neurologist who was one of the top neurologists in Florida. He hadn't heard about it, but said: "Let me look into it for two days and I'll get back to you." He did research and called me back two days later and said: "It looks good, and there are no bad side effects – let's give it a try."

Within a month of taking the LDN, I started walking on my own and within two months, I was out of the wheelchair. It took away most of my symptoms. After that, I got pretty much back to normal. I still had some symptoms, but as long as I didn't overdo it, I was fine. If I did too much housework at one time, then I would pay for it for a day or two. I would get pain and numbness and tingling back. If I was out in the heat for too long, my eyes would start to go blurry. Other than that, I was living a normal life again.

I started out on 3mgs of LDN once a night, between nine at night and three in the morning. Back then, that was the protocol, because I started taking it in 2005. I wanted to wean myself off the *Vicodin* to start the LDN, so the first night I took the LDN, of course I was in a lot of pain. When I took the very first pill of LDN, it took all the pain away.

I waited five months (because it takes time for your body to get damaged, so it takes time for your body to heal) to go up to the 4.5mgs, the maximum dose. My neurologist saw how well I was doing on it, so we just decided to go up to that dose to see how I would do on that. Some people do good on the 4.5mgs and some don't and have to stay on 3mgs. The only side effect I had was weird, vivid dreams, which were good dreams, not bad dreams, and a little bit more insomnia, which people with MS get anyways. Within two weeks, those things went away and I've been fine since. Since taking LDN, it's taken away all my symptoms and it's stopped or slowed my progression down.

I saw the neurologist in Florida for about a year. Once he saw how good I was doing on it, he started prescribing it to other patients. I had ten lesions on my brain, so after about a year of taking the LDN I went and had another MRI done and all the lesions had gone, but the mass in my spine was still there.

5 Low Dose Naltrexone is the off-label prescription of the FDA approved drug *Naltrexone*.

6 http://www.lowdosenaltrexone.org

There are times, if I overdo it, the MS will bother me a little bit, but not like before. All the symptoms that I had – the 'MS hug', the drop foot, talking, swallowing, all of the back pain, muscle spasms, numbness and tingling in my legs – have gone now.

LDN also helped with the fatigue, spasticity in my legs, tremors in my arms and gave me more energy. I had more strength in my arms, so I could drive again, do the household chores and pretty much everything. I could concentrate better too.

I still have good days and bad days, but I'm pretty much back to normal. I have a video on YouTube[7] that my friends Cyndi and Adam Lenz did about a year after I started LDN.

After I was diagnosed, I started my own website to be able to help other people. When I started researching for myself, I had to look through tons of websites to get any information, so I decided to put everything on one website so that people didn't have to go to ten million different websites to get information.

I started a LDN support group on Yahoo, and from there I started taking over the doctor's list for my pharmacist (doctors from all over the world that prescribe LDN). When people contact me I email them a doctor's list for their area and other information. I spend a lot of time on my website and the support groups. There are support groups on Facebook too. I get tons of emails every day, from people asking for lists of doctors or asking me questions. If I don't feel comfortable answering their questions, I send them to either my pharmacist or somebody who knows the answer. I spend a good half of the day doing that, but it makes me feel good helping other people, and saving other people's lives. A lot of them email me back and tell me how they're doing, and a lot of them make me cry. There have been so many people with different diseases – different types of cancers, Crohn's disease, fibromyalgia, Lupus, Irritable Bowel Syndrome, problems with thyroid, HIV AIDS, Parkinson's disease, autism and Alzheimer's.

I have improved throughout the years. Since I have been on LDN, I have had one cold in seven years. Everybody that I meet would never guess or know that I have MS. I have no symptoms now. I am stable and I may even be still improving, but it has either stopped or slowed my progression down. I just went for another MRI on the seventh of this month and everything came back normal. The only thing that they mentioned was that I had two bulging discs in my neck from an accident that I was in years ago, which I already knew about, but they said everything else was great. The mass in my spine had gone too.

For me, it's getting the doctors to prescribe it. I had a hard time getting the doctors here in Pennsylvania and the doctors in Arizona to prescribe me LDN, because they always kept telling me that there's no proof that it works. I tell them: "Well, I'm eight years proof that it works, and if you do your research online, you'll see that it does work, because it covers so many different diseases and cancers."

7 http://www.youtube.com/watch?v=6R1GAZ6L9rk

I went to a new GP on June 27, 2013, and he didn't know about LDN, just *Naltrexone*. He checked it out and saw that it was prescribed off-label,[8] but had no problems prescribing it to me. After he checked me all out, he said: "For someone that has MS and transverse myelitis, you sure look pretty healthy." It was a big relief to finally find a doctor in Pennsylvania that was open minded. I thanked him for being so nice, and he said: "Well, you treat people how you expect to be treated." And I was like: "Exactly!"

People who want a doctor to prescribe LDN have to keep looking until they find one. The doctors who prescribe it are awesome. There are doctors that I have been to who didn't know anything about it, but when I gave them information and taught them about it, they've started prescribing it to other people. I would have helped thousands of people over the past eight years. That makes me feel good.

There is a list on my website of different compounding pharmacists that make the LDN up. Skips Pharmacy in Florida is one of the cheapest and best. There are also vets who are starting to prescribe it to animals.

I myself know that it works – I'm proof. Doctors need to be more open-minded in helping their patients, instead of putting them on medications that make them worse. It's not a cure, but until there is a cure, or something better, I'll stay on LDN.

Harvard educated Bernard Bihari, MD (1931-2010), discovered the clinical effects of FDA-approved Naltrexone *using low doses (Low Dose Naltrexone or LDN). In 1985-86, he conducted a groundbreaking clinical trial on patients with HIV/AIDS. Doctor Bihari says that the immune system normalising effect of the drug application he discovered applies to a wide range of autoimmune diseases.*

Research trials can be found at http://www.lowdosenaltrexone.org/ldn_trials.htm

79-minute interview with Doctor Bihari: http://www.youtube.com/watch?v=x54Jc-cr8GT879

Crystal Nason's website is http://crystalangel6267.webs.com

8 Off-label is the use of a pharmaceutical drug for an unapproved indication.

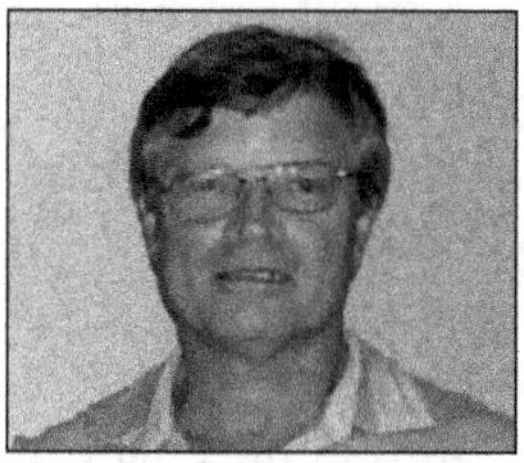

Steve Newport, 63 years

Florida, USA

Diagnosed with severe Alzheimer's disease at 56 years

Interview with Doctor Mary Newport, Steve's wife

I am a neonatologist, which is a physician who cares for sick and premature newborns. I wanted to have children as well as be a doctor, which meant that I would need to be on call. Someone needed to be there to care for our kids, so from early on in our marriage, we decided that Steve, who was an accountant, would stay at home and be the caregiver for our two daughters. That suited our family. Steve did the accounting for my practice from home, paid great attention to detail and performed quite well at this job for many years.

When he was about 51 years old, he started forgetting things. At first he would miss appointments that he was supposed to take the girls to, even if I called him half an hour before he was supposed to leave. He would hang notes from a long piece of tape in a doorway and sometimes he would still forget. At first, I thought it was a guy thing. I mentioned this to one of his sisters and she said: "You know, I'm like that too." It struck me as odd, because I didn't think that I would forget those things.

Then he started making payroll mistakes, and they were whoppers – several thousand dollars difference on someone's pay check and not noticing it. (*They* would notice it though!) It happened several times, so I started sitting down with him while he was doing the payroll. We didn't know what to blame it on at that point. Maybe our practice was a little bit larger and more complicated, but he also started procrastinating. He just couldn't seem to get organised, and he was missing tax deadlines.

All of this was new behaviour that crept in over a year or two. He started having problems remembering if he had been to the bank or the post office – that was when I thought that this was clearly not normal. At the post office he would pick up the mail from my practice and then he would misplace it, leaving it in the garage, or in his truck. Then he couldn't remember if he'd even been there, so we didn't know if there was mail to go looking for or not.

Our younger daughter was entering the terrible teen years and she was giving him a very difficult time. He was depressed that he had given up having a possibly more interesting career outside of the home to take care of her and that bothered him a lot. So we saw a neuropsychiatrist, who mentioned the word 'dementia' at that point, but he also said: "I really don't think that's what it is. He's depressed, and depression can affect memory, so we'll put him on antidepressants and see if that helps." So Steve went on those.

A year later, we moved an hour north, so that I could open a newborn regional care centre and that made everything much more obvious that he had a problem. He couldn't find his way around Spring Hill, which is a very small town, and he couldn't remember which street he was on or which direction he was going. He had to go to the dentist one day and he couldn't find his way there. He phoned up and they had to talk him in and then I had to spend 45 minutes on the phone with him to get him home.

The garage was a disaster area, because he was a hoarder. He would spend hours and hours in our garage looking for something. If he couldn't find something, he would just go out and buy it again. When we moved from our house, there were truckloads of stuff and we ended up with three storage units, because he couldn't part with any of it. The sad part was that when we did finally have a use for something, it would have a part missing that would make it unusable. It was really kind of a nightmare. It was very frustrating for him, and for me too.

Steve's accounting skills were still deteriorating. He couldn't finish more complex things like an annual tax return anymore and we had to start going to a CPA.[1] We shouldn't have had to do that, because he had been doing it for 20-plus years. I was really worried about Alzheimer's, so I set him up for a test with a neurologist. He took a 30-point test for memory. If you're normal, you'll easily get 30 points. This was in 2004, he was 54 years old and he scored 23 points. The doctor did several other tests – an EEG[2] and an MRI[3] and all kinds of blood work to rule out other causes.

The doctor didn't want to call it dementia at that time. Six months later, when he came back, Steve had already deteriorated to the point where he said: "I do believe he has Alzheimer's." So he started him on *Aricept*,[4] that increases one of the neurotransmitters in the brain. I didn't really notice any difference from that, but we kept him on it. The doctor said that once you get on one of these drugs, you can't come off of it. That's what the pharmaceutical companies tell you – if you come off of it you may worsen very suddenly and if you restart it you don't get back to where you were before you stopped taking it. They scare you that way. It could be true, but I don't know.

By 2006, Steve was clearly continuing to get worse. He couldn't use a calculator, do simple math or any accounting at all. He would get very, very lost when he was driving. He was supposed to be following our daughter

1 CPA – Certified Professional Accountant.

2 EEG – electro electroencephalogram measures the electrical activity of the brain for up to 40 minutes.

3 MRI – magnetic resonance imaging is a medical imaging technique used in radiology to investigate the anatomy and function of the body. MRIs are widely used in hospitals for diagnosis, staging of disease and for follow-up, without exposure to radiation.

4 *Aricept*, the trade name for donepzil, a common drug for Alzheimer's, can help improve cognition and behaviour, but does not alter the progression of the disease.

home from Tallahassee and took a wrong turn and ended up three hours away from home. Luckily, he had a cell phone and could remember how to use that, so we got him home. Shortly after that he had to stop driving – it was too worrisome. He couldn't even work out how to operate the windshield wipers.

We took him to the Byrd Alzheimer's Institute in Tampa, associated with the University of South Florida. They tested him fairly extensively and agreed that he most likely had early-onset Alzheimer's disease and suggested he start *Namenda*,[5] so then he was on the two common drugs that are used for Alzheimer's.

At that point, he was turned down for a clinical trial, which was extremely disappointing. It was the only available trial with a drug that was supposed to help reduce inflammation in the brain. In that particular study, it turned out that it didn't do anything, so we didn't really miss out on anything, although at the time it felt like it. He didn't qualify for the study because he had a history of depression. That was bothersome, because this man understood and comprehended that he had these memory issues – who wouldn't be depressed?

We muddled along for a couple of years watching him deteriorate. By early 2008, he started having tremors in his hands. He had trouble finishing his sentences. As he was trying to find the words, his jaw would tremor. He stopped reading. He had always read novel after novel, but they were just piling up. He had lost a lot of weight. He used to be able to find food and make dinner for himself, but I got very busy in the neonatal ICU[6] every night and he had basically stopped eating and had lost ten pounds over a few weeks. I had to have one of our daughters come and make sure he had lunch, or if I was late, dinner as well.

He really had to have someone with him while I was working. All kinds of crazy things would happen. He left the propane gas on the gas stove on a couple of times and I came home to the smell of propane in the house, which was frightening. He locked himself into a little area out in our courtyard, outside in the very hot weather. Luckily, I decided to stop at home quickly and found him there.

In May of 2008, a new clinical trial became available, so we took him to the Byrd Institute and were shocked to see that he scored only 12 out of 30 on the test and he needed 16 to qualify. It was devastating, because he qualified in every other way. They had taken depression out of the criteria, but now his score was too low. The drug was an intravenous vaccine that was supposed to very quickly remove beta-amyloid plaque from the brain. The working theory at that time was that if you remove the beta-amyloid plaque, the patient should get better. For him not to qualify for that study almost took our last hope away. So our doctor said to come back in a couple of weeks so he can try again. He suggested that I prepare him and go over some of the basics like the day of

5 *Namenda* is the trade name for memantine. Research is showing that it has little effect on Alzheimer's disease symptoms.

6 ICU – intensive care unit.

the week, the season, where we were going and things like that. Then he said: "Well, if he has Alzheimer's, he won't remember any of that." We thought: "We're not going to give up and we're going to keep trying."

In the interim, another drug became available, also to remove beta-amyloid plaque. I booked the screenings for two days in a row. The night before the screening, I got on the internet and thought: "What if a miracle happens and he gets accepted for both studies and we have to pick one of them?" I happened upon a press release for *another* medical treatment that I hadn't heard a thing about yet, called 'AC1202'.[7] It was called *Ketosyn*, which later became called *Axona*.[8]

I thought that was intriguing, because it said that it improved the memory in about half of the people with Alzheimer's who took it. You don't read about *any* medications that claim to improve the memory – they only say that it possibly slows down the course of the disease in some people. So I looked up 'AC1202' and found the patent application. It was a complete and an utter fluke that I came across it. I learned that Alzheimer's was a type of diabetes of the brain and this patent application explained it in great detail. A group at Brown University, led by Doctor Suzanne DeLaMonte,[9] had looked at the brains of people with Alzheimer's who had died and who did not have Type 1 or Type 2 diabetes. Every brain had insulin resistance and insulin deficiency in it, so they coined the term 'Type 3 diabetes'. They published another paper in 2008 and found that this insulin resistance of the brain was present in the very early stages of Alzheimer's and that it became more progressive until it was very severe and widespread.

Glucose needs insulin to get into cells and is used as the primary and preferred fuel for the brain. When people go into starvation, they use up the glucose stores in their body within 36 or 48 hours, after which they start breaking down muscle and using amino acids to make glucose. Then you start breaking down fat, which is converted in the liver to 'ketone bodies'. The brain quickly and easily switches over to using ketones.

Newborns are chubby – they use their fat and go into ketosis for the first 36-48 hours, which tides them over until the breast milk comes in. The mother more easily goes into ketosis too, when she's pregnant – it's a survival mechanism. It's really part of what has helped us 'make it' through our evolution, in that we're able to switch over and use alternative fuels such as ketones when needed.

The idea that an alternative fuel such as ketones could bypass a problem like insulin resistance in the brain is based on work done by Doctor Richard Veech at the National Institutes of Health near Washington DC. In the 1990s, Doctor

7 *Study of the ketogenic agent AC1202 in mild to moderate Alzheimer's disease: a randomised, double-blind, placebo-controlled, multicenter trial* Henderson S et al www.ncbi.nlm.nih.gov/pubmed/19664276

8 *Axona* is a medical food marketed for the diets of patients with Alzheimer's disease that contains a preparation of coconut oil (caprylic triglyceride). The basis of this prescription is that during digestion, caprylic triglyceride is turned into ketones, which provide an energy source other than sugar for the brain, due to people with Alzheimer's being unable to utilise sugar as a fuel source for their brain.

9 *Alzheimer's disease is type 3 diabetes – evidence reviewed* http://research.brown.edu/myresearch/Suzanne_delaMonte

Veech[10] needed something new to study. He decided that ketones seemed important and to find out what they can do. He found that more neurons survived in cell cultures with a ketone body containing beta-hydroxybutyrate, when they were exposed to substances that caused Parkinson's and Alzheimer's disease. This was in 2000, and he put out several hypothesis papers, that ketone bodies appeared to be neuro-protective and that a lot of diseases have a problem with insulin resistance and insulin deficiency. Providing someone with a ketone that you could drink would provide an alternative fuel for the brain and help Alzheimer's, Parkinson's and other diseases.

When he published this research around 2000, Doctor Sam Henderson, from a different lab, filed a patent application for 'AC1202', which later became *Axona*. His idea was that low-level ketones from medium-chain triglycerides (MCTs) could act as an alternative fuel for the brain. It was found *in the 1960s* that MCTs are converted to ketones in the liver. Even if you eat a high sugar diet, if you take MCTs, you will convert part of them into ketones, which the brain will quickly take up and use. Doctor Henderson's patent was for *MCT oil.*

I didn't think it was so brilliant that he was trying to patent it and make a medical prescription food out of it. I was kind of upset, because the patent application was in 2000. They had done a study in 2004, when Steve was having problems, but still had a normal MRI. If I had known about this four years ago, he might not have gotten so much worse. I felt they had kind of hidden this information and tried to protect it to make money out of it. Nevertheless, it was a brilliant idea. If I hadn't come across the AC1202, none of this would have happened for Steve, so in some ways I owe a lot to them.

Back in the late seventies and early eighties, we were adding MCT oil to the feedings of our smaller preemies[11] to help them gain weight faster. It was tolerated very well by the babies and I knew what it was. What I didn't know was that it was available over the counter! In the patent application, it mentioned that the MCTs were extracted from coconut oil. That was the "aha!" moment, because I had seen coconut oil on the supermarket shelf.

It was 1am and Steve was set to be screened for the clinical trial at 9am. Obviously I didn't have time to run out and buy coconut oil. We went to St Petersburg for this screening and Steve scored only 14 out of the 30 points. He needed 16 points, so again, he didn't qualify. The doctor asked him to draw a clock – a standard Alzheimer's test. He just drew a few little circles and a few numbers and it wasn't organised anything like a clock. I was really taken aback; that what he thought he drew was a clock was devastating. The doctor said that he was on the verge of severe Alzheimer's. You know, you live with a person every day and you see them deteriorating, but you don't realise how severely they're affected.

10 Doctor Richard Veech is a biochemist MD and PhD from Oxford University in the UK who conducted studies on ketones. He worked with Hans Krebs, the biochemist who delineated the Kreb's Cycle. Doctor Veech knew about ketones from the 1960s and 1970s when it was first discovered by Doctor George Cahill's lab, that during starvation, the brain uses ketones as alternative fuel.

11 Prematurely born babies.

I could just see our life deteriorating right in front of our eyes and once again, the hope factor was quickly vanishing. So on the way home, I thought: "What do we have to lose? We'll pick up some coconut oil and I'll just learn everything I can about it when we get home." It turned out that it's everywhere in Spring Hill, in healthfood stores.

I got onto the internet and learned everything that I could about coconut oil, ketones, MCTs and that coconut oil had close to 60 per cent of MCTs. *Axona*, or AC1202, had used 20 grams for their dose in the clinical trials, which is 20mls, which converted to a little over two tablespoons of coconut oil. So the next morning I put two tablespoons of coconut oil in Steve's breakfast.

The screening for the next trial was scheduled for early that afternoon. On our way down to Tampa, we went over and over what the day of the week was, but he just couldn't remember that it was a Wednesday. He couldn't remember that it was Spring, or the *word* 'Spring', so I didn't think he was going to do very well. When we got there, he was taken away by the nurse and he came back and he said he didn't think he had done very well. The nurse came back, took his blood pressure and started taking blood from him. I asked: "What's going on?" "Oh," she said, "didn't he tell you?" He got 18 and he's qualified for the trial." It was about four hours before that he had taken the coconut oil. We were just overjoyed. We found out later that the ketone levels usually peak at around three hours after taking coconut oil.

It was a very unusual stroke of fate that all that happened on those particular two days. At that point I didn't really know if it was just good luck, or if it was the coconut oil. I thought: "What harm is there in continuing this? He has Alzheimer's." There's all this mythology that coconut oil raises cholesterol, it's artery-clogging fat, but *his brain is dying*. What if it did raise his cholesterol? That would take years. Doctors have made so many people frightened of it.

I found out about a cook who worked in an assisted home. She was raised in Africa and had used coconut when she was growing up. When she started using it in her cooking in the home, she said that the residents became more talkative and had more energy. Then the doctor came in and said: "No, no, you're going to raise their cholesterol," and wouldn't let her cook with it any more. I thought: "Jeezle Pete – these people are happier, more talkative and they have more energy, and you're going to take that away from them, because you're worried about their cholesterol?" Personally, I think I'd rather die of a heart attack than of Alzheimer's disease. [*laughs*]

Steve did much better on the test that day. Then the next day, we started seeing him doing better. I decided in the morning that I was going to make sure he gets 35mls of coconut oil every morning and start cooking with it too. Bruce Fife[12] has written several books on coconut oil. I found his cookbook and his book 'Coconut Cures.' His information is very interesting, well researched

12 For books by Bruce Fife: http://www.coconutresearchcenter.org/books.htm

and very well documented.

The day after that, Steve was a different person. He came out from our bedroom alert, talkative, happy and his sense of humour was back. He had been very sluggish in the morning, and wouldn't talk at all. He couldn't find utensils, or figure out how to get water out of the front door of the refrigerator. By the fourth or fifth day, I felt like I had got my husband back. I remember sitting there having breakfast, and both of us feeling like our life had changed for the better. He said that he felt he had gotten his life back and he felt happy again.

That was just amazing, because I felt like his wicked stepmother before that. I was making him eat, making him take his pills and he didn't want to do any of it. Our relationship had changed from husband and wife to caregiver and patient. I felt like I had gotten him back and it was just a wonderful time.

After about two weeks, when the improvements continued, I felt like I had a new mission in life – to get this message out to other people. It was going to be another year before *Axona* came out and I felt very strongly: "Why should people have to wait?" It was on the shelf in the form of coconut oil and you can get the MCT oil over the counter. I had gotten some MCT oil from a company that was providing it to *Axona*, who weren't even making this themselves! The company was actually purchasing it from another company and making it into a product that would be patented as a prescription medical food, so I didn't really feel too bad about busting them [*laughs*] and letting everybody know they can just buy it online or from a healthfood store. And it's cheap – MCT oil in the United States is only $14 a quart – equivalent to a month and a half's supply. They charge $100 a month for *Axona*. If Steve improved, then other people out there are going to improve too. All I could picture was millions of brain cells dying – I felt like I had a moral obligation to tell everybody dealing with Alzheimer's disease about this.

Steve continued to improve over the next year. His weird gait went away. He was walking normally and he could actually run again – he hadn't been able to do that for two years. One day Steve said, "Well this is weird, I can read now." He explained how he had not been able to read because the words would go into 'pixels' on the page and move around, so he couldn't focus. The words were literally moving and he couldn't read because of it. That symptom has never come back. Being able to walk normally and run has never gotten worse again and now we're almost five years later.

I hear from a lot of other people that they see an improvement in quality of life. If you have cancer, it's a major breakthrough if a company comes up with a drug that gives you three or four extra months to live – it's all over the news.

About six weeks after we started the coconut oil, we went to see our family in Cincinnati. The year before, Steve didn't remember a lot of their names and conversations didn't really make a lot of sense. Everybody was just blown away that he was participating in the conversations, understanding jokes and laughing. He remembered his brother-in-law's and his niece's names.

He had drawn a clock two weeks after he had started the coconut oil and then 37 days after. I showed both drawings to the family. They all thought that it was incredible and that there really was something to this. Then I wholeheartedly decided to try to get this message out in a big way, so I wrote the article *What If There Was A Cure for Alzheimer's And Nobody Knew?* in 2008.[13]

I tried to take this article to an Alzheimer's Association conference, where there would be 5000 researchers from all around the world. My hope was that I could interest some of them in doing research so that they can investigate it. I thought that these people were intelligent enough to make up their minds if this science makes sense or not. A lot of them are young PhDs trying to get grant money for various projects related to insulin, nutrition and that kind of thing. There were 2000 poster presentations there and I tried to talk to as many of them as I could and give them a copy of my article, even though I was banned from doing that. [*laughs*] All I wanted was a table in their exhibit hall, but they didn't let me have one and I was really upset about that. At first they accepted, but a few days before the conference they told me that I couldn't have a table. If anything, they should be embracing this idea – it's just food. They think that only a medication is going to work. They have huge donors that are pharmaceutical companies and the coconut oil industry is not one of their big donors.

Steve helped me so much with getting the word out about coconut oil. I started passing out information to local healthfood stores and they started inviting me to do talks. Steve would come with me and answer people's questions and explain the thing about his visual disturbance, reading, how he couldn't run, how much better he felt and how his depression had gone away. It was pretty neat. Over a year, Steve's conversational skills improved. He was able to comprehend and remember what he had read, then tell me about it a few hours later, which was infinitely better than ten months before. One evening, he commented that the unusual colours of the sunset in the sky might be related to a volcano that had affected air traffic in Europe about a week earlier, which we heard about on a newscast.

In the fall of 2008, a reporter from the *St Petersburg Times* caught onto it and decided to run a story about us. They were brave. [*laughs*] When I was at the Alzheimer's Association meeting, I tried to get a reporter from *USA Today* interested in doing it, but her editor wouldn't let her run the story. They were afraid. This is coconut oil – it's dangerous stuff!

Steve got into a clinical trial about two months after we started the coconut oil. The company decided to let him in, in spite of all that, because coconut oil was just a food and how could that spoil the results? I thought: "Gee, if we could just get rid of the beta-amyloid plaques from his brain,[14] maybe we'll have him around for a long time and he won't die from this disease." He had extensive testing, which

13 http://www.coconutketones.com/whatifcure.pdf

14 The drug in this trial was designed to remove the beta-amyloid plaques in the brains of Alzheimer's sufferers.

was another one of those things that seemed too coincidental – he improved on this 75 point cognitive test by six points during that year. In the 78 point daily living activities test he improved by 14 points. That's really pretty remarkable, because people with Alzheimer's are going to deteriorate over one year. We later found out that Steve was on the placebo for the first 12 or 14 months. Other people who were on the placebo dropped by an average of over six points over 18 months.

Steve improved for the first year on the coconut oil, and then he had a year while on the trial where he was quite stable. After that, he got into the crossover phase of the trial where he was on the drug itself, for between five and seven months. At the end of that time, we started seeing some worsening. He had more confusion, trouble finding his clothes, taking a shower and he needed more help.

I was mystified as to what was going on, because he'd been sailing along really well and been so stable. He'd had a little cold around that time. We'd gone to Greece and he caught an intestinal virus there. People with Alzheimer's often have a setback after they've had an infection. At that time, I thought it was most likely related to the infection that he'd had, but then I thought that he might be having side effects from the clinical trial drug. Being a doctor, some people in the trial who thought they were on the drug told me that they had gotten much worse over the last year because of the side effects.

Steve had wounds that wouldn't heal for a month – it was strange. He'd just nick himself shaving and he'd bleed day after day after day. Then he fainted, which he'd never done in his life. He had a high CPK,[15] which could have been a heart enzyme. They were worried about the heart with this drug, so we decided to take him off of it for a day or two before we went to Greece. We found out a few months later that they had stopped the study because they found that the drug had made people worse, faster than the people on the placebo and accelerated the course of Alzheimer's disease in them. I think that is most likely what happened at that point, because he'd been on that drug for around seven months.

After that, I started questioning beta-amyloid and what the role of it is. I saw this paper that said beta-amyloid was antimicrobial and how there's herpes simplex virus in the plaques. Maybe removing these plaques is questionable. They didn't have the amyloid plaque scan available at that time, so we don't know if Steve's were removed by the drug. It was an irony that coconut oil had helped Steve improve his scores so he could get into this clinical trial that then may have made him worse. It was just unbelievable, and it's sad, you know?

After that Steve improved again and was quite stable for another eight or nine months. Then he developed gout and went on prednisone.[16] Boy, that

15 CPK – creatine phosphokinase is an enzyme found mainly in the heart, brain and skeletal muscle.

16 Prednisone is a synthetic corticosteroid drug that is used to treat inflammatory diseases, but has adverse effects. Because it acts as an immunosuppressant, people who take it are more susceptible to infection.

did a number on him – oh my gosh! We know now that he is so sensitive to medications. Last year he had a very serious problem from *Valium*,[17] which is supposed to help calm you down.

We had gotten him with a new doctor and he was doing quite well. They had filmed him vacuuming and putting dishes away for the 700 Club[18] and he looked very good there. Shortly after they filmed him, we saw this new geriatric specialist with very strong credentials and lots of Alzheimer's patients. Steve was coming into our bedroom saying: "This isn't my place – you need to take me back to my place." This would go on for hours sometimes, when it was the middle of the night. So this new doctor suggested giving him half of the lowest dose of the *Valium* to relax him and help him to sleep easier. It seemed logical to me and didn't strike me that it could cause a major problem. He was fine for about three weeks of taking it, then one day when we were having lunch with our daughter, he broke out in a dripping sweat. The next day he started pacing, much like he did when he was on the prednisone, talking to himself like he was hallucinating that somebody else was there. He also broke out with a fever blister. I thought that maybe he had a herpes simplex infection flaring up in his brain. He'd be with it for a while, and then he'd start pacing and talking. One night, after he kissed me, hugged me and told me that he loved me, he went to bed, then woke up with a terrible night terror. He was getting aggressive, took a lamp and threw it. He had never been like this before. We ended up taking him to the hospital, where they gave him some anti-psychotic medication and then he reacted to *that*. He got worse and worse and they kept giving him medications. I couldn't convince them that he was reacting to the medications. I asked the nurse to please not to give him more medication, but they kept giving it to him. He got sicker day by day and he wasn't allowed out of bed.

I ended up taking him home, because I thought he would die if he stayed there. He was used to being out of bed and walking all day long. He was so weak when he left hospital that he couldn't even stand up straight and was bent over at 90 degrees. That all happened in a relatively short time. Our daughter and her fiancé came to help us. Within a matter of days of taking him off the medication, he was much better again. But it really took him a couple of months to recover. That turned out to be a pretty serious setback for him. It was a horrible ordeal.

I really wanted to try to understand what had happened in the hospital, so I got his chart afterwards. They stopped his Alzheimer's meds suddenly and started giving him these anti-psychotic medications. The drugs he was given have warnings that they're not to be given to elderly people, or people with dementia, because they have a very high risk of adverse effects. Steve developed symptoms of Parkinson's disease, where he had these strange movements and his hands flapped so loud you could hear them. I talked to his doctor and said that I was

---

17 *Valium*, or diazepam, has a relaxant effect. It is used for a range of mental anxiety disorders, muscle spasms and alcohol withdrawal.

18 The 700 Club is a television program of the Christian Broadcasting Network, which airs throughout the US. It features a range of topics with live guests. It is available on CBN.com internationally. http://www.youtube.com/watch?v=ZZOR-Qd3QSg.

pretty sure it was the side effects of *Haldol*,[19] but he insisted that it wasn't. The nurses said that it couldn't be, because it was 24 hours since his last dose. They weren't listening. He started having massive sweating episodes, just soaking the sheets in his bed. I found out that *Haldol* can cause neuroleptic malignant syndrome, part of which is sweating, shock and fever. There's a 20 per cent mortality from that if it's not treated. When we took him out of hospital, those symptoms stopped and he got better, but it took a toll on him. So many people who are put into assisted living have some behaviour problems and are put on *Haldol* or some other anti-psychotic. I've talked to a number of family members who have said that their relative was walking and eating when they went in to assisted care and they died a few weeks or months later.

We still don't know what causes Alzheimer's disease, but what I have seen with Steve is that he will have long stable periods and then he has an infection, gets medication and that's when he has a setback and deteriorates. The second edition of my book[20] describes what has happened to Steve this last year. I also added a whole lot of material about medications that can cause, contribute to, or worsen Alzheimer's disease.

My secondary message is about medications and Alzheimer's. Family members have to be really careful and recognise what's going on. A whole lot of over-the-counter medications, called anti-cholinergic drugs, counteract the effects of the Alzheimer's medications. They are simple things, like antihistamines and cough medicines. One of the problems with Alzheimer's sufferers is that they don't make enough acetyl-choline. *Aricept, Exelon*[21] and drugs like that are to prevent the breakdown of acetyl-choline so that more of it is available. These over-the-counter medicines are anti-cholinergic, so when somebody with Alzheimer's has over-the-counter meds for a cold or whatever, it's completely counteracting their medication. They can actually cause confusion, hallucinations and delirium in people with Alzheimer's. Some people are on multiple medications like this. One lady, who came into an Emergency Room hallucinating and delirious, was on six anti-cholinergic medications. When she stopped taking them, she got better.

It's now coming up to five years since we started the coconut oil. Physically, Steve is still in great shape. He can still run. Cognitively, he's down from where he was at his peak. He's happy, and he's very loving – he tells me a couple of dozen times a day he loves me and he gives me hugs. He wants to be with me. I do feel like I still have my husband. To have had extra good years with him has meant everything to me.

Mary T Newport, MD, grew up in Cincinnati, Ohio, attended Xavier University for pre-medicine, and graduated from the University of Cincinnati College of

19 *Haldol* (haloperidol) is an antipsychotic medication used for schizophrenia, acute psychosis, mania and other nervous system disorders.
20 Doctor Mary Newport's book, *Alzheimer's Disease: What If There Was a Cure?* is now in its second edition.
21 *Exelon* is a cholinergic drug used for mild dementia and Alzheimer's disease.

Medicine in 1978. She trained in Pediatrics at the Children's Hospital Medical Center in Cincinnati, and completed her fellowship in neonatology, the care of sick and premature newborns, at the Medical University Hospital in Charleston, SC.

She has practiced neonatology in Florida since 1983 and has served as founding medical director for two newborn intensive care units. She is currently in full-time practice as a neonatologist in the Tampa Bay area.

Doctor Newport has been married to Steve Newport since 1972. They have two daughters and a grandson.

Her article What If There Was a Cure for Alzheimer's Disease and No One Knew? *relays her family's experience with this disease and her research into a dietary intervention that may benefit persons with Alzheimer's and other neurodegenerative diseases.*

September 27, 2011, marks the date of the release of her book, now in its second edition, Alzheimer's Disease: What If There Was A Cure? *Her website is http:// www.coconutketones.com*

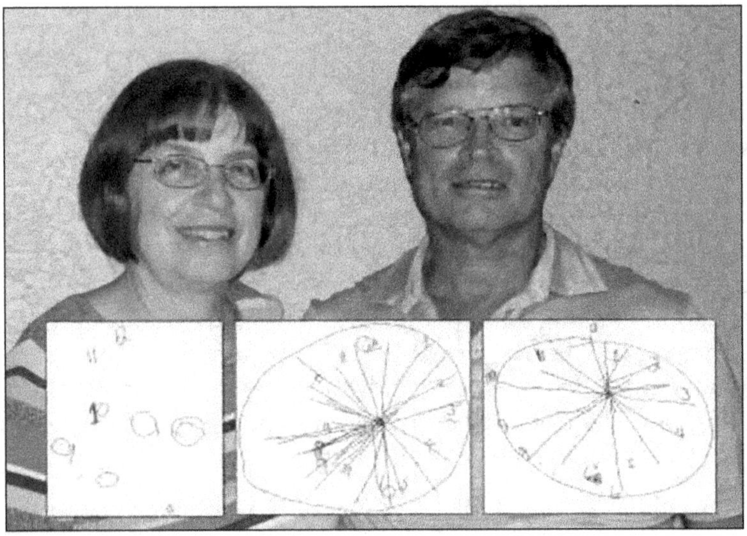

Steve and Doctor Mary Newport. The inserts show the progression of clock drawings after taking coconut oil.

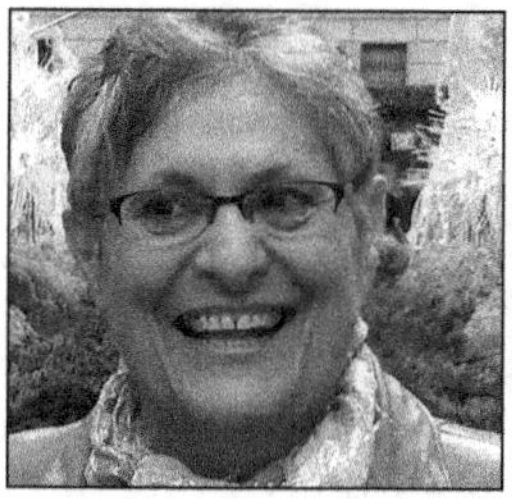

Raphaela Savino, 74 years

Lakewood, New Jersey, USA

Diagnosed with ovarian cancer at 52 years

I've just celebrated 22 years as a survivor of ovarian cancer. Just before I was diagnosed, I was working as a nurse,[1] having a busy, stressful working life. Shortly before I discovered the cancer, I had started to get into a more healthy way of living and eating. When you get to a certain age you realise that you're not going to live forever.

I never paid much attention to my health in the past. You know, I was young and crazy and didn't pay attention to anything. You get into cigarettes and alcohol and everything else. It was hectic, but I was starting to be more careful and cautious about what I was eating and starting to go more for natural, healthy and more organic eating. Not that I ever ate bad, bad. I'm from Italian heritage, so we always ate good food. I wasn't taking a lot of medication or anything like that.

It was in January 1992, right after the holidays, and I was looking at my weight. Not that I was ever really fat, but I was never a skinny Minnie. I was laying in bed one morning and I usually feel my waist and abdomen to see just how far out it would protrude. I'd say: "Oh man, if I can't feel my pelvic bones, I know I'm too fat." I felt a lump on the left side of my abdomen and I said: "Now, what is this?" I didn't feel it on the right side and I got really nervous and scared. The very next day, I got on the phone and started talking to some of my friends and colleagues and they said: "Oh, it's probably a fibroid in your uterus, or something like that."

I had a friend who was working as a resident at Bellevue Hospital and she happened to be in obstetrics. I called her up and said that I needed a good gynaecologist, so she referred me to a woman that she trusted and was working at Bellevue. I made an appointment as soon as I could. I got in to see her and she did a pelvic exam. When she finished, I felt that she suspected something unusual because she had this look on her face. I don't remember the things she said. At that time, I realised that you don't go to the doctor alone. She said: "I'm going to refer you to a gynaecological oncologist and I'm going to send you over for a pelvic ultrasound right now. And I'm going to take a blood

1 Raphaela is a registered nurse.

sample right now." She took blood and did a CA 125[2] and it was very high. All this happened to me and nothing made sense. I said to myself: "Oncologist? Why would she be sending me to an oncologist?" Nothing was connecting and nothing made sense to me. I was so scared.

I had the ultrasound, and of course the technician didn't say anything to me. Then I went to see the oncologist and he told me that there was a large neoplasm[3] and recommended surgery right away. He said that we won't know until we get in and do a biopsy, whether it's cancer or not. I was just blown away by the whole thing.

I had the surgery, then the surgeon told me that it was a very large malignancy and he thought he got it all out. Part of it had adhered to my ureter and they were very lucky that they managed to hold on to the ureter. In the hospital, he of course put me on the track for chemotherapy. They sent in the staff to explain the various forms of chemotherapy that I was scheduled for. No-one asked me if this was what I wanted – it was an automatic thing: "You're going to have chemo[4] and that's that." Being a nurse, I knew that that was a terrible route to go. This was 20 years ago when the effects of chemo were just dastardly. I mean it was horrendous, because I'd seen what it did to people.

A friend came to see me in hospital. This is what I see as divine intervention. Her father had recently died of pancreatic cancer, but before he died, she had done extensive research on alternative treatments to try to save her father. Pancreatic cancer is a death sentence, of course, and it's a rapid one. She had read about Doctor Nick Gonzalez – he was the only one who was having success with pancreatic cancer. It was too late to save her father, but it was fortunate for me that she had his name and number and all the information on him. She said that this was something that I could do.

I was torn and they were pushing me and I'm surrounded by western medicine; the doctors, the nurses, my friends, my colleagues: "You have to do the chemo." Part of me said, "No, I don't want it." I was discharged from the hospital with an appointment and I was supposed to go to the chemo ward that Saturday. I didn't show up for the chemo at NYU[5] hospital and they started calling me: "Where are you, Raphaela, why didn't you come?" I didn't have the courage to tell them that I wasn't going to go and that I was going to try something else. I knew that they would be upset with me and I was in this vulnerable position.

I went home and I called Doctor Gonzalez's office. The first appointment I could get was two weeks from that day. My rationale at the time was that I can give this a try, and if it doesn't work, there's always chemo. I went to see Doctor Nick Gonzalez and started on the program immediately. Then I had a post-op appointment with the surgeon to check me out and take out the sutures and so on. I went to his office and he gave me such a blasting out for not going to the

2 CA 125 (Cancer or Carbohydrate Antigen 125) is a protein tumour marker present in ovarian cancer cells.

3 A neoplasm is an abnormal growth of tissue in the body, usually cancerous.

4 Chemo – chemotherapy.

5 NYU – New York University Hospital.

chemo. He said, "You have to go to the chemo." He pretty much said that I'll die if I don't go. I told him that I was doing alternative treatment with this doctor, who happens to be located on Park Avenue, not far from where the surgeons are! He said, "You can't trust these..." He really put him down. He didn't know anything about him, but he was closed to any idea other that what he was trained to do and what he believed in. I felt terrible that he felt that way. I shrunk up. I think anybody else would have just given in. I don't know what gave me the courage and the strength to disregard what he said and go on my way.

Doctor Gonzalez was very positive that he could help me. He explained the program to me – it was going to be a lot of work. I was given the overall metabolic treatment program, which consisted of diet, supplements and detoxification. It was a daunting experience to know that it was going to involve taking 150 supplements a day, that I would have to eat all organic food, that I would be doing this detox[6] that would clear out my liver and all the cancer cells would be destroyed through a natural, holistic way. It rang true for me. I don't know how to explain it, but it made sense to me and I wasn't afraid to do the work. I knew there was a lot of self discipline involved. I'm a former nun – I was in religious life for 12 years, and that was not an easy thing to do. I guess I should have told you that in the beginning! [*laughs*] When I went in, in the sixties, it was still with the old-fashioned habit. You left your family, you left your home. Entering the religious life meant leaving the old world behind and going into a life of sacrifice and discipline. It wasn't like I hadn't been down this road, so I didn't shy away from that.

Doctor Gonzalez interviews you about what your belief is – in a way, your spiritual belief. You have to believe in the choice you make. If you don't have faith in it, it's not going to work, so that's a big part of it. I connected with it, it felt good to me and it was certainly worth a try. He recommended that I leave work to just concentrate on the program. I said that I couldn't leave work, I was self-supporting. I proceeded to try to be super, super-woman and made sure that I got all the food shopping done to eat organic, which was not an easy thing to do in Brooklyn. I had to go to Manhattan to shop for the organic, healthy food, bring it home, prepare it and cook three healthy meals a day. Then sort out 150 pills so that I would have a packet for the morning, a packet for lunch and a packet for dinner, for ten days. Then I would make sure that I prepared the packets for my pancreatic supplements. After that, I had to prepare on the five-day break, one of the detox programmes, which also required buying certain items and having them ready. And at the same time, work full-time. He kept saying to me, and this was his theme-song: "The body heals best when it's at rest. You're body's going to be working really, really hard to break down the cancer cells and get rid of them and you can't do that unless your body is resting." I said: "I know, but I can do it." I did it for three months.

6 Detox – detoxification.

The people at work, even though they thought I was crazy for doing this, and thought that I should be doing the chemo, didn't laugh at me to my face. I had to bring my own lunch because I couldn't eat what they were eating. I would take out my packet of pills for my lunch and they'd say: "You're going to eat all those pills?" Every time they turned around and looked at me, I'm swallowing more pills!

I lasted for three months and then I pretty much collapsed. I was so exhausted, I had to give in. I called up work and said that I had to take a leave of absence and I had to take three months off. Nick was expecting that I would do that sooner or later. It was much easier for me to be able to stay home and rest while I was healing.

The leave of absence turned into one full year. I had applied for social security disability, which I was entitled to, but when I submitted my medical review, I was turned down. They didn't believe that, because I wasn't doing chemo, I was an authentic ovarian cancer survivor, medically ill and doing this program. So I had to get an attorney to appeal the decision in court and explain why I was doing what I was doing and that it was real and authentic. I had to bring all my medical records, and for the program that I was on, and I had to prove everything. I won, but it was a year later. For that year, I had to struggle without the income, surviving on savings and borrowing from friends, and it was really a rough road. Then at the end of the year, I was ready to go back to work, and that's when I got the cheque. [*laughs*]

I got checked every three months, and my cancer rate slowly came down, came down, came down. Pretty soon people were saying: "Gosh, you look good." I knew that if I had destroyed my immune system with the chemo, I never would have been able to battle the illness. My immune system was getting stronger and stronger with all the supplements and the detox that I was doing. I could feel myself getting so much better.

When I went back to see the gynaecologist, she assumed that I had gone on for chemo. She asked me how I was doing, and I said that I was doing great. She said that I looked wonderful. When I told her that I wasn't doing the chemo, her face went white. She was shocked and couldn't accept it. She shook her head. She wouldn't believe it and made some weird comment. I was shook up when I left her office, that it couldn't even enter her realm of understanding that I could survive without going the traditional route. The same thing with the surgeon, he just couldn't accept it. I got no support from any of the western doctors.

I returned to work and I continued to stay on the program and see Doctor Gonzalez every six months. In my follow-up program, I continued to get an ultrasound every year or two. I'd do mammographies, and I'd do gynaecological exams. I also did lab work. I'd get CA 125s when I got my blood work in addition to Doctor Gonzalez's hair sample, which is a guide that tells me what my cancer rate is. Within a year, everything came down to normal.

One doctor who read my recovery story said that the reason I was cancer-free was because I had everything removed by the surgery, but when they did the surgery there was evidence of some cancer in the liver. That was in the operative report. Even though they take out the primary lesion, you never know how much cancer is your body. From the ovaries, the cancer can go to your breast, then it's in your lungs, then it's in your brain, it can just be anywhere. Doctor Gonzalez knew this and that's why he was concerned about my sticking to the program and doing the liver flush[7] and all of the protocols. Now I have the greatest liver! You should see my liver blood work. My doctor says that my blood work is like a young person's. [*laughs*]

My physician now is a pretty open-minded one – thank God I have one. She's young, female and she knows what I'm doing and that I see Nick every six months, which obviously is not harming me. I had to have a support group – you know, find people that were supportive of what I was doing – and stay close to them.

It breaks my heart when so many friends and relatives I know could be helped, if they would be willing. It seems easier to lie down and have an IV[8] put in your arm once a week or whatever and think you're going to be cured. If people hear about this protocol, they're not interested. It's very sad, because you know what's going to happen. If people had the courage to look into different ways of healing themselves, they might find that it would be so much more satisfactory. Compared to traditional methods that you see people suffer from, you feel good, you feel healthy and stronger. If they stepped out of the box, they might be pleasantly surprised.

Now I am not working and am enjoying retirement. I have rediscovered oil painting. I did it intermittently during my working life, but now I can devote a lot more time to it, so I've been painting, drawing, doing water colour and enjoying the art a lot. I am in good health – it's like a miracle. If people only worked hand in hand, a lot would get done, wouldn't it?

For all types of ovarian cancer, the five-year relative survival rate[9] is 44%. Women diagnosed when they are younger than 65 do better than older women. If ovarian cancer is found (and treated) before the cancer has spread outside the ovary, the five-year relative survival rate is 92%. However, only 15% of all ovarian cancers are found at this early stage. (American Cancer Society 1st November 2013 www.cancer.org)

---

7 The liver flush – first used in the 1920s to improve liver function www.townsendletter.com/Dec2007/livercleanse1207.html

8 IV – intravenous drip.

9 Survival rate indicates that the patient is still living at five years after diagnosis, irrespective of the level of health and quality of life.

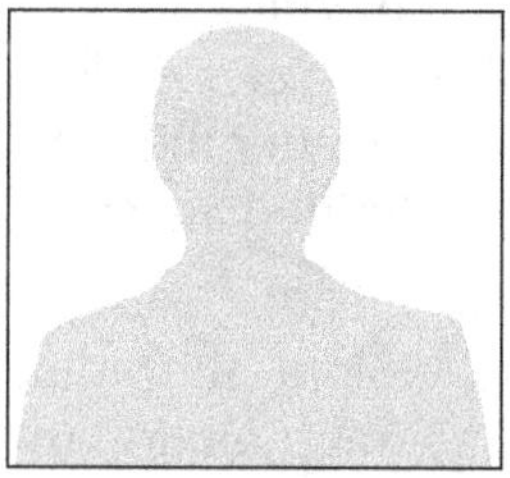

John Scott, 67 years

England, UK

Severe asthma, food and environmental allergies, plus sinusitis in childhood, followed by Crohn's disease and ME (myalgic encephalomyelitis/chronic fatigue syndrome) in adulthood

When I was four, I remember being admitted to hospital with abdominal pains that the doctors never got to the bottom of. It was probably the beginning of Crohn's disease, which didn't surface again until much later, but it was a strange episode. Psychologically, it was very damaging, because I was separated from my parents for a week. In those days in the UK, parents only got to see their hospitalised children at specified visiting times, which were infrequent and strictly limited.

My asthma also started fairly early and was pretty bad. I remember often struggling to breathe. The only relief I got was from some horrible little yellow tablets that I had to hold under my tongue and not swallow. They tasted absolutely vile! There were no inhalers in the early 1950s, so asthma could be extremely debilitating and for a child, very frightening.

Fortunately, I began to grow out of the asthma in my early teens, when I also began looking at alternative approaches to health and began weight training. In those days, this was considered a very bizarre practice and people thought I was a nut-case. My doctor even told me that I'd give myself an enlarged heart by using weights, such was the state of medical understanding about resistance exercise in those days! I actually became very fit doing this. When I went to college to train as a teacher, I started the college's first physical culture club. The PE[1] department didn't even have any weights when I arrived, and it was quite challenging persuading them to obtain some.

A few years after leaving college, getting married and starting work as a teacher, my nasal problems got really, really bad. An ear, nose and throat specialist wanted to enlarge my nasal passages with a hammer and chisel, a prospect that prompted me to go off and do some research! There was no internet in those days, so it was a matter of going to the local library and hoping that they had the books you wanted. I discovered that milk can cause all the nasal problems that I was having, so I cut out milk completely and this solved the problem. There were no more nasal issues for quite some time after that.

I had a successful career and became a head teacher at the age of 36. But, after

1 PE - physical education.

I had had that job for four years, my health fell apart. It was a very stressful job. Not only was the school that I ran a special school for children with a wide range of special needs, but the behaviour of some of the youngsters was extremely challenging. Also, due to long-term industrial action by teaching staff, there was a period of many months when I was left to look after the entire school every day during the midday break with only a few untrained assistants. It was at that point that my health finally caved in.

My food intolerances began to escalate and I would get violent abdominal pain after eating certain foods. Then I was struck down by a viral infection that never went away. Even though I took an unprecedented seven weeks off work, I never fully regained my health. Normally with a viral infection, a couple of weeks would see me right, but this time I just couldn't get going again. I really struggled for the following four years, only managing to continue by spending every evening and weekend resting.

Even though my health got progressively worse during those four years, at no point was I given a diagnosis. If I'd been told at the outset that I had ME,[2] I would have stopped working earlier, but I kept hoping that it was something I would get over.

I tried everything to help improve my health – even buying a bike in a vain attempt to get fit, but found I couldn't get much further than the end of the road I lived on. Nothing else worked either, and in the end, my doctor insisted that I would have to retire, which was the last thing I wanted to do, because I loved my job. In spite of the many challenges, it really was the best job in the world.

Only after I officially retired did I hear a doctor mention the words "myalgic encephalomyelitis". It was a relief to finally get a diagnosis, even though, at that time, this condition was dismissed by most doctors, and I didn't get much sympathy from anyone in medicine.

The process of obtaining invalidity benefits proved to be a minefield for someone who was profoundly exhausted, and I had to fight all the way to get what I knew I was entitled to. After my first benefit application was turned down, I had to go through a gruelling appeals process, which, like most of the others with ME who were forced to go through this same process, I eventually won.

My food allergies and intolerances continued to worsen. The first food I had reacted badly to was sweetcorn. Every time I ate it, I got such violent pain that I would be rolling around on the bathroom floor in agony between attempts to make myself sick, which was the only strategy that gave me any relief.

The doctors couldn't get their heads around my situation at all. They scoped me but could only find a small amount of inflammation in my stomach, so concluded that there was nothing wrong with me. Left to my own devices, I found that the only way to deal with these episodes of violent pain, other than making myself

2 ME – myalgic encephalomyelitis or chronic fatigue syndrome (CFS) is a severe, complex, acquired illness with numerous symptoms related to the dysfunction of the brain, gastrointestinal, immune, endocrine and cardiac systems. ME has been classified as a neurological disorder in the World Health Organisation's International Classification of Diseases since 1969 (ICD 10 G93.3) http://www.mecfs.org.au

vomit, was to take a large dose of Epsom Salts[3] as soon as a reaction started. This flushed everything through my system. Although it gave me diarrhoea, it always brought blissful relief after about four hours. In the absence of any help from the medics, I carried on using the Epsom Salts treatment for many years.

Gradually, more and more foods began to cause this reaction. Eventually, I lost all the fruits and all the vegetables, and then other foods as well, until there were only a handful of foods that I could tolerate. Some of these reactions were diagnosed as allergy and others as food intolerance. One allergy specialist told me, after doing a few tests, that there was nothing wrong with me, implying that it was all in my head – a diagnosis I'd become accustomed to hearing. A gastroenterologist also said there was nothing wrong with my gut and advised me to "go away and eat a normal diet".

After going through all of this for many years, it seemed obvious to me that my immune system must be the root of the problem, so I saw an immunology consultant. Unfortunately, he immediately dismissed the possibility of it being an immune reaction; said it was all in my head and that I must change the way I thought about how food affected me. I asked him to tell me how I might do this, or to refer me to someone who might be able to help in this regard, but he ignored this request. When I suggested he admit me to his ward and observe my reactions after eating normal foods, he replied: "Oh no, we're not going to do that," and left me completely on my own again.

Gradually over the years, the food intolerances became so severe that they threatened my survival, and I had to resort to living on hypoallergenic semi-elemental feeds.[4] It was while I was hospitalised, due to a severe reaction to a new vitamin tablet, that I began using the special feeds. The consultant, in whose care I was placed on this occasion, recognised my reactions to food as real and introduced me to a variety of special medical feeds. When I left the hospital, I had a couple of carrier bags full of the feeds they had given me, and my local GP continued to prescribe these until I eventually became intolerant to *them*. At that point, my GP and I began to experiment, with me exploring what was available and the GP prescribing whatever I found that didn't upset me.

Once I was on these feeds, I stopped losing weight and could even add weight if I wanted to, just by having more of the powder, which is very easily digested. However, one of the downsides of using these special feeds was that the nasal symptoms I had suffered as a teenager returned with a vengeance. Even the feeds that didn't use proteins derived from milk still produced the nasal symptoms, which once more became a constant problem.

After having identified a couple of semi-elemental infant feeds that I could tolerate, and I had been reaction-free for a while, I experienced a return of abdominal

3 Epsom Salts – magnesium sulphate (MgSo4) is an organic salt traditionally used as a component of bath salts. Medically, the salts are used for aches and pains, to remove splinters and internally as a saline laxative.

4 An elemental diet is where a patient is fed liquid nutrients, sometimes through a tube, made up of amino acids, fats, sugars, vitamins and minerals in an easily assimilated form. It lacks whole or partial protein, due to its ability to cause allergic reactions.

pain after eating and started passing black tarry stools. A new gastroenterologist ordered a barium follow-through X-ray, which amazingly I had never had before. When I returned to see him, he held the X -ray up for me to see and showed me the swelling above a stricture. It was almost the size of a second stomach – a situation that he described as very serious and requiring immediate surgery.

When I met the surgeon, he told me that the enlarged section of intestine "could explode at any time" – a rather frightening revelation! He put me at the top of his operating list and the offending section was soon removed. A biopsy confirmed that Crohn's disease was the cause, and the gastroenterologist said that he was very surprised nobody had spotted it before. He also thought that this surgery would solve my problem with adverse food reactions and that I would no longer need to use the special feeds, but this wasn't the case. My extreme food sensitivities were all still present, and continued until I eventually got worms.

Not long after the first intestinal surgery, I again developed abdominal pain, which further surgery revealed was caused by a phytobezoar – a solid ball of plant material that was stuck above another, new stricture. The phytobezoar was four and a half centimetres in diameter – about the size of a golf ball. The surgeon who removed it said that it had made his day, because he didn't see these very often!

My sister-in-law was employed in a department at Nottingham University where Professor Pritchard[5] and his team were working with hookworms. She sent me a press cutting about their work and I phoned Professor Pritchard, who was surprisingly helpful. He said that he couldn't supply me with any hookworms, but having been made aware of this potential treatment, I then kept my eyes and ears open. When the Hookworm for Crohn's disease trial[6] was eventually publicised, I jumped at it, although I almost failed to qualify.

After I filled in the application form, the researcher said that I hadn't scored enough points. I commented on the difficulty of accurately quantifying one's symptoms with Crohn's. For example, should one respond in terms of a good day or a bad one? This led to me being given another chance to complete the form, but with my worst days in mind, and this enabled me to get into the trial. The problem was that I didn't have many of the symptoms that others with Crohn's have. While I did have the stricturing, I didn't get the diarrhoea, and some of my test results were normal.

Once the trial began, I found the regular traveling to the university for blood tests hugely stressful, due to the ME/CFS. At that time, a normal day for me consisted of dragging myself out of bed in the morning, parking myself in a chair, watching some TV, falling asleep quite a lot of the time and then climbing back into bed at night. So having to travel 15 miles by taxi to get to Nottingham University was a huge strain and I had to summon every ounce of willpower in order to manage it.

---

5 Professor David Pritchard BSc Zoology, MSc Immunology, PhD Immunology. MRC Postdoctoral Researcher at University of Nottingham, Lecturer in Immunology. Chair in Parasite Immunology, School of Pharmacy, 1998 www.nottingham.ac.uk/pharmacy/people/david.pritchard

6 http://gut.bmj.com/cgi/content/meeting_abstract/59/1_MeetingAbstracts/A2

When you get hookworms, they're microscopic larvae contained in a few millilitres of clear liquid. They have been incubated from the faeces of someone else who's got worms and then cleaned. You put this liquid onto the pad of a bandaid dressing and apply it to the inside of your arm. Within minutes, the larvae burrow into your skin and a strong itch typically develops within ten minutes. Before they enter the host's skin, the larvae slough off their skins, a bit like snakes do. These 'cuticles', as they're called, are left behind and cause a rash when the immune system reacts to them. The worms then enter a capillary and are carried by the bloodstream to the lungs. There, they burrow through the alveoli, or air sacs, in the lung. They follow the debris that the lung hairs remove from the airways up to the top of the trachea (windpipe)and into the lower part of the throat, then transfer to the oesophagus. From there, they travel to the stomach and finally set up home in the jejunum of the small intestine. There, they take about three weeks to mature, then attach to the wall of the intestine and start to feed by drawing a small amount of blood.

Once the worms attach, the immune system registers their presence and starts trying to fight them off by causing inflammation in the gut, which results in transient symptoms for some people. The worms respond by secreting molecules to reduce the inflammation. For the next eleven weeks or so, the immune system and the worms continue to challenge each other until they reach an 'agreement', at which point any early side effects resolve.

I had more severe initial side effects than most people experience, with intermittent diarrhoea for 19 weeks, but I was already getting many benefits while suffering from the 'runs'.[7] My nose was much clearer and I was able to breathe through it easily for the first time in years, so I really didn't mind the diarrhoea!

Once the worms are established at around 12 weeks, you can start to get some benefits. Not everyone does, though – one guy with allergies and asthma had to wait for 19 months before he started to see any benefits. Then he suddenly went into remission.

By 11 and a half weeks, just before the end of the trial (which was only for 12 weeks), I found I could eat some normal foods again, so I asked for an extension. I was silly really – I should just have said that I didn't want the worms to be terminated, but I was so exhausted by the whole process of making repeated trips to the university that I wasn't thinking straight. Instead, I asked them if my worms could have a stay of execution. They agreed to give me an extra three weeks, so my worms were left in place for a total of fifteen weeks. In the extra three weeks, I was able to eat a number of normal foods without any difficulty. When I obliged the researchers by taking a pill to kill off the worms, they said that they would give me some fresh worms outside the trial. I therefore went back to my gastroenterology consultant to ask him to refer me to get more worms, which he was happy to do. However, when I returned to see the trial researchers, they said that they couldn't give me any more worms until the trial was completely finished.

7 'The runs' – frequent diarrhoea.

The trial was only about half way through at that time (it took three or four years for it to be completed). I realised that it was going to be a long time before I would actually get any more worms from them, so I went online and got my own.

Once I got my new worms, there was nothing further I needed to do. It was just a matter of gradually watching the transformation as the worms began to work their magic.

The really bizarre thing was that after I'd had this new dose of worms for 11 and a half weeks, I had a dream – a really vivid dream – the kind that I've only had two or three times during my life. In this dream I was in a Chinese restaurant, looking at the menu on the wall. At that point, I heard a voice in my head say that there were three foods I could eat. I can't now remember exactly what they were (my memory has been terrible since I developed ME/CFS), but they were low-allergy foods like rice, so these were the foods that I started with. After finding that I could tolerate these, I began to try other foods and found that, gradually, over the next 18 months, I was able to reintroduce all foods, so that I could once again eat anything I wanted.

The immune system responds to the worms during the first 14 weeks. Any side effects occur mainly in the middle of this phase, when the immune response is at its maximum. Once you've had the worms for 12 weeks, you can add more and continue to do this till you have a colony of around 140. Experience has shown that this is an ideal number for therapeutic purposes in an average-sized male. Once you have a colony of approximately 140 hookworms, you may not need any more for several years. A few people who have a robust immune response to helminths[8] and therefore see off their worms more quickly, need to add more as often as every six months in order to keep their disease under control.

Some of us with Crohn's disease, and also a few who have ulcerative colitis or coeliac disease, fall within this category and need to take supplementary doses more frequently. If I don't add more worms every six months, I start to get symptoms coming back. My nasal symptoms are the first to return and I lose my ability to tolerate cheese, which is a nuisance, because I really like blue cheese! If I forget to top up my colony on time, I start to get migraines after eating cheese. This and the returning nasal congestion alert me to the fact that I need to get more worms.

Crohn's disease is arguably a helminth deficiency disease that only arises in susceptible individuals because of a lack of the worms that the body needs to keep its immune defence troops busy and stop them from indiscriminately attacking other targets, like the gut. There's a graphic showing the parts of the world where hookworms and helminths in general are endemic and those are the parts of the world with the lowest rates of autoimmune disease.[9] The parts of the world where helminths have been eradicated, like the UK and America, have huge pandemics of autoimmune disease and allergies.

8 Helminth is another term for a parasitic worm; a flatworm, tapeworm or nematode.

9 http://static.cdn-seekingalpha.com/uploads/ 2012/5/12/1122334-13368327296724055-Iggy-Igette_origin.jpg

The trial that I took part in at Nottingham University was never reported, because it was only a safety trial. However, they're now running a new study for people with multiple sclerosis (MS).[10] This time, they're giving the subjects 25 worms instead of the ten that I was given, and they're leaving them in place for nine months. It will be very interesting to see how this trial works out, and I believe that they will certainly have successes. The people who have bought worms online to treat MS have shown an almost 100 per cent success rate.[11]

It is generally easy to obtain therapeutic helminths, which are supplied by several companies. Unfortunately, the US authorities have classified hookworm as a 'biologic drug' and issued an import alert in respect of them, so it is more difficult to get hookworms in the States, but there is one company that will ship them to US citizens.

The attitude of the American FDA to helminthic therapy is really nonsensical, because intestinal worms are clearly not drugs. Hookworms are simply one of the thousands of symbiotic microorganisms that humans have co-evolved and cohabited with for millennia. In the case of helminths, we have got rid of them in the last half century as a result of improved hygiene and sanitation. What those of us who are using helminths as a therapy are doing is simply putting back something that's gone missing because of our modern lifestyle. It's not only the obvious immune-related diseases that are helped by correcting a helminth deficiency. Nobody's tried helminths yet as a prevention for cardiovascular disease, or the other diseases of old-age like Alzheimer's, but there is evidence that all these conditions are associated with inflammation, which helminths are very effective at controlling.

Doctors are very resistant to the idea of reintroducing helminths to treat, let alone prevent, disease. Those of us who frequent the online helminthic therapy groups[12] regularly see people posting reports saying that when they've mentioned this to their doctors, the medics have gone ballistic, telling their patients that they're fools and they'll harm themselves by having these dreadful things inside them. Interestingly, we have a number of medics in the helminthic therapy community, many of whom are using helminths to treat their own intractable conditions. But it will no doubt be several decades before the majority of doctors open their minds to this idea.

I was forced to retire years ago due to my illness, but now that my health is so much better, I'm able to spend most of each day working, either helping others who are using helminthic therapy, or researching for the *Foods Matter* website[13] – a huge database and portal for allergy-related conditions. I've just completed a Human Helminth Care Manual explaining how people can best look after their worms, and there are many more projects waiting for me

10 http://www.nottingham.ac.uk/research/groups/clinicalneurology/trials/wirms.aspx

11 http://blog.autoimmunetherapies.com/blog/2011/05/01/ multiple-sclerosis-and-helminthic-therapy/

12 https://www.facebook.com/groups/htsupport/ / https://groups.yahoo.com/neo/groups/helminthictherapy/info

13 http://www.foodsmatter.com

to tackle. My laptop goes pretty much everywhere that I go, and I've even modified my exercise bike so that I can work on my laptop while cycling!

Myalgic encephalomyelitis is an illness with many names. Within the UK National Health Service it is commonly called Chronic Fatigue Syndrome. ME is a long term (chronic) fluctuating illness that causes symptoms affecting many body systems, more commonly the nervous and immune systems. Symptoms are persistent fatigue or pain.

(http://www.actionforme.org.uk/get-informed/about-me/what-is-me)

John Scott has written a number of articles on the Foods Matter *website http://www.foodsmatter.com*

- 300 Helminthic Therapy Success Stories for More Than 70 Different Conditions
- Helminths Give Chronic Headaches the Old Heave-ho
- Don't Let Worms Give You the Squirms!
- Hookworm Timeline
- What to Expect After Inoculating with Hookworm
- How I Maintain a Vibrant Hookworm Colony

plus

- Human Helminth Care Manual – how to protect human helminths from substances that might adversely affect them *https://www.facebook.com/groups/htsupport/652789044777054/ (requires group membership)*

John Scott's blog Gut Buddies *is at http://gut-buddies.com/wordpress/*

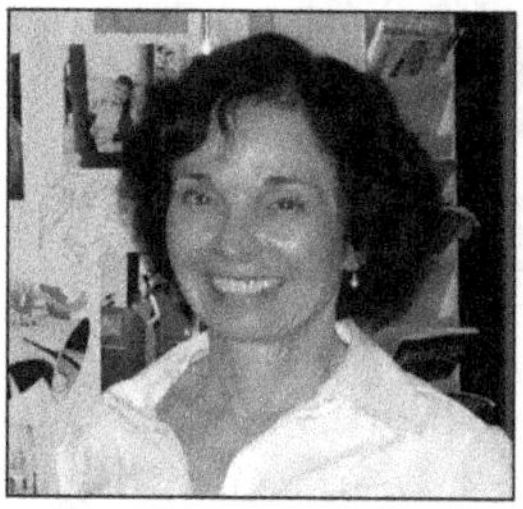

Mary Jo Siegel, 61 years

California, USA

Diagnosed with Stage IV Non-Hodgkin's Lymphoma at 40 years

I was diagnosed about 21 years ago now. I had these terrible stomach attacks, so I went to a gastroenterologist. I went through all these tests, CAT[1] scans and MRIs,[2] but nothing showed up. He told my husband that there was nothing there. Even on a blood test it didn't show up, so they were telling me and my husband that it was in my head. Someone said it was my diet. We knew it was not my diet, because we were very aware, even then, of diet. I had gone to the emergency room in pain on two separate occasions and they just sent me home. I didn't know what I had.

I went to UCLA[3] and then USC.[4] It wasn't until the third time I went to the emergency room that I was diagnosed. The doctor there suggested doing a CAT scan while I was in pain. It showed that my pain was due to a tumour that somehow only showed up while my intestine was twisting. Then they were able to do a biopsy and that's when they found out I had lymphoma. It was a low-grade lymphoma, meaning that it grows slowly, but I was told that even that was always fatal. Even though lymphoma is a blood cancer, I had tumours above and below the diaphragm, as well as in my bone marrow, so that put me at a stage IV.

I went to many lymphoma specialists, and they all told me I was going to die. I was 40 years old. I already had a distrust of doctors, so when I was diagnosed, my husband and I decided to do a lot of research, because what was prescribed for me was a bone marrow transplant. We did the research on that and it was horrible. The bone marrow transplant consisted of high-dose chemotherapy and massive radiation. The radiation would be the same as one mile from ground zero at Hiroshima. That is exactly what the doctors told me, so high-dose chemo[5] and massive radiation would attempt to save my life.

1 CAT scan, also known as a CT scan, or Computed Axial Tomography is a diagnostic medical imaging procedure that examines cross sections of the body allowing a three dimensional view of specific areas.

2 MRI – magnetic resonance imaging is a medical imaging technique used in radiology to investigate the anatomy and function of the body, using magnetic fields and radio waves to form images of the body. MRIs are widely used in hospitals for diagnosis, staging of disease and for follow-up, without exposure to radiation.

3 UCLA – University of California, Los Angeles.

4 USC – University of Southern California.

5 Chemo – chemotherapy.

They would bring me as close to death as possible and then rescue me. One out of ten people died of the procedure – and you're never the same after that. The bone marrow transplant would give me some years, but how many would depend on how I responded. I was still going to die of this disease.

They wanted me to do this procedure in Boston. My husband and I travelled there to talk to the doctor who would do it. I got to go to a transplant ward and see the people in there. I almost fainted looking into the room, because these people were in so much pain. There were three people in there who were in the foetal position with so much pain they couldn't have a blanket on them. It was a horrible sight. I made my mind up right there, that if it was my only, only hope, then I would do it.

They gave me a disclosure to sign that was a quarter of an inch thick, of all the things that could happen after this procedure. One of them was that within five years, I had a 50 per cent chance of getting another cancer.

So we decided to do some more research. It's kind of interesting – bone marrow transplants, then and now, are not FDA[6] approved. As of a few years ago, it was not approved and I'm pretty sure it's still not approved by the FDA. Doctors get insurance to pay for it.

The doctor said to me: "Don't worry about it – we'll figure it out." They wanted me so much for their research. They were very, very nice to me and my husband – I was their best friend at that point. They told me they were going to give me baseball tickets. The doctor wanted to take us to a baseball game the following night. It sounds ridiculous, but I know now that it's a research thing. They make it seem that this is your hope. I'm just so grateful that I didn't do that.

I was very fortunate – my husband was very supportive. Twenty one years ago, there was no internet, so my husband and I went to the UCLA library over and over again to learn about lymphoma and it was very scary. We poured through medical books and that's how we learned about exactly the type that I had. I knew that we couldn't just do nothing.

Somebody in my cancer support group said to me that they had heard about this Doctor Burzynski. She had stage IV ovarian cancer and had written a letter to him and asked him if he would help her. He wrote a letter back to her saying that he had not done the research on ovarian cancer yet, but told her to keep up her search. She said to me: "Look, I'm stage IV ovarian. Any quack or fraud would tell me to come on down and he did not." That told me a lot. Right after she told me that, my husband and I made an appointment and flew to Houston.

I started treatment while I was there. I came back and told my oncologist that I was doing this. He was quite upset about it, but I knew I was doing the right thing. I felt really good about Doctor Burzynski, and the treatment

6 FDA – US Food and Drug Administration is an agency of the United States Department of Health and Human Services, responsible for protecting and promoting public health.

was non-toxic. I could always do the toxic treatment if the non-toxic one didn't work. I'm talking 20 years ago (it's a little different today), but the best thing about Doctor Burzynski's treatment is that his antineoplaston treatment is absolutely non-toxic.

Antineoplastons are taken either as pills or an infusion. When I first started, I asked to go on the pills, because it was so easy, right? I was on them for three months, then the tumour in my neck started actually getting larger. I flew back to Houston and I asked Doctor Burzynski about it – you know, we got so scared. He told us that it was either the tumour breaking down, or growing. He recommended that I go onto the infusion, which I did. My very next CAT scan showed reduction. I had a catheter implanted in Houston and I took the infusion home and learned how to put the bottle into a plastic bag. It was a real procedure to do it 20 years ago and it had to be sterile. I had my own little place set up in my room and I did it twice a day. Nowadays, it comes in the plastic bag already. The work that it involved kept me busy and that was a good thing. The way I looked at it was that this was making me well, and I had to do the work, you know? Sometimes it's good for patients to do some work to get well.

I wore a fanny-pack (some people put them in a backpack) and I just lived a totally normal life, except filling the bags and all that. I was able to go swimming – I'd just tape everything up. I'm telling ya, it was just a wonderful treatment – the fact that you're not sick and throwing up with your hair falling out and all that.

I was on treatment with the IV[7] infusions for about nine months when I was pronounced "in remission". I stayed on the treatment for three months more, then I went off it. From the time I started antineoplaston treatment, every CAT scan I had showed reduction.

I had CAT scans every three months for many years. I've had way too many scans in my life. From every three months, it went to every six months, once a year and then it went to once every other year. I had my last one about three years ago. I feel that I do not want them any more, but I'll probably have one every five years or more.

Other people have benefited from antineoplastons too. One little girl was the youngest baby ever diagnosed with this brain tumour at three months old. At nine months she was crawling and her father put the fanny pack on a skateboard. It was so adorable – she would crawl around with her medicine behind her.

In the second Burzynski movie, there's a lady from the UK[8] in her twenties with a brain tumour – and they show her doing her procedures. She had the most horrible brain tumour, it was so aggressive. It gets to a certain point and then doubles every so often. The brain tumour that she had is always fatal and she is totally cancer-free right now. There's another lady from the UK on the treatment too. They're both doing so well.

7 IV – intravenous.

8 UK – United Kingdom.

Some people may think antineoplaston therapy is costly, but chemotherapy is more expensive than antineoplaston treatment. It's just that insurance will pay for chemotherapy and in most cases will not pay for antineoplaston therapy. I just talked to a man who told me that his chemotherapy is running him $60,000 a month. His insurance company is paying it, but he could never pay that.

My brother-in-law, who recently passed from melanoma, made a conscious decision – he and his wife did not to go to Doctor Burzynski because they felt they couldn't afford it. For melanoma, there's nothing out there. He tried everything, nothing worked and he went through hell. Then his doctor said to him: "There's a newly approved melanoma drug – 'Ippy'[9] for short. It was $120,000 for three injections. These three injections were not to save his life – just to give him maybe another two months. He could not afford that, but the insurance paid for it and it didn't help.

It's incredible that people bring up this argument. I do know how expensive Doctor Burzynski's treatment is, but not compared to chemotherapy. If his drug is approved, then insurance companies will have to pay for it. That is our goal.

When I was being treated, Doctor Burzynski would treat children for free when he could. Things are different these days, with all of the lawsuits he's been through, but the money that he makes goes back into his research.

There was a trial in 1995. Even before the trial, there were hearings where the Texas State Medical Board would call Doctor Burzynski and bring him before the board. I do not work for the clinic, but my husband and I set up our own website. We decided to organise the patients, because we felt he needed some support.

If you could see all the people that antineoplaston treatment has already helped, it just isn't right that the FDA says, "You can have it," or, "no, you can't have it." It's arbitrary and it's horrible, so we're going to get the word out to everybody. I thank God every day that I found Doctor Burzynski.

Mary Jo Siegel continues to work on her website http://www.burzynskipatient-group.org

Burzynski – The Movie *was awarded the Humanitarian Vision Award at the Newport Beach Film Festival in 2010. It is available on Netflix, or free on http://www.burzyn-skipatientgroup.org*

A second movie, Burzynski – Cancer is Serious Business, *was released in 2013.*

www.burzynskiapt.org is a website that was created by patients who have achieved remission with targeted drug protocols from the Burzynski Clinic.

9 Ipilimumab, marketed as *Yervoy*, is an FDA-approved drug used for the treatment of cancer, including melanoma. It works by activating the immune system.

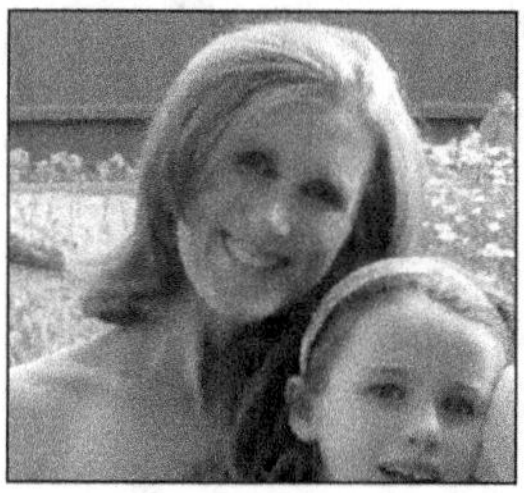

Debra Surman, 43 years

Australian Capital Territory, Australia

Life-long asthma and sinusitis

I've had asthma since I was very young. As a child I was in and out of hospital a lot for severe asthma, in the pre-*Ventolin*[10] days, when there really wasn't much medication available for children. I was given an inhaled medication for children called *Intal*.[11] Then *Ventolin* came along and after that, the first wave of steroid preventers.

Dust mites and animal hair are particularly bad allergens for me, and some environments are worse than others. I was on inhalant steroids from my early teens, or maybe a bit younger. I grew up in Brisbane – the whole time I lived in Brisbane, I used the preventer.

In my early twenties, I moved to Asia. All of the time I lived there I didn't need any asthma medication at all. I put it down to a climate that was hot, humid and very constant. I'm always well in those types of environments. Later, when we moved to Canberra, my asthma symptoms got completely out of control. They were seasonal and very severe. My allergies caused sneezing, sinusitis and bad asthma.

I was spending a lot of money on medications – about one hundred dollars per month. The change of seasons was when I was most vulnerable, and the onset of winter was just disastrous. I was using a general anti-allergy tablet, a high-dose inhaler that combined a preventer and Ventolin in a single spray, plus a nasal spray for sinus. I really detested the amount of medication I was taking and it wasn't always keeping my asthma under control anyway.

Because I've had asthma all my life, I know how to manage it fairly well. It was certainly not life-threatening, so I don't want to be extreme, but having chest tightness all the time drove me insane. It impeded my physical activity level, which I found distressing. I wasn't depressed, but was certainly down psychologically, having to treat myself to the extent that I was. Steroid medications leave you with a dry mouth and there are lots of other effects.

I can't remember what the words were that really caught my eye when I saw an advertisement for a Buteyko course in the local paper. At the time, we were

10 *Ventolin* is the trade name for salbutamol, a bronchodilator drug that is inhaled to enhance breathing during asthmatic wheezing.

11 *Intal* is the trade name for cromoglicic acid, which is an inhalant drug that prevents the release of inflammatory chemicals like histamine to reduce the allergic response to asthma.

actually thinking about moving away from Canberra with our two children, who were five and seven years old, because I felt so sick all the time. That's pretty drastic isn't it? I felt that I would do better living closer to the coast, because inland there are more extreme changes of temperature.

Initially, I did the Buteyko course because I was quite desperate about finding something that would make me feel better. I was very sceptical at first and didn't really believe that it would work. I had not breathed through my nose for my entire life, so it was hard to believe the whole idea that: "anyone can breathe through their nose". At the same time, it was such a carrot for me. What if I really could breathe through my nose? Before I was even half-way through the course, I knew that it would change my life.

Prior to the course, I had a consultation with a Buteyko practitioner. She showed me some exercises to help me to breathe through my nose, so I had practised that before I did the course. By that time, I was quite eager.

The course goes for five days and it's quite intensive, because you have to practice the method three times a day at home, but I was 110 per cent committed.

My capacity to be able to breathe through my nose and fill my lungs did take a while. I can tell, because I'm a runner. When I first started, I couldn't really run with my mouth closed.

By the time I finished the five-day course, I was pretty much asymptomatic. I was holding my breath for up to a minute at a time, which is what you're aiming for. I was using carbon dioxide to relax my airways quite efficiently.

After the course, I reduced my medication over a six-week period. During that six weeks, I slowly discarded the *Ventolin* and steroid combination medication and I used only a preventer. Then I slowly cut that down.

I have not taken *Ventolin* in the two years since I did the Buteyko course. If I ever have severe asthma, I've learned to use a preventer to manage my acute symptoms rather than *Ventolin*, which is a stimulant. The way *Ventolin* acts is not aligned with Buteyko. In Buteyko, you try to calm the asthma attack by relaxing the smooth muscle in your lungs. Even though *Ventolin* does open your airways, it actually doesn't relax the muscles. If you give the preventers a chance, they actually do the same job as *Ventolin*, but they just take longer.

Now, I only use a preventer maybe twice a year for three or four days each time. I went from spending one hundred dollars a month at the pharmacy to zero. I don't take any medication now! It has been an incredible success and it has literally changed my life.

There are a lot of smaller health benefits of not mouth breathing – I don't have a dry mouth anymore. I sleep in a different way and breathe through my nose, which is beneficial for my dental health. If anything happens to my nose and it blocks up, I know how to unblock it. I haven't exercised with my mouth open for two years.

Imagine being on medication for your entire life for a condition that you were told: "You were born with it, you'll always have it and you'll always need medication for it." I was 41 by the time I did this course. For 41 years I didn't breathe correctly. I had never had the experience of being able to control my breathing, to breathe through my nose or use breathing to heal myself. Now I can do all of those things and I'm really healthy.

I still practice the Buteyko technique, mostly through the exercise I do. When you exercise with your mouth closed you're practicing Buteyko, because you're building carbon dioxide levels in your bloodstream – it's the carbon dioxide that acts as a smooth muscle relaxant. The only time I consciously practice Buteyko is when I feel any chest tightness, which I can get when I've been talking a lot (you lose a lot of carbon dioxide when you're talking), when I've been sick, or when there's a change of season, which is when my asthma usually becomes acute again.

I don't know what the statistics are on asthma, but the proportion of asthmatics in Australia is so high. Imagine if even half of those people could have the same results that I've had – Buteyko could help so many people. We need to ask really powerful questions, because I am a life-long chronic asthmatic who's had my life completely changed. Why hasn't someone picked this up?

My asthma is not cured. I still get seasonal asthma, but I manage it by practising a *natural breathing method* – that's very different for me. I was not a slight asthmatic, I was a severe asthmatic. The enormity of managing it without medication just leaves me breathless.

For me, there's a place for a standard GP[12] who gives medical advice and then there is a role in my life for natural remedies as well. I don't have a prejudice against either.

I wish that I had exposure to something like Buteyko 20 years ago. I'm fitter now and I exercise better. Prior to Buteyko, if I had a bad session of asthma, it affected my immune system, because I was more likely to get sick. I have also made some nutritional changes. I actually can't remember the last time I was really sick. For me it's been so fantastic.

Now I'm the biggest advocate of Buteyko – I tell everybody about it. When anyone talks about asthma or sinus, I literally say: "You have to go and do a Buteyko course!" Every asthmatic in the world should do one.

The Buteyko Institute Method (BIM) is a breathing training program which may provide significant improvement of symptoms for many people with asthma, sleep disordered breathing and other breathing-related conditions. The Buteyko Institute Method is scientifically based on the standard medical principles of respiration, the normalisation of breathing and the Bohr[13] effect. (http://www.buteyko.info)

12 GP – general practitioner.

13 Bohr effect – Danish physiologist Christian Bohr described haemoglobin's oxygen binding affinity during respiration in 1904, where increased carbon dioxide concentration results in haemoglobin proteins releasing oxygen and vice-versa.

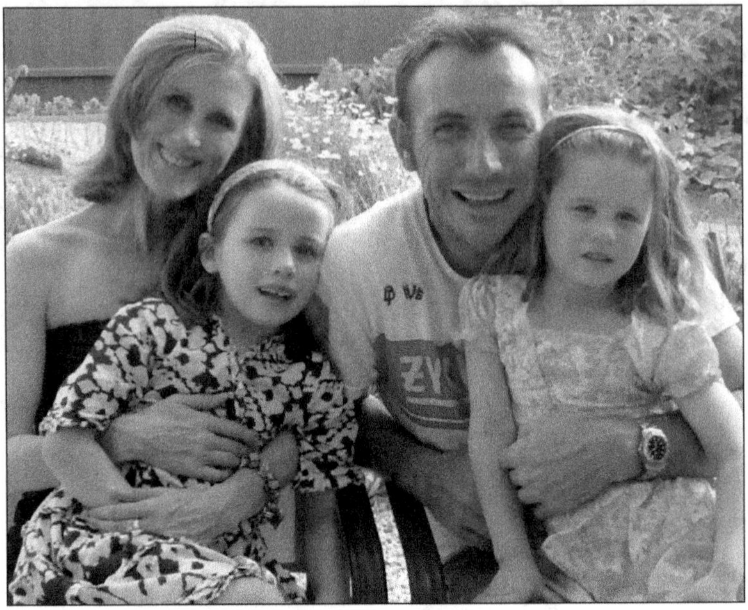

Debra Surman with her husband and two daughters.

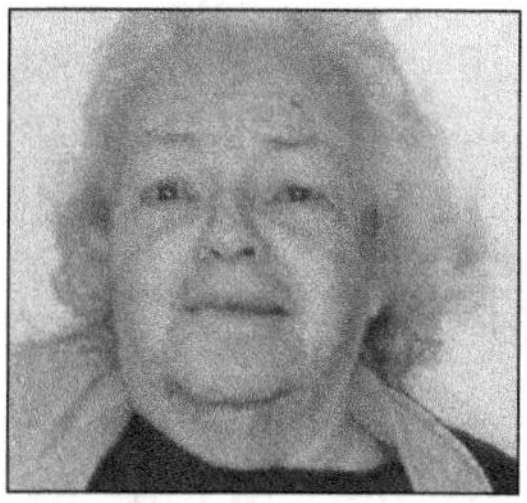

Arlene Van Straten, 77 years

Shiocton, Wisconsin, USA

Diagnosed with pancreatic cancer and liver metastases at 46 years

Well, I had three jobs and five kids, so I was a busy girl. One night I had fixed supper, sat down to eat and I ate too much – I ended up in the bathroom at two o'clock in the morning. I got the shakes and I couldn't quit shaking. I got my husband out of bed and he took me to the hospital. I was there 17 days, didn't eat anything and I never lost a pound. They couldn't figure out what was the matter, so they told me they were going to operate to remove my gall bladder and I would have a four-inch incision on my right side.

They didn't remove my gallbladder, because they found lumps on the liver – now I have a 19-inch railroad track across my belly. When I came out, I asked: "What is the matter with my stomach? It hurts so bad." They said, "Well, you'll have to talk to your doctor." I said, "Well, what time will he be in?" They said, "About 5.30 this afternoon," and this was at 9.30 in the morning.

When they came back at about five o'clock in the afternoon, the doctor told me: "Do you know what an organ looks like?" I said, "Well, of course." "Well," he said, "Your pancreas is like a wet sponge." I said, "Meaning what?" He said: "Well, you've got cancer in it and it's metastasised to your liver." Of course, they had taken biopsies of both, and my doctor informed me that I had six months to live. Well, I was mad.

When I was in hospital I was so bored. My doctor came in and I said: "I've got a bone to pick with you, just sitting in this hospital. That's for the ill. I need permission to get out and walk – this is driving me nuts." He said: "You can't do that." I said: "Why can't I? I'm not doing anything here. You let me walk in the halls – why can't I walk outside?" He thought about it for a couple of days and came back and said: "Permission granted – but you can't be any more than an hour away." I said: "I won't be." So I'd go out and I'd walk for a couple of hours and I'd come back. You've gotta do something, other than sitting in a hospital. I wasn't ill.

When I came out of Appleton, I went to a doctor in Marshfield who ran all kinds of tests, just like they'd done in Appleton. He also told me I had six months to live and that I should go home, have a nice vacation, and enjoy what good days I had left. Now I was really pissed. I came home from Marshfield, then I got on the phone to Mayos[1] in Minnesota. It takes eight weeks to get an appointment out there. I got an appointment and they did all the testing and X-rays that everybody else did, and told me that now I had three months to live. I was supposed to go home and put my financial affairs in order. I said to the doctor on the way out: "You know, I've got just one thing to say to you. Only the good die young, so I'm going to stick around a long time. You haven't begun to see how angry this gal can get." He shrugged his shoulders and walked out.

Well, there was no help. There's no chemo,[2] no radiation – nothing will help the liver. So what do you do? I had three jobs and five kids, but I found time to go shopping and went to the healthfood store and found a book for three dollars. The name of it was *One Answer to Cancer* and it was written by a Doctor Kelley. There was this Doctor Kelley in Grapevine, Texas. So I called him and asked them about an appointment. The girl on the other end said: "Well, just hang on a second." Then she came back and said: "You don't have to come to Grapevine. We have an office in each state that works with us." Who it was in Wisconsin, was Doctor James Kolmer, a chiropractor at Stevens Point, so she gave me his phone number. When I called him, he said: "We'll see you tomorrow at ten o'clock in the morning."

So we went to Stevens Point. He saw me come down the hall and he said: "You are not going to die from cancer." I said: "Well, that's what they told me," and he said: "They don't know what they're talking about. You do what you're told to do, and you're going to live a long life." Just like that. He proceeded to do some blood work and got me to fill in the book that had – I'm going to say, hundreds of questions. I never did count them, but the book was an inch and a quarter thick and there was everything in there from: "Did I have ridges in my fingernails?" to: "Did I have callouses on the bottom of my feet?" and: "Was I having trouble with my eyes?" Just one thing after another and everything pertained to something. I don't have a clue what, but it all did. I went back with the blood work, samples and he mailed it in to Doctor Kelley in Texas. In about two weeks, I got the book back from him, it had a list of the pills I was going to take – how many a day and all the rest of it, the foods I was supposed to be eating, recipes, how to cook it and how to fix it.

I was to take 357 pills a day and there was not even an aspirin in it. You're talking about volumes of pills. They were all vitamins and minerals. You name it and it was in there. I was taking 10,000 units a day of vitamin C and there were 90 pancreatic enzymes a day – they did the work of the pancreas so it could heal itself. There was also $1,800 for the pills. I paid that only once and they were cheaper after the first time. There was a discussion with my husband and I said: "Well, I'll take it out of savings this time and I'll put the money back – I'll work it off. If it don't help, I won't order them no more. If it helps, you won't be able to stop me."

1 The Mayo Clinic is a not-for-profit medical practice and medical research group based in Rochester, Minnesota.

2 Chemo - chemotherapy.

I never took chemo, never had no radiation. They said it wasn't going to do any good, so I made up my mind – I didn't need either one of them. I said: "Me and the good Lord – this is between us. If I'm meant to be around, I'll be here. If I'm not, I won't."

By the time them pills were about three weeks in, I could eat without throwing up and I had energy up the kazoo. I was working 20 hours a day out of 24. I helped people remodel their houses, I helped old women – I went in and fixed their curtains for them. I did landscaping, helped buy a couple of houses, bought furniture for houses and re-did the rectory, which hadn't been painted in years. The furniture there was really crass, so I had to buy furniture for there too.

My husband's aunt was a nun, and she got the whole Franciscan nunnery down there praying for me. We had a real good friend that was a priest, and he started saying Mass every day for me too. I told the good Lord: "I can do a lot of good down here – I can't do nothing upstairs, so if you need me here, tell me what you want me to do and I'm open."

I was never sick in bed – only the good die young! My youngest daughter is deaf and I did a bus route for handicapped kids. We had a wholesale ice business as well as a gas station that I did the bookwork for, and I ran the work crew, so I had my hands full. I never did quit working – I just slowed down some.

Every six months I had to go back and have blood redrawn and then they would re-evaluate and send me back the pills. People would look at me take my 357 pills and say: "Where do you find time to do that?" And I would say: "Lady, if I don't take them pills, I will have nothing but time, because I'll be dead."

I was on the pills for five years, then Doctor Kelley disappeared. I didn't know where, why, or how, but he was gone – unavailable. No telephone, mail – nothing. I found out that the medical association had run him out of Texas and he went underground. They came in with guns and started taking files and papers and saying: "You're going to be out." I couldn't find him anywhere in the United States. Five years I was on them pills and I couldn't get any more.

I was watching television one day and I heard this name, 'Nicholas Gonzalez', and I thought: "I recognise that name." Doctor Kelley's understudy was Doctor Nick Gonzalez. I listened to it – it was from New York. When I called him he recognised my name because I had signed a piece of paper years ago that gave him permission to use my story in a book. He said: "Well, I haven't gotten to writing the book yet." I said: "What's taking you so long?" He said: "Well, you know how it goes." I said: "No, I don't know how it goes, so where is it?"

I never went back to a doctor – I felt so good I just kept going and kept working. I'd go back and see Jim Kolmer and kept in contact with Nick Gonzalez. When Nick called to see how I was doing, I'd say: "Fat'n-tastic." He said: "Well, that's good." And I said" "No it's not. I weigh 230 pounds and I'm afraid to go on a diet because I don't want to screw up my pancreas." I didn't know what to or what not to do, or just to die fat.

I'm healthy as a horse. I eat good and I retain my food. The last time I had blood work was five years ago. My only other health problem is that I'm fat. When I had cancer, I weighed 220 pounds. Now I'm 231 pounds so in thirty years I've put on 11 pounds.

Between you and me and the gatepost, I know that there's four kinds of cancer that chemo would help, but they use it on everybody. All it is, is money. They don't do it for somebody's good, they do it for money. The health program in the United States is an abyss – it's a mess.

When you go to the doctors and they tell you that there's nothing they can do – no chemo, no radiation, nothing's going to help – where do you go next? You're going to die? I didn't like that option. If that's what my options are, I'm going to try something else. I wasn't done with life – I hadn't seen none of my grandkids.

Now, I have to tell you, I have 14 beautiful grandchildren. Most of them have graduated from college. The baby of that crew is 22 and studying audiology – her mother is my daughter who's deaf.

When you've been given six months to live, it's better to take matters into your own hands. I'm not saying you should disobey your doctor, but I'm not saying you're supposed to believe him either. It ain't the doctor that's going to be the result of your demise, it's going to be you.

Comment from Doctor Nick Gonzalez:

I've known Arlene Van Straten now since 1986, when I first interviewed her by phone as part of my investigation of Doctor William Donald Kelley's therapy and patients. At that point, she had already survived for four years with stage IV pancreatic cancer – a remarkable survival even then, with biopsy-proven liver metastases all confirmed at the Mayo Clinic in Rochester, Minnesota.

Told she had no conventional options that would be of any use to her, she searched for an alternative approach and managed to find a copy of Doctor Kelley's 1969 book *One Answer to Cancer* at a local healthfood store. The rest is history. Under the guidance of a wonderful local chiropractor in Wisconsin trained by Doctor Kelley, Arlene began the Kelley nutritional therapy and survived. She continues to survive, now more than 31 years from her original diagnosis.

I remember so well my first conversation with her – she was smart, feisty, determined and had no use for the conventional medical doctors who told her she would be lucky to live six months. She has proven them all wrong, following her own instincts and ignoring their dire predictions, to her life-saving benefit. Today, she remains as feisty as ever, though she might be slowing down just a bit.

How unusual a patient is Arlene? As an academic researcher at heart, with a particular interest in pancreatic cancer, I follow the conventional literature on the disease closely. To this day, I have been unable to find a single similar case in the world's literature, of a 31-plus year survivor of stage IV pancreatic cancer, with biopsy-proven liver metastases. Not a one, other than Arlene. She is truly unique, truly that remarkable, and remains a credit to Doctor Kelley and his nutritional approach to cancer.

To put her case in perspective, in 1998, the FDA[3] approved the chemotherapeutic drug *Gemzar* for the treatment of pancreatic cancer, based on a controlled clinical study of 126 patients. Not one of these patients lived longer than 19 months, yet the one-month improvement in average survival over previous chemotherapy, from 4.5 months to 5.6 months, was considered such an "advance", the FDA approved the drug, which is now a billion dollar a year industry. Meanwhile, Kelley's successful but unconventional treatment has never achieved any mainstream recognition.

Patients like Arlene make my work today wonderful and we continue to see many successes with this specific and terrible disease, as well as with cancer in general. Certainly, Arlene deserves credit for ignoring the experts and choosing her own path and Kelley deserves credit for his contribution to cancer treatment.

Nicholas Gonzalez, MD
New York, February 2014

Doctor Nicholas Gonzalez has been investigating nutritional approaches to cancer and other degenerative diseases since 1981, and has been in practice in New York since 1987. Doctor Linda Isaacs has been working with Doctor Gonzalez in his practice since 1985. They use aggressive and individualised nutritional protocols to work with many types of cancer and other illnesses such as allergies, autoimmune disorders and chronic fatigue. Lectures by Doctor Gonzalez about his work and research are available at http://www.dr-gonzalez.com

3 FDA – US Food and Drug Administration is an agency of the United States Department of Health and Human Services, responsible for protecting and promoting public health.

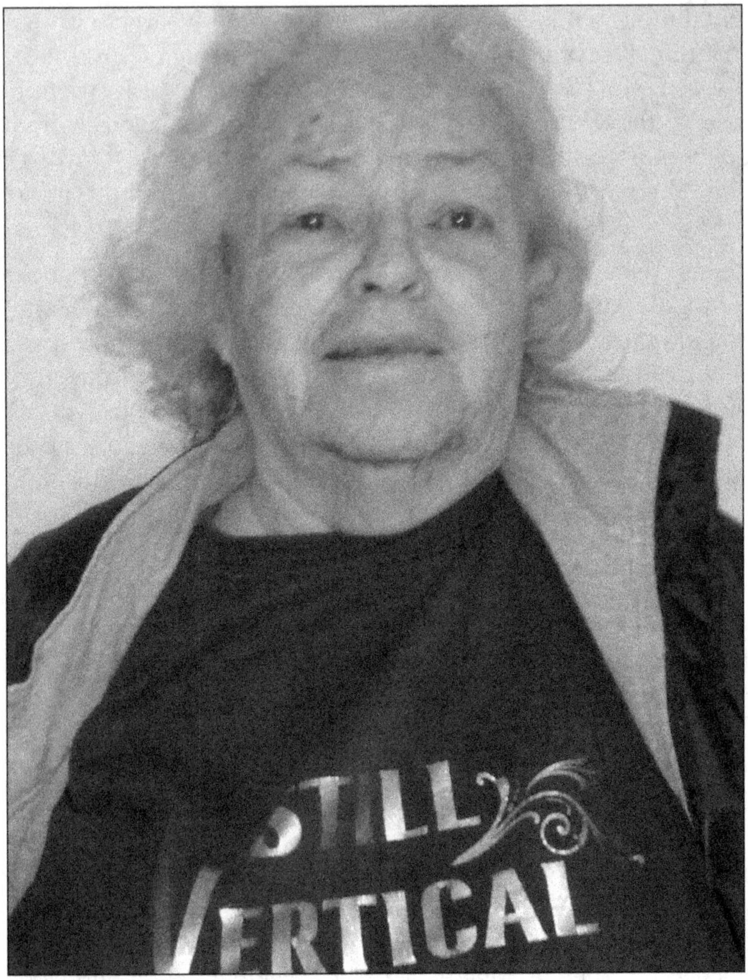

Arlene Van Straten, 77, the longest known surviving pancreatic cancer patient in the world.

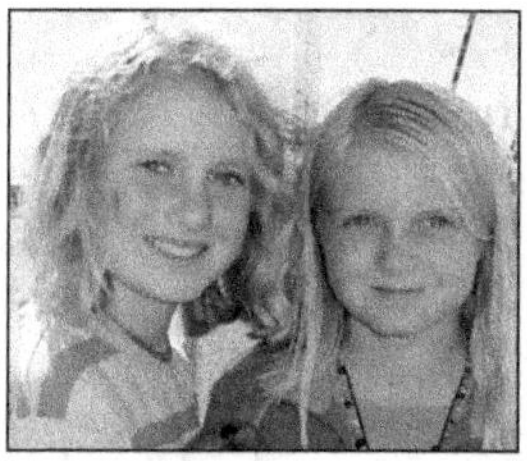

Alice and Annie Walker

Hamilton, New Zealand

Alice, diagnosed with autism at 2 years
Annie, diagnosed with kryptopyroluria at 5 years

Interview with Sam Walker, Alice and Annie's mother

Alice is my first child and she was always a little bit different from other kids. At our coffee group (a group of mums who met at antenatal classes, still going 12 years later), she would always be the child who didn't need her mum, whereas all the other kids were more clingy.

She did everything out of sync compared to normal children. At seven weeks of age, she was sitting up in a high chair, holding a carrot and pretending to chew it – we just couldn't believe it. When she was only a few months old, she would pick up the phone and say: "Daddy, hello." We would think: "Gosh, you can't really talk." She didn't crawl, but walked very confidently at nine months.

When people offered to look after Alice for an hour, I'd say: "Well, you need to do all these things..." They'd say: "Don't be so silly. I've had three children and I know what I'm doing." Then within seconds there was chaos, because Alice was different.

When she was nine months old, at her first Christmas, we gave her a plastic pizza tray, with velcro, so she could 'cut' it. She loved it, but then she had no interest in anything else. She was an only child, so we gave her lots of presents. I had wrapped all these presents and then I had to unwrap them all. On her birthdays, if something arrived in the post a day or two later she would say: "No Mummy, it's not my birthday. Save it until next year, when it's my birthday," or she would say things like: "No thank you, I've had a birthday present, I don't need anymore."

When Alice was about 18 months, we went to South Africa. While we were there, she lost all her words, then she gained all these new words. Then when we went back to England, she lost all those words. That's what would keep happening – she'd have words, then she would just lose them again.

The child minder she went to said to me one day: "Do you think there's anything wrong with Alice?" I said: "Yes, there's something different about her, but I don't know what you would call it." Then, at 18 months, she asked me directly what I thought was wrong with her. I told her that she didn't play with her toys – she lined them up, or stacked them. Also, she would only watch one video, *Noddy*, over and over again and had no interest in television. When I asked her what she thought, she said: "Autism."

I dashed her down to the doctor (her diagnosis was done in England). First of all, they test for deafness. I took her to a private doctor, because I was so desperate for an answer. He asked me if she could point, which she definitely could, so he said: "Well, she cannot have autism." Of course, I went away, saying: "Oh, that's fine then." Very poor, after the appointment.

When Alice was 18 months old, we made the decision to have her MMR[1] vaccination done. If you look at her photographs as a very young baby, you've got happy, happy, happy. Then from the day she had her vaccine – bam, all her photos change. She goes from happy and smiling, to a blank face.

Unfortunately, at the same time as the MMR, she developed chicken pox. She had the worst chicken pox that the doctors had ever seen and they almost hospitalised her. I talked to Paul Shattock[2] from the University of Sunderland, who tested her urine for gluten and dairy a couple of times. He said that the viral overload from the chicken pox, plus the MMR, along with a genetic disposition, tipped her over into autism. There is definitely a genetic disposition in the family, even though no-one in other generations has had a diagnosis.

Her autism really was full-blown. During the day, Alice could run around talking, but as soon as five o'clock came, her arms would move strangely and she would lose all her words, so that there was no speech at all. Her arms would be flailing and all she could say was: "Arrrgh, arrrgh." If she had an accident or got stressed, she lost her words and couldn't communicate at all.

It took six months to get Alice diagnosed. Between eighteen months and two years, she was assessed twice by an autism specialist at the Royal Berkshire Hospital in Reading, where she got her formal diagnosis of Autistic Spectrum Disorder. She was two years and two days old. The paediatrician just said to me: "This is the number of the Autism Society. They might put you in touch with a support group, but there's nothing you can really do." It was like: "Bye-bye, that's it."

I was one of those parents who just went: "Thank God I know what it is, because now I can deal with it." I set-to on the internet and found out what I could do. I found an incredible nutritionist who had just trained with Patrick Holford in London. She did a blood test, which came back saying that Alice needed to be on a gluten-free and dairy-free diet. She put Alice on Aloe Vera, probiotics and a number of supplements. We were pretty much dairy-free anyway, because my father has Crohn's disease (which is linked to autism). I don't react to milk well either, so we had very little dairy in the house. That didn't freak me out, but gluten-free was new.

---

1 MMR – measles, mumps and rubella vaccine.

2 Research by Paul Shattock and Kalle Reichelt, MD, led to the widespread use of the gluten-free, casein-free diet in treating autism as a metabolic disorder. See end note.

I'm not the kind of parent to go in slowly, so it was all-out. All gluten and all dairy were gone immediately. After three days of hell, we had a different child. Alice was more alert – she was 'with' us and she was completely different.

We were still getting meltdowns though. Although we lived a vegetarian, organic lifestyle, we didn't know enough about colours and additives. There were some gluten-free, dairy-free sweets we used to buy her and she would go absolutely off the scale within minutes of having them. She would cry and you couldn't get through to her, like the naughtiest toddler you can imagine. It was my ex-husband who noticed the connection.

We realised there was no point in disciplining Alice traditionally. When she was two, she was very difficult to walk with. By this time, I had a baby as well, so I had to employ a nanny, because I couldn't safely walk with both of them in the street. Once, when I had taken them swimming on my own, Alice ran off in a carpark. All carparks are bad, but English ones are particularly terrible. I grabbed hold of her hand and I smacked her bottom and I said: "You mustn't do that!" She just looked at me really seriously and said: "Why did you smack me?" There was no association between the fact that she'd just run off and done something that I perceived to be naughty. At that point, I realised there was no benefit whatsoever in disciplining this child like other parents did and she never got a smack again. She was on her own planet – 'Planet Alice', we called it.

Between two and three years, we were doing the diet and some supplements, but were still struggling with her speech. We did an EarlyBird[3] programme with the National Autistic Society,[4] which taught us how to speak to her so she understood every word. If we wanted her to put her coat on, we'd say: "Alice, come." We would wait until she came to us and then say: "Alice, coat." You'd give her one instruction, wait until she'd done it and then move on. I remember going to a party when she was about four years old and this woman turned to me and said: "Why do you talk to your child like a dog?" I burst into tears and ran home. The doctor had given me antidepressants and I started taking them that day. It was awful to be judged like that for doing what we thought was right.

Along with the EarlyBird programme, an autism lady would come around to help her. At preschool, she had a worker to help, and we used to do *Makaton*,[5] the sign language. When we were out, the noise was often too much, but you could say in *Makaton*: "Alice, careful. Alice, do you want to go to the toilet?" Or, "It's time to go home." The actions were what she could understand. We also had her doing picture cards and we made a picture timetable for each day. Preschool and the nanny also did that, so everybody was helping.

As well as being on the full gluten-free, casein-free diet, Alice was having lots

3 EarlyBird is for parents of children with an autism spectrum disorder (ASD) of pre-school age http://www.autism.org.uk/earlybird

4 National Autistic Society http://www.autism.org.uk

5 *Makaton* is a language programme designed to provide a means of communication for people who cannot communicate well by speaking.

of supplements. She couldn't take them as tablets, so they were all broken into non-dairy yoghurts. One doctor in England eventually let us have gluten-free products on prescription. People with coeliac disease are entitled to this, but not children who haven't had a bowel biopsy. He thought I was completely neurotic. It was like he didn't believe that my children were autistic – he didn't have a clue. It became: "I just want to get rid of your family – you are too much," so he finally gave me a prescription. Before we travelled to South Africa, I asked him if there was anything I could give Alice to keep her calm. His reply was: 'If you're calm, your child will be calm."

As long as she stayed on her diet and supplements and wasn't given any food colourings, Alice was pretty much as normal as other kids and we considered that she was recovered. She was doing music, ballet classes and swimming lessons. None of her teachers had any problems with her, or knew she was different. We had to still do a lot of planning and prepare food ahead of time, but as long as we prepared Alice, we didn't have problems.

We had to do a lot of role-modelling though. When we moved house, there was preparation involved, like driving her to the new house every week. When we emigrated, we drove her to Heathrow airport and took her to the big simulation area where you pretend to go through the X-ray area and sit in the chairs on the plane.

The only thing we couldn't get quite right was her sleep. We had to have a massive routine from four o'clock in the afternoon onwards and that couldn't really change. Every six months, my ex-husband and I would have to go to a hotel around the corner – literally, to get a night's sleep. Before we left, we'd have to write a timetable in pictures and at the bottom we'd have to show: "Mummy and Daddy are coming home." Otherwise, she'd think we were never coming back again. We had a very restricted lifestyle, but if we kept to our timetable, we had a relatively normal life.

Between ages three and four, Alice went through patches where she didn't talk. Riding for the Disabled[6] took her on and we went horse riding each Wednesday for one hour. After horse riding, Alice would talk non-stop all the way home and it was a one-hour journey. She would tell me everything about the week, all her news, what was going through her head – it would all come out. As the week went on, her talking would wear off again. Horse riding was the biggest thing for this child. Now, she rides every week, but if she goes through a bad patch, we say: "Right, you're going to the horses."

There's something magical about horses and autistic kids. I'm the sort of mum who will try anything and I'd heard about horse riding helping. It was just incredible to watch. From no speech, going horse riding, then bam, talking all

6 Riding for the Disabled (RDA) is a worldwide movement represented internationally by the Federation of Horses in Education and Therapy International (HETI). It is a charitable organisation which provides opportunities for anyone with a disability to enjoy safe, healthy, stimulating, therapeutic horse riding and horse-related activities.

the way home. Riding for the Disabled was one of the most crucial elements to bring Alice from her world to the world that the rest of us live in. There was an autistic boy who did horse riding with Alice who it didn't make much difference to, but he wasn't doing the diet. A combination of therapies helped us.

When she was a baby, Alice's nappies were different – a lot of autistic kids have diarrhoea. It wasn't severe, but she was constipated. She had chiropractic treatment or cranial osteopathy every week. Both helped her and everything became more normal. Her constipation improved, she slept better and had a better disposition – she was happier all round. There was no way I would have paid to go every week if I hadn't noticed a difference. When things physically improved, there were mental improvements as well, and we started to get the words. Whether it was the motion of horse riding, going to the chiropractor, or swimming, there was always a difference when we'd done something physical.

She needed to run a lot. One of the key reasons for us moving to New Zealand was to buy a place with space. That gave her the opportunity to keep running and keep being physical. Alice and her younger sister Annie are both very physical children – they're always outside running around. They're not TV addicts and it really does make a difference. They have an old-fashioned children's joy in running around with chickens and dogs and cats. That simple joy and exercise every single day really does benefit them. They very rarely get sick.

When we came to New Zealand, Alice was four years and nine months old and a very happy, normal child. My ex-husband came over to set up the house and I followed a month later with a three and a four-year-old. That's an aeroplane journey I won't forget in a hurry. I had all their special food and three carry-on bags. At Heathrow airport, something got into Alice's eyes and that was it – she cried and cried and it was absolute chaos. The airlines were supposed to help me, but they didn't. We got to Singapore and I just needed sleep, so I booked into the hotel there for six hours. I was so tired I just fell asleep and I thought the kids would too. It was Christmas time and I had taken a whole lot of Christmas presents to keep them amused on the journey, all of which involved glitter. When I woke up, they had glued and glittered the whole room.

When we got to our house in Hamilton, we just had to eat whatever we could get. There were additives in everything – it was terrible. Even a packet of crisps contained dairy, wheat and additives. In England, crisps were potato, oil and salt, and you could give your kids a treat when you were out. I still struggle here with the food.

The first six weeks in New Zealand was hell. I watched their behaviour start to dissolve. Alice went backwards first of all, with tantrums, not sleeping, in her own world, not understanding and just running around. Then Annie went backwards. They both fell apart and went into their own worlds. Everything was unfamiliar, I didn't know where to get things from, or where practitioners were.

What I did then was sit on the computer and research. I could research for 18 hours a day. I remember sitting in my kitchen one night, with a very large gin and tonic, tears pouring down my face, saying: "This is the state I'm in – this is what has happened to my daughters. I don't know what to do now." What happened to them was horrific.

I found the Autism Biomedical Group[7] in Australia and it saved my life. I got support through knowledge – finding products and finding practitioners. I also attended the MINDD[8] Forum in 2007, which introduced me to lots of wonderful people who were to become crucial in helping me with my children's health.

One of the first people I found through that group was a general practitioner in New Zealand who treated autism. She sent me a list of trained practitioners and I found a doctor who was just six kilometres up the road. Even though his practice was full and he wasn't taking on any new patients, he allowed Alice and the rest of the family to join his surgery. He had an interest in biomedical treatment for autism and Alice was one of the first children with autism that he treated. He went over and above what you would expect of a doctor. He was always there for us, and still is.

This doctor really transformed Alice, by getting rid of gut parasites and all these things that hadn't shown up as an issue in England. Between him and a paediatrician here in New Zealand who treats autism, Alice had a lot of blood tests, stool tests and urine tests. She was tested for so many things. They went through it step-by-step, giving her what she needed.

She had an X-ray of her abdomen to see if she had faecal impaction – which she did, so she was given laxatives. We tightened up the diet, introduced bone broths and fermented foods. We took away all the phenolic foods[9] for a while, then reintroduced them very slowly. The supplements – oh my God, the supplements she had to take were just astronomical.

By the time Alice had turned five, she had given up talking again. She had a lot of mercury, lead and arsenic[10] showing up in her tests, so we were trying to get those heavy metals out of her system. We used bentonite clay baths, which were brilliant. What a difference when Alice had a clay bath. We also used detoxifying foot patches to get rid of her heavy metals. The first night I used the foot patches on Alice, she literally got up the next morning and started talking. It was like she had been storing words. She was speaking in sentences even more than age appropriate. My younger daughter, Annie, and I also put the foot patches on, but we woke up feeling really sick with terrible headaches. For us, they pulled too much out too fast, but for Alice they were fantastic. I

7 Biomedical Autism Group is an Australian email forum majoring on biomedical protocols and treatments for children who have autism and those who are somewhere on the spectrum; ADD, ADHD, PDD-NOS, Aspergers.

8 *MINDD Foundation* (Metabolic, Immunologic, Neurologic, Digestive Disorders) www.mindd.org

9 Studies by Doctor Rosemary Waring, PhD, revealed that many children with ADD/ADHD and autism are deficient in the PST enzyme (phenol sulfotransferase). In the late 1960s, Doctor Benjamin Feingold, MD, discovered that after eliminating all artificial phenols, plus naturally high phenol fruits and vegetables, up to 50 per cent of children with allergies and ADHD significantly improved.

10 Mercury, lead and arsenic are heavy metals that are toxic and affect brain function.

forgot the crucial lesson: 'Go low, go slow.'

We did foot patches and bentonite baths at the same time. Alice's brain was working better and she was so much more alert. She was less confused and could follow instructions more easily. Whenever I meet parents with autistic kids who are struggling to speak, I say to them: "You've got to invest fifty dollars in these foot patches and try them," because for me, it was one of those miracle things that happened.

Infra-red saunas were phenomenal too. After two terms of saunas, she was just incredible. She needs to be in the sauna for the full half-hour to break a sweat, but what a difference when she does it. This child has gone from never wanting to read a book, refusing to even do the ten minutes reading for school at night, to walking along the street with her nose in a book. She devours books now. About a month ago, after she had been having saunas twice a week, I said: "You know Alice, I don't think there's one little bit of autism left in you – I can't think of anything." She said, "I know, Mummy."

We saw a chiropractor and a homeopath every month. We also had an autism assistance dog who helped Alice with social skills and to reduce her anxiety when we were out. We were doing six nights a week of Epsom Salts baths[11] and one night a week of bentonite clay baths.

Now that Alice is 11, she'll actually verbalise what she wants. She'll say to me: "Mummy, I need my bentonite clay bath now, I've started to get confused again. I feel better when I've had it." Plus, the other day she said to me: "Stop, Mummy, you've just given me too many instructions and I'm getting muddled up. So hang on a minute – what was the first thing you wanted me to do?" How brilliant that she can manage herself and say: "Whoa there, lady!"

When we see the signs of autism creeping back, it will be because she's very tired – at the end of the school year usually. She has a very strict bedtime routine, because she needs 11 hours sleep a night – still. If she hasn't had her 11 hours sleep for a few days running, then we notice symptoms coming back. If she's been exposed to gluten, because the other kids haven't been careful enough, or someone accidentally gave her some, then we see signs coming back. Last year, when she went to stay with a friend, she accidentally had a few sips of cow's milk and some normal toast crumbs and she came home screaming. She couldn't think – it was just awful, so she had to detox again. It cost us thousands of dollars to put her right.

Alice is excelling at everything she tries. She plays piano and guitar, she sings and she horse rides. She does really well in athletics at school as well, so she has become an 'all rounder'.

11 Epsom Salts – magnesium sulphate (MgSO4) is an organic salt traditionally used as a component of bath salts. Medically, the salts are used for aches and pains, to remove splinters and internally as a saline laxative. In biomedical treatment, Epsom Salts are used as a detoxifying agent.

When we stick to our lifestyle and we're in charge of it, Alice is so well. We've managed to take her to England, South Africa, Kuala Lumpur and Singapore this year and we've had no reactions. In fact, in other countries, she's really, really well, to the point that when we were in England, we took her off some of her supplements. Unfortunately, over here, in the Waikato area in particular, it's very toxic to live in. Doctors have done lots of blood tests on autistic kids and the Waikato kids have got a lot more heavy metals in their bodies than the kids in Auckland – especially mercury. The levels on blood tests should be 0-20 and they were all getting levels just over 20. They sorted that problem out by changing the normal range from 0-50 – so, no more problems with mercury!

We try and do everything right, but although we live on a section with tank water, eat mainly organic, and have a salt pool, Alice can still get symptoms. When she wasn't very well a few weeks ago, I rang the council and asked them if they had sprayed my front garden, because it looked really dead. They said that they had, but they hadn't told us. I had guessed by the way my grass looked and the way my daughter was behaving. We can't eat the olives we're growing, because of the sprays they used. We've told them not to spray anymore.

I'm really glad that Alice got her diagnosis in England when she was two. It meant that I was able to get in there and help her. In New Zealand, it's so hard to get a diagnosis of autism, which means children can't get the help they need. If I'd been in this country, we possibly would still be battling to get a diagnosis. I have friends who have had to wait until their kids were over ten to get a formal diagnosis – then they've lost all those years of intervention.

Annie, my other daughter, got her diagnosis much later. Where Alice had autism, we didn't know what Annie had. She did not utter a word for the first two years of her life, other than 'Mamma'. She only wanted to be with me, one of my closest friends, or our nanny. When her dad came home, she would go to him, but other than that, it was pretty much only women. She cried at everything and clung to us. We knew she was different from Alice, and we also knew she was not autistic. We didn't realise until she finally got her diagnosis of kryptopyroluria[12] when she was five, that she was on the autistic spectrum.[13]

Annie's a much milder case, so we haven't had to do the same level of intervention, but she has the same food allergies as Alice and needs all the same supplements. She had a blood test done that showed she is intolerant to gluten and dairy. She also has heavy metals.

Annie was a lot easier to fix because we'd done it once already. Her kryptopyroluria is managed with zinc. She came to horse riding with us and fell in love with horses too. Everything was easier, except for the anxiety. That's where Alice was able to be the big sister to Annie. I couldn't even park

12 Kryptopyroluria is the result of abnormal haemoglobin metabolism. When bound to kryptopyrrole, zinc and vitamin B6 are excreted into the urine as pyrroles, causing a wide range of symptoms.

13 The autistic spectrum includes a wide range of mental, emotional and behavioural disorders ranging from mild Attention Deficit Disorder to severe autism.

the car in front of a shop and go in. She would sit in the car with silent tears and shake with fear. Now, we very rarely see signs of her anxiety, but we know it's still there. She can't watch any bad types of films or bear any cruelty, unkindness or injustice in the world.

Annie is so different from Alice. She likes to eat things separately – she doesn't like any of her food to touch. If we put out a roast dinner, she'll put the cauliflower on the plate and eat it. Then she'll put the peas on the plate and eat them. I still have to puree some of her food, because she won't eat anything with lumps in it. With a lack of zinc, kids don't want to try new foods. She is an absolute nightmare for trying new foods, so I have to blend them up, because she just can't bear some textures in her mouth.

I let the girls take their own supplements now. They know what they're supposed to take. I know from their behaviour when they've cheated and I'll say: "You haven't taken your zinc for a couple of days, have you?" And Annie will say she's forgotten. She has to keep her zinc levels up.

People are really reluctant to have their kids labelled. I know a lot of people here who will say: "My child's not autistic, they've got Asperger's." I feel like saying: "Asperger's is on the autistic spectrum. Your child has Autistic Spectrum Disorder." But of course you can't, because it's like 'autistic' is some really dirty word. In their mind, Asperger's just means they're really intelligent. I make a point of saying: "Alice, you have autism." We're not going to dress it up. She's proud of who she is, and so am I.

Diets for autistic kids are often in the 'too hard' basket for parents. It's stuff they've never, ever heard about and it is really challenging to change your diet. I hear parents saying: "I know colouring is not great for them, but that's okay, they'll run it off at school." Even for me, who ate organic, was vegetarian and knew about dairy intolerance – I thought I was onto it, but when I was told to go gluten-free, I felt like I was completely stupid. I had no idea where to start and I panicked. I had to ask lots of questions. Some parents just don't have the money to do these things and, sadly, a lot don't know how to find the help. It is just too hard, especially where both parents have to work. They're so tired and already doing all this stuff. Then you throw in this major curveball to change their child's diet dramatically – they mentally and physically can't do it.

If you've got an autistic kid and you want to recover them, you have to have money. There's no two ways about it – poor people can't do it. The medical bills are and always have been astronomical. When my ex-husband and I were married, we were on a really good whack with his wages. If we hadn't had autistic kids, we could have had a fantastic lifestyle. He'd get paid every two weeks – the day he got paid, I'd pay all the bills, then we might have a hundred dollars left. The kids come first – the better they are, the better they can be educated and the better they can be in the future. It's not negotiable.

If I was to take Alice to a paediatrician now, they'd tell me I had a really healthy, intelligent child who was excelling above what you would expect from most children.

Paul Shattock, a retired pharmacist and parent of an autistic son, was Honorary Director of the Autism Research Unit (ARU) at the University of Sunderland. He is Chairman of ESPA (Education and Services for People with Autism) and was President-Elect of the World Autism Organisation 2010-2014. His research investigates the theory that autism is a consequence of a metabolic disorder. Along with Kalle Reichelt, MD, from the Paediatric Research Institute in Norway, his research led to the widespread use of the gluten-free, casein-free diet in treating autism. In 1998, he was made an Officer of the Order of the British Empire (OBE) for his more than 30 years of services to the autism community. (Food and Behaviour Research http://www.fabresearch.org/548)

The Global Autism Collaboration website provides information on the biomedical treatment of autism http://www.globalautismcollaboration.com

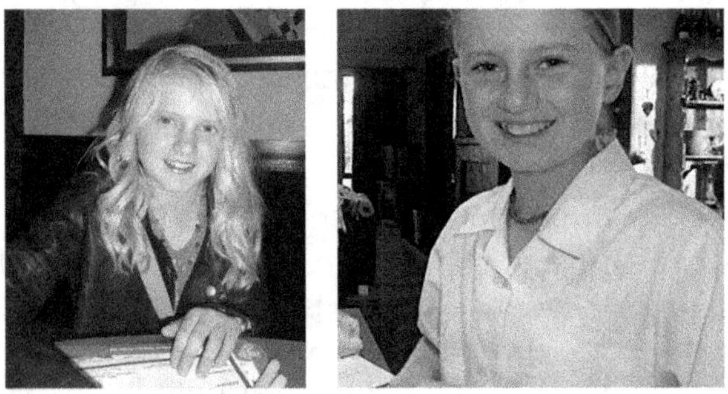

Alice (left) and Annie Walker in 2014.

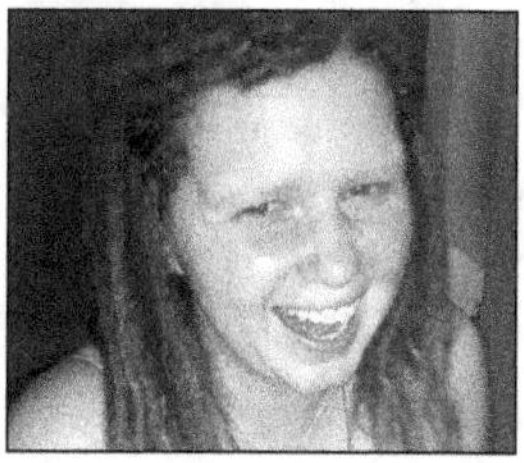

Emily Wall, 17 years

New Jersey, USA

Diagnosed with epilepsy at 12 years

When I was in sixth grade in 2006, I started having these episodes called 'blank-outs.' It's very hard to describe, but it's kind of like you can't think and your cognitive ability shuts off. I could see, but I would stare off into space. I was always afraid that I was going to be called on during class, because I couldn't do anything or say anything to anybody, and then I would snap out of it.

It was happening every now and then and eventually I told my mom. My mom's a nurse, but she didn't know what it was, so she brought me to my doctor. My doctor actually has epilepsy and has been on medication his whole life. He said he didn't know what it was and told me it could be migraines or something like that. He also thought it was more like daydreaming, or that I drifted off into space because I was bored in class. Not to brag about myself, but I'm an A student, I'm involved in school and I'm ahead in my class. He was really saying that it was nothing and didn't do anything about it, but said if I started to get the episodes more regularly, to come back and see him.

Then when I was in seventh grade, in February 2007, I was sitting in religion class taking a test, and all of a sudden everything went black. When I woke up I couldn't speak. Emergency Medical Technicians (EMTs) were around me, my mom was there, and nobody else was in the classroom. I remember being carried down the school stairs and into an ambulance. My mom was saying: "Emily, do you know who I am? Can you say my name?" I knew in my mind who she was, but I couldn't vocalise it. I couldn't say, "Mom, Mom." They let me go home from the Emergency Room that night.

When I went to school the next day, of course everybody was like, "Oh my gosh, what happened? You had a seizure and everything." I got the test that I was taking when it happened back, and it just said '100' on the top, even though I only answered two questions of it and there was scribbling all over the bottom. [*laughs*]

Some people have one seizure and then it's done – they never have another one again, because they grow. I think I grew six inches that year, so they thought that was why I was having seizures, but I knew that those blank-outs had something to do with the seizure. I always had a little blank-out before I blacked out.

I continued to cope with the blank-outs. I used to sit in class and stare up into space to just deal with it and pray that teachers wouldn't call on me when I was having one. If they had, I would not have been able to speak and then somebody would know what was going on and say, "Emily, why aren't you talking?"

Six weeks later to the second, I had a grand mal[1] seizure in the same class, doing the same thing, which was opening the Bible. It was quite odd for somebody who had red hair, because everyone was definitely thinking: "Oh my gosh – the exorcism?!"

Again, I woke up with EMTs surrounding me. My mom was there and again I was brought to the hospital. I was falling in and out of sleep, because I get very tired after my seizures and the grand mal really wiped me out. One thing I do remember from the hospital is that at the time, I was the only kid in my class without a cell phone and my mom was like: "We have to get her a cell phone, she's going to be going through seizures and you never know, somebody might not have a cell phone, so she will have a cell phone on her." And I was like, "YES!"

I always had to be with somebody – for the first year after I started having seizures I had to take somebody to the bathroom with me! They would have to stand outside the stall to make sure that I was okay.

We went to a neurologist in New Jersey, who suggested that we continue to wait to see what happens and not put me on medication. My mom thought that wasn't what we should do, because I expressed to her that I thought that the blank-outs had something to do with the seizures. Overall, my mom did not think that the neurologist was doing her job correctly. We had a friend who was a brain surgeon in Louisiana, who suggested that we go to the New York University Medical Center and see a neurologist there.

The neurologist put me on *Trileptal*.[2] I did fine on it for a few weeks, but then I started to have absence seizures, when I had an aura before a blank-out. My aura was buzzing in my ears and I couldn't think or talk. My aura got worse and I started to feel like a man was chasing after me and it started to get scary. So every time I would have an aura, I would tell my mom, she would call the doctor and he would say: "Okay, up her medication," or, "she's to come in for an appointment," or, "she needs to come in and have a test," which was usually an EEG,[3] where they try and induce a seizure.

1 A grand mal seizure (great sickness) occurs where there are violent muscle contractions with a loss of consciousness.

2 *Trileptal* (oxcarbazepine) is an anticonvulsant drug used primarily for the treatment epilepsy, anxiety, mood disorders and tics.

3 EEG – electroencephalogram is a recording of electrical activity along the scalp, used to help diagnose epilepsy.

During an EEG, it is dark. They ask you to open and close your eyes, then they flash a light in your face and ask you to hyperventilate for three minutes. I always failed those tests and so it was always: "Up the medication again." You couldn't tell that I was seizing visibly, but I could always feel that I was having an absence seizure and my doctor could see it in my brainwaves.

We got to the top dose of *Trileptal* that my body could handle for my height and weight. The side effects were really bad – I was very sleepy. Surprisingly, my grades were never really affected. I was always an A/B student and my doctors were amazed by that. They were always like: "How are you doing this? You're having absence seizures at school every day and you're still able to take notes and getting As on tests and everything!"

I was taken off *Trileptal* and put on *Keppra*,[4] which started my second medication trial. I was on that for six months without seizures of any kind. I was probably the happiest girl in the world. It was just before I was supposed to get a permit for my drivers license, so I was very happy. I had a boyfriend at the time and I thought I was in good shape.

Then one night I was doing homework in my room and an absence seizure came on. I called my boyfriend and said: "I just had a seizure," and he said that I had to tell my mom. I said: "But I told *you*." He said that if I didn't tell my mom, he would call and tell her. I burst into tears and said that I didn't want to tell her because I wanted to get my license on time. (You have to go a year seizure-free before you can get your license.) He told me: "Your health is more important than your license. You'll eventually get it if you figure out what's going on." It turned into a fight and I said that I wasn't going to tell my mom.

So he called my mom and said: "Emily has something to tell you." My mom came into my room and sat down and said: "Emily, what do you have to tell me?" I burst into tears and said: "I've just had a seizure after six months of going seizure-free. It wasn't a big one but it's *back*." So that was a pretty huge moment. Again, we went back to the doctor, took an EEG test, and again I failed. They just continued to up my dose of *Keppra*, because I kept having seizures. They upped my medication every month-and-a-half to two months, even though I was having seizures every single day. They didn't want to up it too quickly.

By December 2011, I was at the top dose of *Keppra* that my body could handle, and I was still having seizures. So my neurologist said: "We're going to add some *Zonegran*[5] on top of the *Keppra*." I was okay with that. I was perfectly fine with taking pills. In the beginning, I wasn't. I used to have to stick them in food and everything, but by then I could just throw a handful

4 *Keppra* is a trade name for levetiracetam, an anticonvulsant drug used to treat epilepsy.

5 *Zonegran* is a trade name for zonisamide, a sulfonamide used as an adjunctive therapy for a range of seizure types in adults.

back and chug water – it was fine. The first night after I took the *Zonegran*, I had seizures, and after three days I was still having seizures, but they weren't big ones.

Over the course of my medication trials, I had four bigger seizures – no grand mals, but bigger ones, where I was shaking. My mom never took me to the hospital after that, because she didn't feel that it was necessary for us to pay hospital bills when she knew how to deal with it. She let me rest afterwards and then she would call the doctor. Obviously, she would watch me closely.

When the *Zonegran* failed, my mom called the neurologist and said, "Can we please do the ketogenic diet?"[6] And he said, "No."

My mom found out about the ketogenic diet through *The Charlie Foundation*[7] when I first started having epilepsy. In the United States, you have to go through three medication trials before you can try the ketogenic diet. Even after you have been through three medication trials like I had, most doctors don't want to do the diet, because they say there's not a lot of information to back it up. So when we first went to a neurologist and asked about the ketogenic diet, he said that we couldn't do it because of having to do the three medication trials. When my third medication trial, which lasted two weeks, also failed, my mom called the doctor and asked again: "You said we only had to do three medication trials, so now can we do the ketogenic diet?" His answer was: "Well, I don't really think that would be the best choice, I think maybe we should up this medication and see how it does."

At that point, my mom said: "I'm done with this medication. I can't put her on this medication for the rest of her life. She can't do this anymore – I don't know what the long term side effects are. I want her to be able to bear children. I don't want her to have to deal with this when she gets older."

My mom and I went out to breakfast. As I was eating chocolate-chip banana pancakes, which I miss *so* much, she said: "Emily, your seizures are getting pretty serious and it seems like there's never an end to this problem." I said: "I know Mom, I've been dealing with them for four years." Then she told me: "All of our family have been researching this diet that could possibly work for you." She never told me that it was the ketogenic diet she asked about. I didn't even know what it was.

I was very apprehensive, because I was the pickiest eater you could possibly imagine. I would eat bagels, french fries, pasta, chicken fingers, pizza and bread. I would never stray away from what I usually ate or try anything new. My mom was persistent and explained the diet to me over breakfast. By the end of the meal, we were both in tears. She said that it would be very hard and that she might have found a doctor who would be open to it. She

6 The ketogenic diet is a scientifically tested, high-fat, low-carbohydrate, adequate-protein diet that has been used in medicine since the 1920s to treat epilepsy in children.

7 *The Charlie Foundation* www.charliefoundation.org

stressed she really didn't want the long term side effects of the medications to affect me in the future when I was making choices and that I'd been taking those meds for a while, and she was very scared. She didn't want me to have to remember to take them when I woke up every morning and every night.

That was the thing – we had to take my meds everywhere. It was always a stress and in the back of my mind. If I'd forgotten to bring them with me, we'd have to leave somewhere to go and get my meds. She didn't want that for the rest of my life and she didn't want me to go to college having seizures.

We ended up switching to a female doctor who was a little more open to the fact that we wanted to try the ketogenic diet. When we went for our first appointment, we were very nervous. We went to her office and listened to her talk. She said that brain surgery was an option, because I only had the seizures on one side of my head. When my mom asked if we could we try the ketogenic diet, she said that brain surgery would take about three months to approve, so yes, in the meantime we could try it.

Just at the same time, the New York University Medical Center got a dietician for the ketogenic diet in the same office that we were in. When our new doctor told us that we could try it, me and my mom were so happy we both started crying. Seriously, it was the best feeling ever. I was told that the diet worked for everybody. You have to start out with three days in the hospital, and everybody makes it seem like it's going to work.

When I went into the hospital, Courtney, my dietician, said that my mom was the best prepared patient ever. Usually, Courtney had to go to grocery stores and get ingredients that patients are supposed to bring themselves. But not my mom – 30 meals were already cooked. [*laughs*]

In the hospital, they try and get you into a state of ketosis.[8] Some medical students came around to see me and interviewed me. One of them asked me what I thought I would do if it failed. "If it failed? What do you mean? I thought it worked for most people." He said that there is a percentage that fail at this diet. It really opened my eyes that this may not work and I would have to rethink my options.

In the first few weeks it was hard, because you're starving all the time. You don't get to eat what you normally eat. I lay in my bed in a foetal position, crying my eyes out, because I was hungry. It wasn't because I was truly hungry though, it was because I was missing the foods that I couldn't eat.

My body needed to be acclimated to the fact that it was running on fat. I lost 15 pounds and I was weak. On one very hard day, my mom came into my room and said: "Emily, you're 17 and you have the choice not do this if you

8 Ketosis is a state of elevated levels of ketone levels in the body that can be used as energy.

really don't want to." I really thought about not sticking with it, but honestly, it was the longest I'd been without seizures and I knew I would never have forgiven myself if I gave up.

It's hard on my family, I know it is. I have two brothers and they give up a lot for me. We don't eat dinner as a family as much anymore, because I can't eat at the same time as they can. They don't like to eat in front of me, because I finish my meal very quickly. We used to go out to dinner as a family all the time and now we can't do that. I'll let them go, but we miss out on a lot of family time. A lot of conversations revolve around my diet and my mom spends a lot of time cooking for me. My dad has said to me, multiple times, that I need to start cooking. I know I need to do that, but finding the time to do that is hard too. Without the support of my family and my community, this couldn't have been possible. It's amazing what people have done to help me overcome this.

I really turned to God during this. I went to a Catholic grammar school when I was little, and I believed in God, but I didn't pray all the time. Now I go to church a lot and I definitely look towards the church a lot more than I used to. It's something to lean on and I lean on my parents a lot more also.

I'm at the point now where this diet is just something that I have to deal with – and I am approaching my first year seizure-free. As my body started to acclimate to the diet, I started to regain my strength, the weight I lost, and now I feel normal. I'm used to what I have to do. It's just like anything, or any other diet – the first few weeks are always hard, but I haven't had one seizure. They haven't even tried to bring up the brain surgery again.

I don't even remember what before felt like. I don't even crave the food like I used to. I still have to acclimate to certain things, like last night when I went to my cousin's wedding, I had to bring my own food. It's hard to explain to people, like when the server came over to put food on my plate, I had to say: "I'm sorry, I'm not eating, because I'm on a diet." When you say diet, people look at you and they're like, "Oh, a diet?" Then I say, "Oh, no, no – a medical diet. Like, I have epilepsy," and you have to explain it to them.

When I first did my diet at school, people didn't understand it either. I was lucky enough to have a chemistry teacher who had a fridge in her lab she said I could use whenever I wanted, so I could bring certain meals in. It's amazing the support that I've gotten from people around me. Honestly, without it, I seriously couldn't have done it.

They're trying to get me to come off my medications. So far, my medication has been reduced twice. When you start the diet, they don't just take you off your medication, because then obviously it won't work and they don't want to see me fail.

At my last appointment, I had an EEG. It was the first EEG I have had where

I passed without any seizures at all. Me and my mom both started crying – I could almost cry talking about it now. It was the happiest moment ever, to know that this could be out of my life forever.

The path ahead is to keep slowly reducing my medicine. If we go too fast, I could have a seizure and then we'd have to start over again. I'm just happy that it's being reduced and I'm taking less pills in the morning and at night. It's nice – so nice.

I've convinced myself that hunger is a state of mind. It really is – you just have to talk yourself out of it. Over the summer, I fell out of ketosis, because I was having too many snacks and I wasn't doing any exercise. My ketones were down, so my dietician said that I needed to take away two of my snacks for a few days just to get me back into the correct ketosis. I don't think I've ever cried so much about food. Then I took a look at myself and said, "Emily, you're crying about food. Food!" [*laughs*]

Through this whole experience I've been writing a lot and keeping track of everything. I wrote a lot about that night I was mad. When I look back, I would never remember that I was that mad about food. It's great to look back on those feelings.

I really hope that I can get my story out there and get people to look at this diet. Actually, my mom's friend, whose son is three weeks apart from me, started having epilepsy this summer. My mom said that they should find a doctor that will escape the medication and go right for this diet, because, seriously, it works.

I also really hope that it becomes a first choice for so many doctors; where medication is not the first option and people don't have to dig and delve to find out what the diet is. Medication might work for some people, but it's horrible to take pills every day – it really is. If food can change that, that's great. It really makes me take a look at what I eat and it makes other people take a second look at what they eat. My mom has definitely changed what my brothers eat – no sugar or anything like that.

The thing that's hard about the ketogenic diet is that it can be expensive for families that don't have the income to do it. We had to buy a separate freezer for me, so my mom could cook a bunch of meals and put them in the freezer. Then I could just take them out and warm them up myself. The ingredients aren't exactly cheap, because they're all organic. Insurance doesn't cover food, it only covers medicine. I feel like that's another reason people turn to medications, because of the expense. They need to realise that the diet works and it should be a first-choice treatment.

At the time of her interview, Emily was a senior high school student interested in travel and photography. She is looking forward to going to college and is as yet undecided in her major.

Two uplifting YouTube clips Emily has made about life on the ketogenic diet:

- Count Blessings, Not Problems
  http://www.youtube.com/watch?v=wEMbYcqpcj4
- A Year In the Life of a Keto Kid
  http://www.youtube.com/watch?v=K_rGACQCMto

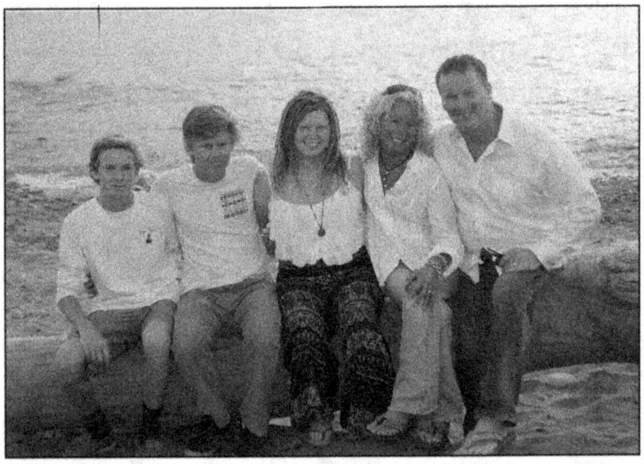

Emily (centre) with her family - brothers Cahill, Robert, mom Tara and dad Rob.

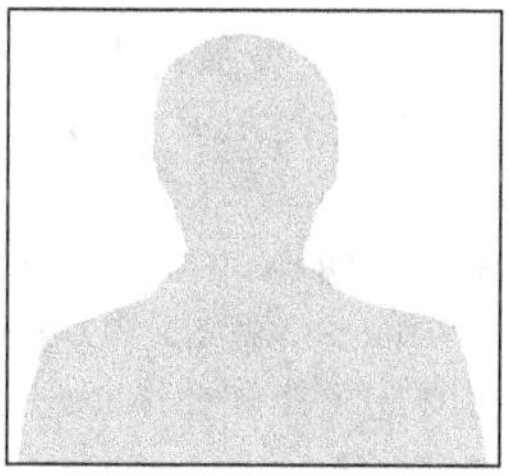

'Dawn', 45 years

Minnesota, USA

Diagnosed with rheumatoid arthritis at 37, multiple sclerosis (MS) at 38 years

Prior to my diagnosis, I was having a lot of balance issues. Everything was spinning around me. I didn't have a ton of symptoms, mainly balance and my equilibrium was off. The room was moving all around me when I was sitting perfectly still. Heights didn't usually bother me, but all of a sudden I thought I was going to fall down the stairs. I had jello legs – they would just give out on me at any moment.

One of the symptoms I had for about two months before my diagnosis was this horrible itching feeling under my skin. The doctors at the time didn't know what it was – they just kind of wrote it off. I had tests done on it, but they couldn't find anything. Meanwhile, I was practically scratching my forehead raw, because it was such an irritation.

We didn't know what the symptoms were for about a year. About a month after I was diagnosed with MS, I had my first and only big flare,[1] where they put me on about five days of prednisone. My legs would completely give out on me while I was walking. I would spend most of my time on the couch, because my sleep was just horrible. My speech had slowed down. My mouth couldn't keep up with my brain. My memory got progressively worse. I had times where I would stop mid-sentence and completely forget what I was going to say.

I lost about 25 pounds during the flare, probably as a result of the steroids. Nothing tasted good in my mouth. Everything felt gross and tasted gross. While it was good to lose the weight, it wasn't the way I wanted to lose it.

After the prednisone, I was home from work for about two months. I couldn't drive. They never did find optic neuritis or anything in particular wrong with my eyes, but I could not drive safely. My eyes would go in and out of focus. Thankfully, I didn't have to drive for anything. My husband would do the errands if we needed anything.

They started me on *Rebif* [2]– the injectable medicine for the MS, which was three times a week. I did that for about two and a half years and then I stopped it. I got sick of having really red welts two inches in diameter, all over my

1 A flare is a worsening of multiple sclerosis symptoms, caused by inflammation in the central nervous system.

2 *Rebif* (interferon beta 1a) is an approved medication for the treatment of patients with relapsing forms of multiple sclerosis.

body from the injections. I got tired of trying to find places where I could give it to myself. It gave me terrible headaches and I felt like I had the flu – it was horrible. I would take the shot before I would go to bed, which is what they suggest, only because they say that it will give you flu-like symptoms. Sure enough, I would wake in the middle of the night wanting to throw up. I was really hot and I just felt awful. They would tell you: "Well, pop a couple of *Tylenol*[3] before you do it." Okay, fine, but I was never really able to take it symptom-free. It always gave me some kind of yucky feeling and I did not like it. Anything that's supposed to help you really shouldn't do that.

Eventually, I woke up and said to myself: "You know what? This is stupid – why am I doing this?" [*laughs*] One of the things I felt negative about was how much they were charging my insurance company every year. It was like $45,000-50,000 a year for a medicine that I could not tell was making any difference. *Rebif* is one of the first medicines that a lot of doctors will prescribe to people with MS. When I tried to get an opinion from my doctor about which drug I should use, she said: "Well, the *Rebif* is only three times a week as opposed to daily, and it's the thinnest needle that you're going to find." I thought: "Okay, that's all you have to tell me. It's got a tiny needle and it's fewer times a week." I realised that drugs aren't necessarily the way to go. I didn't have any more flare ups when I was on it, but I didn't have any more flares when I stopped it either. After that I went for about a year drug-free.

I didn't even know what MS was when I was diagnosed. I've done a lot of reading and got a lot of information from other people that had MS who are either recently diagnosed, or had it all their adult life. Some people did say that they had fewer flares or that they had more minimised flares from taking the *Rebif*, but most of them were still having flares. Had I had to pay out of pocket for that drug, I would have quit it a lot sooner than what I did.

The biggest symptom that has been there all along is short term memory loss. That's something that I had really hoped that by now would have eased and corrected itself. Advancing age doesn't help the matter and I've got a family that's continually pointing out how bad my memory is getting!

I found out about LDN[4] when I hopped online. One of the first websites I went to was *Patients Like Me*.[5] It's an incredible website and I'm on there daily. It's just so good to get feedback about how other patients are dealing with all their symptoms, what they're doing, things they're trying – how they are handling their illness. You get people from all areas of the spectrum – people who have been recently diagnosed to people who have had it for years. It's a great thing. I have been on the LDN since March of 2011, so about two and a half years, not quite.

3 *Tylenol* is a US brand of acetaminophen, also known as paracetamol, used to reduce fever and pain.

4 LDN – Low Dose Naltrexone is the off-label prescription of the FDA approved drug *Naltrexone*.

5 *Patients Like Me* www.patientslikeme.com

I had a really hard time finding a doctor who was willing to prescribe the LDN. The first doctor that I found who would prescribe it was one that did phone consultations. He was on the East coast, a thousand miles away from me. It wasn't a good arrangement. Every three months I would have to call up and check in with him on a particular date at a particular time and I kept forgetting the appointment. Then he would charge me for the appointment. So I had to stop that because it was costing me too much money for missed appointments. I only had the LDN from that doctor for about a year, then I took another year off with no meds at all. It took a long time to find a neurologist who would prescribe it. I'm lucky. She's very open-minded and it's about a half hour drive from here, so that's a good thing. My past three or four neurologists wouldn't touch it. They were hell-bent on these drugs that drug companies were telling them were going to help their patients. They wouldn't even discuss it.

To watch me walk most days, you would never know I had any disability. I have also got rheumatoid arthritis. I was diagnosed with that about a year before my MS diagnosis. It would come and go for about six or seven months, but it got to the point where it just hurt like crazy. I could barely walk on my right leg. I could have handled it more if it was a shoulder or an arm, but the knee is kind of an important part of the body for getting around! I could not do stairs. Thank goodness we've got strong hand rails and my arms are so strong, so I could grab those and stop myself taking a tumble. After getting up out of a chair, I had to be really careful, because the pain would kick me right back down to the seat where I was sitting. I was doing a lot of grabbing furniture after the first couple of steps. I was popping pills – you name it, I was trying it, but you take enough of those and they start to hurt your stomach. Right before I started the LDN, the pain had gotten ten-fold worse. Thankfully, two days after taking the LDN, my arthritis just disappeared. I'm getting a double bonus – the LDN is taking care of my MS plus I haven't had pain in my right knee since I started it.

Have you heard about that term CCSVI?[6] About three years ago, they found out through a lot of studies that most MS patients have stenosed[7] jugular veins and three years ago I started having head-splitting headaches. They gave me medicines for the headaches, but they just knocked me out and only took care of the headaches for a while. Finally, I went in to a neurologist – their answer to it was: "Well, it's just the MS." Again, through *Patients Like Me*, I got in touch with an interventional radiologist. He did all kinds of scans on my jugulars. About six months after I went to him, I went in and had a procedure. It's like an angioplasty, but it's called a venoplasty, because it's with the veins. My headaches disappeared immediately after I had that procedure and my balance was perfect. Unfortunately, it was just temporary, but I felt amazing immediately after I had that procedure. Again, that was something that my

6 CCSVI – chronic cerebrospinal venous insufficiency is compromised blood flow in veins draining the central nervous system, thought to play a role in the cause of multiple sclerosis.

7 Stenosis – abnormal narrowing of a passage in the body.

previous three neurologists wouldn't even discuss. They didn't believe in it and they were very pig-headed. Needless to say, I fired them all and found a good one.

I started seeing my current neurologist about two and a half years ago. She specialises in MS and migraines. I emailed her a couple of times just to find out what she was about and how to make appointments. The way the internet is now, you can get a person's whole history as far as what they treat and so on. You can kind of get a good feel about them before you actually walk into their office and meet them. She said that she liked alternative medicine and that she was open to prescribing new medicines. I found out that she had started prescribing LDN to a lot of people and had such good results. She immediately wrote a prescription for me and I've been good ever since.

LDN has made a huge difference to my sleep. I was having problems sleeping and popping sleeping pills and stuff just to try and stay asleep for more than two or three hours at a time. Immediately after starting the LDN, I would be out like a light for seven or eight hours straight. Even with my husband's snoring, I could still sleep. Then I would wake up in the morning having had interesting, movie-like dreams. I dream every single night and it's very colourful. It's nice. To get eight hours of good solid sleep every night makes such a difference. I'm great for the first five or six hours of the day and then I crash. If there's something I have to accomplish during the day I have to do it in the first four or five hours. I used to take modafinil,[8] but it didn't really make any difference, so now I just drink coffee instead.

My memory issues persist. All my life I have worked. I stopped working due to my memory issues. I would love to go back to work and be a productive citizen again. I had been on antidepressants since I lost my first job. I was falling deeper and deeper into depression. I kept taking the medicine that they told me to take and it was not getting any better. So I stopped taking the antidepressants. Then I started taking these supplements of turmeric with curcumin, which someone else on *Patients Like Me* suggested. It's like this grey cloud has just cleared. Suddenly I don't dread leaving the house anymore, doing errands and just getting motivated to do stuff in the morning. I trust it way more than the prescription-type medicine. It's natural and better than a prescription drug ever was. The fewer drugs and pharmaceuticals you take, the better.

You have to trust your own judgement sometimes and just not be the dog that keeps doing what everyone tells you to do. Sometimes that bites you in the ass, so you've got to move ahead and try something else. I take a whole bunch of supplements now – I have a whole handful each morning with breakfast.

I've gotten a very ugly outlook on pharmaceuticals, just because of this whole MS thing. I used to be very trusting of everything my doctors would tell me before and I did what they said. You start to learn about what's behind a lot of

8 Modafinil is a wakefulness promoting drug for daytime sleepiness.

the things your doctor tells you to do and you get kind of negative. You can find out now which pharmaceutical company is paying your neurologist – in whose hip pocket. It's only been possible in the past two years, where you can type in your neurologist's name to find out.[9] They have to report where their income is all coming from, for the public record. It was an eye-opener when I found out who all my ex-neurologists were getting paid by.

The first thing that they wanted to do when I was diagnosed was: "Here's a choice of all these different drugs you can take – pick one." And that was pretty much it. I was: "Really? Is it going to help? Is it going to make a difference?" When you hear about all the kick-backs the doctors are getting from these pharmaceutical companies, you just get really wary. What can you trust, when my old doctors would tell me and they wouldn't even discuss alternative treatments? There's a big red flag there: 'Let's get out of here!'

Some sensations came back about a month ago – I really thought I was headed for a big flare, but all that happened was my gums went numb and half of my face went numb. My tongue is still tingly, but nothing nearly as bad as the first time I had that happen. I think the LDN that I'm taking has really kept things curbed, I'm really happy with it. I haven't gotten a common cold in the past five years. You read so many positive things about LDN. I really believe it's going to help me in so many ways. I really can't complain about my health right now, if it wasn't for MS written in my files.

9 *Prescriber Checkup: The Doctors and Drugs in Medicare Part D* http://projects.propublica.org/checkup/

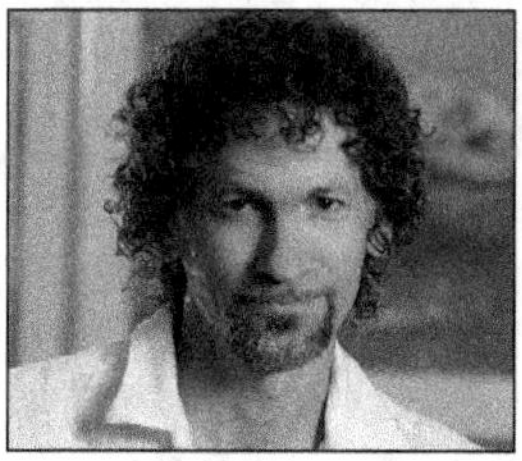

Marc Wishengrad, 47 years

New York, USA

Diagnosed with MSRA (methicillin-resistant staphylococcus aureus) at 40 years

I was the cinematographer on a film in 2007 and we were shooting in an apple orchard in late summer. I needed to pull a vine out from the frame for a pick-up shot that was supposed to match early spring, because there was no green vegetation. I suspected it was poison ivy and pulled a vine out with my middle and ring finger.

That evening I took a long shower and scrubbed my hand with soap, but I already began to feel something under the surface of the skin where I touched the vine. A few days later, my entire finger swelled up. I went to a clinic where the doctor there gave me oral antibiotics and told me to come back if it didn't help. A week later, my finger was so swollen, painful and throbbing that I couldn't bend it.

The antibiotics weren't doing anything, so I went back to the doctor at the clinic and he sent me to the emergency department at the hospital across the street. Being that it was my finger, a hand specialist lanced it to drain the infection. I couldn't believe how painful it was. He gave me a dose of *OxyContin*,[1] which totally took away my anxiety and relieved the pain. Now I was ready to do whatever the doctors wanted, so I was admitted into the hospital and put on intravenous antibiotics. I spent two sleepless nights there and then was discharged with a prescription for oral antibiotics.

I thought that it was all over and was glad to be home in my apartment but the next evening I got a message on my answering machine from a young doctor, saying that I should come back to the hospital. The pus from my infected finger had been tested and the results had come back from the lab. He said that I had no ordinary infection – that it was MRSA[2] – the Superbug.[3] Even though I had already gone through an initial round of IV[4] antibiotics, he said that I should come back for some stronger ones.

So I returned to New York Presbyterian Hospital. It was a place I trusted, because for about a decade and a half I have been a cameraman there, documenting

1 *OxyContin* is the trade name for oxycodone, a narcotic analgesic used to treat moderate to severe pain.
2 MRSA – methicillin-resistant *staphylococcus aureus.*
3 A Superbug is a bacterium that is unresponsive to most antibiotics and known as 'multi-drug resistant'.
4 IV – intravenous.

everything from conjoined twin separation surgeries, to fundraising films about people whose lives were saved by treatment there. I was admitted into the hospital again, but this time to a single room, because my infection was considered to be highly contagious. There had been a recent case of the Superbug that had been on the front page of *The Daily News*, where a 12-year-old boy had died from MRSA. I soon found out what an epidemic this bug has become. MRSA is all over the place. It's spread by skin-to-skin contact and it's rampant. I've read that it kills upwards of 19,000 people a year in this country. In many cases, it has struck young healthy people like football players and wrestlers. Also, people can contract it while they are in hospital for something else.

Even though I work in a hospital environment, they believed that mine was a CA or 'community-acquired' infection. I was treated with intravenous vancomycin.[5] While I was in the hospital, they tested my nose with a cotton swab to check for MRSA. The result came back positive – I did have MRSA colonising there. So at discharge time, they gave me a prescription for some antibiotic ointment to put inside my nose. When I came home, I tried to use the ointment, but found it impossible to take, since it dripped down to the back of my throat and tasted toxic.

I was also given a script for the antibiotic *Bactrim*,[6] orally. After about a week of taking these large, chalky antibiotic pills, I was not feeling healthy. I felt so exhausted I could barely walk down the street and I felt like walking death. My finger had healed for the most part, but the antibiotics had given me diarrhoea and a low-grade fever. I was so weak that I was barely managing to maintain my life, so I stopped taking the *Bactrim*. In order to help recover from feeling so drained, I went to see a Chinese herbalist, who gave me some herbs to detoxify my 'angry liver'.

A month later, I was back to my normal self, and it was Thanksgiving. I went to see my dad, who lived in the Boston area where I grew up. Thanksgiving is a wonderful time to eat a hearty meal and be with family, but being away from my NYC[7] home, I was not consistent with taking the Chinese herbs. While I was riding back home on the bus, I felt my skin was bubbling up or something on the back of my thigh that was in contact with the seat. It seemed to have come out of nowhere – it was bizarre.

The next day, it started to take hold and the whole back of my thigh reddened. There was a dark red dot in the centre that looked like a spider bite and I was beginning to limp. Nothing unusual had happened and I couldn't tell if it was something that got in, or something that was coming out. I didn't realise right away, but it was the return of the MRSA.[8] I didn't want to go back to the

5 Vancomycin is a last-resort antibiotic used to treat life-threatening infections unresponsive to other less toxic antibiotics.

6 *Bactrim* is an antibiotic used to treat a range of bacterial infections, including septicaemia (blood poisoning).

7 NYC – New York City.

8 Recurrent infections of MRSA are common, with rates ranging from 9-18%. Management strategies for recurrent infections remain undefined. (National Centre for Biotechnology Information www.ncbi.nlm.nih.gov/pmc/articles/PMC2861049/)

hospital, because I knew they would give me more vancomycin and more medical bills. I didn't have health insurance and was already looking at owing the hospital upwards of $20,000 from all those specialists that came to see me before. Besides, I felt so unwell last time when I took the antibiotics.

A year before, I had met a trainee homeopath in Hawaii while I was working on a documentary about people coming off diabetes and high blood pressure medication when they followed a macrobiotic diet and lifestyle. I was pretty skinny then and would feel hungry even right after eating, so she had given me some homeopathic medicine for parasites. There was an improvement in my appetite and over time I began to look less gaunt.

We were still in contact and I called her about my situation. She was in Toronto, so she asked me to email a picture to her. She said it looked like an infection and that I should go to the hospital. I wasn't interested in going down that road again, so she told me to look for a homeopath through the North American Society of Homeopaths, so I could find a local homeopath who was recommended by a professional group. From the website, I looked through the list and called a few of them. I left a few messages and spoke to one all the way out in Queens. Finally, Pierre Fontaine called me back. His office was in Manhattan, literally down the street and one subway ride away. I explained to him that I suspected it was the return of the MRSA infection and so he agreed to see me that night. I hopped on the subway and was in his office within an hour.

He examined the area and then started asking all kinds of questions about how I felt and got me to be really specific. He asked me questions that seemed irrelevant to the growing infection in my thigh. After consulting his computer, he came up with a remedy, which he gave me in a small envelope. I left his office at around nine thirty in the evening, feeling very positive about having found someone who would keep a close watch on me. Even though I was limping a little due to the increase in swelling, I felt encouraged that I was going to get through this and that the tiny pills would reverse my condition.

The next day there seemed to be no improvement and it was painful when I moved, but I wasn't taking any narcotic painkillers. The large red area began to centralise into a boil. I photographed the boil and emailed it to Pierre. He realised the severity of the situation and came to visit me at my apartment. I had a little flip camera, so I took a shot of him examining the boil. Then he reached into his leather bag and took out another remedy, emptied a capful of these small round white pills into my mouth and gave me instructions on how to dissolve the pills in a small shaker bottle with a small amount of water. I filmed the whole thing.

In deciding to do the homeopathy, I knew that I was going against conventional wisdom. Even Pierre advised me to go to the hospital. This is not something that people are going to do, because when you get this diagnosis and the doctor says, "Take these antibiotics," you don't argue with him – you do it. He's got a white coat on – he knows what he's talking about!

So I decided to be my own nurse. I was warned that the infection could go up into my heart, but I monitored my temperature and I was talking to my friends on the phone. I kept the area clean. The boil was oozing so much that I had a garbage bag next to the couch to throw the used cotton balls in. It was difficult to move around with this golf ball-size boil embedded in my thigh, but it wasn't throbbing like an angry infection would. I hobbled to the store to buy more bags of cotton balls and bottles of hydrogen peroxide. I kept cleansing, filming and photographing it. I bandaged it up at night and rested on the couch in the daytime. I was concerned for my life, but I was also aware of the bad experience I'd had with the lancing, the extreme pain and all the antibiotics. I didn't feel like I was dying. I wasn't in pain when I was still, so I continued to take the homeopathic remedy and email pictures of my constantly morphing and changing boil to the homeopath.

Because I make videos for the hospital, I had contact with a doctor in the same lab where they originally tested my finger positive for MRSA. Pierre suggested that I get the ooze from the boil in my thigh tested to confirm that it was in fact MRSA. I was pretty sure that it was, but he wanted proof. I went to the hospital by taxi and asked the nurse for a testing swab. I didn't want anyone to see my boil for fear that they would hospitalise me on the spot. I went into the bathroom, swabbed the ooze from the boil, bandaged it back up, then hobbled back and handed it to the nurse and said, "Test this for MRSA." The next day, I called the doctor who did the test. She told me it was MRSA and said: "You gotta get yourself to the emergency room – you need antibiotics." I told her, "No, I'm doing homeopathy." She said, "NO, you can do homeopathy later, you need antibiotics, NOW!"

I continued taking my remedy as instructed by my homeopath. A bit less than a week in, it all came to a climax. One morning after I woke, I went into the bathtub and as I pushed on the boil, it burst and drained completely, leaving a cavity (an age-old method of healing). Most people have never really seen a boil burst, because it's always lanced at the hospital. I emailed Pierre a picture. He called me back and said that I was 'out of the woods'. I continued to photograph and monitor it. At one point, there was some concern that there were some black areas that might be gangrene. Pierre stopped by with a few different remedies. Soon after that, the hole healed. Later, I found out that the remedy he had given me was *Arsenicum Album*.

Two weeks later, in mid-December, I was getting out of the house and back to normal life. I continued to photograph my leg as the area closed up. By the New Year, it was just a healing scar and I no longer needed to put a bandage on it.

Now, in mid-January, a month and half after I had successfully treated the MRSA infection in my thigh without hospitalisation, I made an appointment with an infectious disease doctor. I asked him to re-test me to see if there was any MRSA still colonising in my nose. The test came back negative, I had completely gotten rid of the Superbug. When I told the doctor I had not used antibiotics and used homeopathic treatment instead, all he said was, "Interesting." It didn't shake his world, and that is where it ended.

When treated with antibiotics, an MRSA infection may heal, but the patient can remain a carrier. Any further cuts or broken skin run the risk of a recurrence of an MRSA infection.

The following Spring, while I was sweeping the sidewalk in front of my community garden, I scraped my knuckles on some concrete planters. It felt like the kind of injury that if I still had an MRSA infection, it would have come back, but it was just a normal scrape that got red for a little bit and then healed up. It didn't become angry and hot, like when I had the finger infection. With my leg, the MRSA infection was aggressive and the infection took hold really fast.

I feel great now and my life is non-stop. I'm still making films for the hospital that help them fundraise for their programs. I play the trumpet in a band that I co-founded – the New York City Brass Brothers, which plays New Orleans style jazz, blues and funk. I'm also landscaping a 26-acre permaculture farm in the Catskills.

Recently, I told a doctor friend of mine that I used homeopathy to completely rid myself from the MRSA bug. He could not accept what I was saying. His training told him that the only way to kill that bug was through broad-spectrum antibiotics and without hospitalisation you can't get rid of it. I told him I got tested, and he said: "It must have been a false positive." He thought that either I didn't have MRSA in the first place, or I probably still have it!

At the end of the day, there is no cure for chronic MRSA, so there are inevitably all kinds of recurrences. When it's diagnosed, doctors have protocols to follow. The gold standard treatment is broad-spectrum intravenous antibiotics. I took my healthcare into my own hands and did something that was risky, medically. To think you can use little white sugar pills to treat a potentially deadly infection is unheard of in this country. If I met someone with a MRSA infection now, how could I recommend that they find a homeopath and take care of it themselves? I know I did the right thing for myself, but what I did was beyond the norm.

After losing my mom in 1999 and my dad in 2010, both to cancer, I have a strong desire to educate others about healing ways that have been around far longer than modern medicine. They may be labeled as 'anecdotal' by the scientific community, but they have provided reversal from chronic and terminal diseases for many people. Toward my goal to educate the public about time-tested healing traditions, I have founded a non-profit organisation called The Healing World Foundation.[9]

I have focused my camera on the eyes of countless people who are alive today because they went to the hospital. On the flip side, I have also focused my camera on just as many people who have used homeopathy and other healing methods to completely rid themselves of their disease. I even know someone who had the same kind of cancer that my mom died of, and is still alive today, because she found another way.

Since its first appearance in 1960, MRSA has become widespread in hospitals and the community. In the USA, MRSA infections kill 19,000 hospitalised American patients annually, similar to the number of deaths due to AIDS, tuberculosis, and viral hepatitis combined.

A growing concern is the emergence of MRSA infections in patients with no apparent risk factors. In the United States, four cases of rapidly fatal MRSA infections in children were reported by the Centres for Disease Control and Prevention (CDC) in 1997-1999.

The frequency of methicillin-resistant staphylococcus aureus (MRSA) infections continues to grow in hospital-associated settings and more recently, in community settings in the United States and globally. (Oxford Journals – Clinical Infectious Diseases http://cid.oxfordjournals.org/content/46/Supplement_5/S344.full)

Marc's case of using homeopathic treatment for MRSA was documented in The Journal of Science and Healing *Vol 5 Issue 6 Nov/Dec 2009 by Pierre Fontaine: www.homeopathicservices.com It also appears in a documentary about homeopathy, called* Just One Drop *directed by Laurel Chiten www.blinddogfilms.com soon to be released.*

Marc's not-for-profit organisation, The Healing World Foundation, *has documented traditional healing practices, so that others can learn about them. His website www.wishpic.com includes* The Healing World *documentary and his other films.*

9 http://healingworld.org

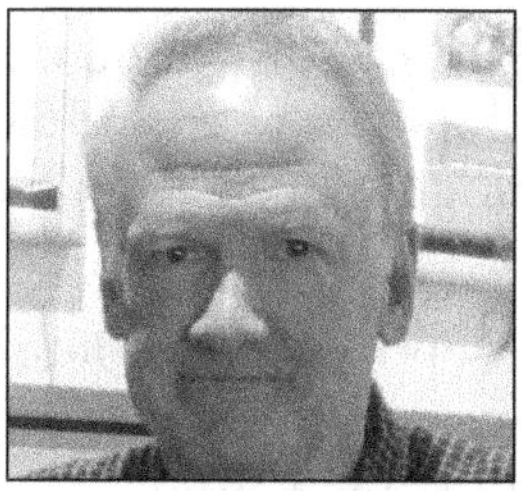

David Yoffie, 58 years

St Louis, Missouri, USA

Diagnosed with stage IV pancreatic cancer and liver metastases at 46 years

I was 46 when I was diagnosed. I own apartment blocks for a living and I had a few hundred units spread throughout St Louis, so I was busy. Because I had acid reflux, I decided to have this laparoscopic[1] procedure, to reduce the acid in my throat.

There weren't any clues to my having cancer. The night before I had that procedure, I was exercising, so I had no symptoms at all, although I felt a little pain in my right side that I didn't normally have. Physically, I was perfectly fine before the procedure and I was fine when I came out. I just got lucky that I ended up going in for that operation, because when they went in, they saw a bunch of stuff on my pancreas and in my liver, so they didn't actually do the operation. They said they'd better biopsy it, so they did, and I had stage IV pancreatic cancer that had metastasised to the liver.

I did do some rounds of chemo,[2] which shrank it a little bit. The chemo affected me some, but I was 46 and luckily it didn't have big effects, like an older person would have. The last round didn't really shrink it any more. There was still a lot of cancer there. My oncologist said: "Well, we can't really shrink it any more," then he told me it's just going to come back, then maybe he'd try another drug, but basically, I was going to die.

My mother did lots of research on alternative practitioners and Doctor Gonzalez's name came up in a number of places. What I like about Doctor Gonzalez is that he probably doesn't take most people as patients. I know people that he has turned down. I asked him, "Why do you turn people down?" He said: "You know what David? If I don't think I can help them, I'm not going to give them false hope and I'm not going to take their money. It's just not the way I work." I respect Doctor Gonzalez's work in that way. You have to send in copies of your medical records and your latest oncologist's report, so I thought I'd give him a try. I almost wasn't a patient of his, because he got the idea from somewhere that I couldn't eat. Once I told him that I could eat, he took me.

1 Laparoscopy is a surgical procedure where a fibre-optic instrument is inserted through the abdominal wall to view abdominal organs and sometimes conduct small-scale surgery.

2 Chemo – chemotherapy.

When I told my oncologist that I was going to see Doctor Gonzalez, he'd heard of him. He basically said: "He's a quack, why bother doing that? He's just going to take your money." I didn't say anything to him, but I thought: "You know what? You're not offering me any help at all, so why wouldn't I try something different?" I guess that's a typical oncologist – not open to different ideas.

I didn't know whether it would work, but I knew I was 46 and I had two little girls of ten and 13 who I wanted to be around for. My parents had already lost a daughter – she died of some kind of heart ailment, without any warning. She was at a party, she stopped breathing, and that was basically it. I didn't want them to lose their son, so I was motivated to try whatever would work.

I started on Gonzalez's programme and it's very time-consuming, the diet. You could have fish, but you really couldn't have much in dairy, meat or chicken. It's basically like a fruit, vegetable, fish and egg kind of diet. You could have soft boiled eggs. That was a change for me, because I wasn't used to eating at home. When you own real estate and you own a lot of it, you're constantly running around and you don't exactly sit down for good meals, you just keep running. That's what I was used to.

On the programme, you're drinking a lot of organic carrot juice and he had you throw in some beets and garlic. I was turning orange, I was having that much carrot juice. I remember my oncologist said: "Well, you can get too much vitamin A from that, and it could be toxic." Doctor Gonzalez commented: "That doesn't happen."

The eating part wasn't the hardest; it was the pills, because there were like 180 or 190 a day. That was a big number and took a little bit of getting used to. I was doing all that while I was still trying to sell my properties.

I got used to the pills, then I thought: "Well, this enema stuff, that sounds crazy to me." Although it sounded crazy, when it was explained to me and when I read about the idea behind it in other places, it made perfect sense. He has you do coffee enemas twice a day: one in the morning and one in the afternoon. The enemas actually made me feel very good. I don't know how to explain it, but it's a very cleaned out kind of feeling. I still like it. I was always a little bit constipated, so that was a nice change for me. You do spend a bunch of time doing it, but you lay out on your side in the tub with your coffee enema and you read a book while you're taking it.

It was interesting, because most people would say, "If you exercise, it's good for you," and all that. But Doctor Gonzalez didn't want me to exercise at all. He said that I was putting a lot of good nutrients in my body and he didn't want me using them up by exercising, because you deplete your body of those nutrients, which was an unusual approach. He also does this hair analysis, where you send him up some pieces of your hair and he sends it off to some lab and they do an analysis of your hair. They come up with probably 30 different things on whether you've had too much of this or too little of that. Some of his pills he bases on that.

After three months on the programme, we did a CAT[3] scan, and the cancer had shrunk quite a bit. Six months after I started this programme, it was totally gone. That was 12 years ago, and we haven't seen anything since.

The cancer was gone after six months of being on the programme, but I've been on the programme ever since then. You never really go off it, but over time you get more and more relaxed with it. I'm not anywhere near as strict as I used to be with myself. I saw Doctor Gonzalez every six months for years, then it went to every year, then every few years. Now it's been years since I've actually seen him.

I continued to see my oncologist in St Louis, only to get CAT scans. I would go back to him and the cancer would be gone, and I asked him, "Well, what do you attribute that to?" He'd say, "It's not Doctor Gonzalez, you just got lucky." I'd say, "Okay then, whatever." [*laughs*] Even with the proof, they don't want to sign off on it.

When people have called me in the past and I have described the programme, nobody seriously considers it. I mean, it's a lot of work, to be honest – it's a real commitment. I think most people probably try traditional treatment and if that's not working, then they try something else. I had no idea if it would work, or if it wouldn't work. To be honest, I didn't really know anything about alternative medicine. I just really had nothing to lose by trying something different. I don't remember talking to many people about it one way or the other, but my parents were pushing it. Traditional obviously wasn't going to work for me.

People approach me. Just about everybody I know who's gone through it do traditional, and then they're looking for some alternative. Well, unfortunately, a lot of times it's already too late for them. Everybody's kind of brought up on the traditional medicine. I guess until you have a problem, you probably don't really know much about other alternatives, but I would certainly encourage everybody to be open to that. You can be open to it before you start with the chemo.

I get a CAT scan once a year. I debate whether to do that or not, because it's been 12 years and they say a CAT scan is like 500 X-rays or something. I don't know that it pays at this point to keep doing them. It gives you some peace of mind, but it's putting your body through a lot of stuff that you probably shouldn't be doing.

Since being on this diet, my reflux has gone. I still take medication for it every day, but after a few months of being on this diet, I stopped eating things that aggravated it and eliminated my reflux.

3 CAT scan, also known as a CT scan or Computed Axial Tomography, is a diagnostic medical imaging procedure that examines cross sections of the body allowing a three dimensional view of specific areas.

I do think there is a benefit to having a positive outlook – I was always very positive. I know people who, once they get cancer, think they're just going to die. You have to open your eyes to a lot of other things.

My parents kept telling me that Steve Jobs should have done what I did. I said to them: "Well, I think he had the money to do whatever he wanted to do." I know he went to Switzerland for treatments. He lasted for seven or eight years after his diagnosis, so that's pretty good for pancreatic.

I understand in older people, once they hear about this type of programme, they're like, "Well, I'm not going to do all that." I don't understand that in younger people though. It's a funny thing – people get hung up on the coffee enemas and say: "Well, that's crazy, I'm not doing that." I say to them: "Well, whatever. You feel good and I could explain the benefits to you, but I don't think you're that interested." People get hung up on little parts of it. They say, "That part's crazy, so the whole thing's probably crazy."

You obviously need a good support system when doing the programme or you're not going to make it through. You need people who believe it will work. One of my secrets is that I have a Jewish mother, and they don't stop looking for solutions. She kept looking for something that would work. She's the one who really pushed me towards it.

I've talked to different people who have done – not the programme I did, but variations of the same thing – and they've had the same results, so there's obviously something to it. It's interesting, because as time goes on, you read more and more from the American Cancer Society what foods to eat and what foods to avoid – it's everything that I was told 13 years ago.

I consider myself lucky. I'm fortunate because my dad's 90 and my mom's 84 and they're both in good health. So based on that, maybe I'll be around for a while.

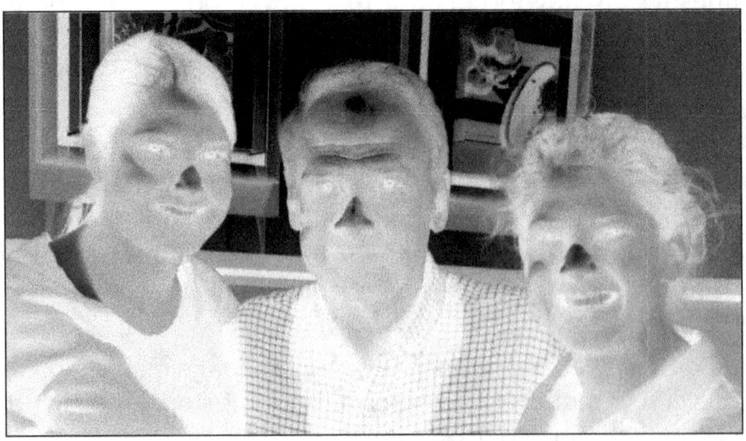

David Yoffie with his teenage daughters.

GLOSSARY OF TERMS

A1C – primary blood test used for diabetes management, which shows average blood glucose levels over the previous three months.

ABA – Applied Behaviour Analysis is an evidence-based, intensive education therapy for children with an Autism Spectrum Disorder.

ACL – anterior cruciate ligament of the knee.

ADHD – Attention Deficit Hyperactivity Disorder – school children who show signs of hyperactivity and inattention which impairs social and academic functioning.

Aesthetician – licensed beauty professional who offers advanced skincare, makeup, and hair removal. Medical aestheticians work in doctor's offices, hospitals and surgery centres.

Allergic shiners – red rings around eyes caused by allergic reactions.

Alpha Lipoic Acid (ALA) – a naturally occurring substance that plays a fundamental role in human metabolism. A nutritional supplement can be given in conditions where oxidative stress is involved. It is also used to treat liver disease.

ALS – Amyotrophic Lateral Sclerosis, Motor Neurone Disease, or Lou Gehrig's disease.

ALT – alanine transaminase, an enzyme that indicates liver inflammation.

AMA – American Medical Association.

ANA – anti-nuclear antibodies found in the blood that help to diagnose autoimmune disease.

Angioplasty – a technique of mechanically widening narrowed or obstructed arteries.

Applied Behaviour Analysis (ABA) – an evidence-based, intensive education therapy for children with an Autism Spectrum Disorder.

APOE (apolipoprotein) – the E4 variant of APOE is a known risk factor for Alzheimer's disease.

Aricept (donepzil hyrochloride) – a common drug used to treat Alzheimer's disease.

Asacol (mesalamine) – an aspirin-based anti-inflammatory drug.

Aspartame – an artificial sweetener, originally marketed as *NutraSweet*.

ASD – Autistic Spectrum Disorder. The autistic spectrum includes childhood and adult mental, emotional and behavioural disorders that range from mild Attention Deficit Disorder, to severe autism.

AST – aspartate transaminase, or serum glutamic oxaloacetic transaminase (SGOT), an enzyme that is elevated in acute liver damage.

Axona (caprylidene) – a medical food for Alzheimer's disease that contains a coconut oil preparation. During digestion, it releases ketones, an alternative energy source for the brain.

Azilect (rasagiline) – a medication for movement disorders caused by Parkinson's disease.

Azathioprine (*Imuran*) – an immunosuppressant drug used for autoimmune diseases.

Bactrim (sulfamethoxazole and trimethoprim) – an antibiotic used to treat a range of bacterial infections, including septicaemia (blood poisoning).

Betaseron (interferon beta-1b) – an injectable drug for relapsing multiple sclerosis.

Biomedical treatment – the process of addressing the anomalies in a patient's biochemistry by using specific nutrients. It is based on the pioneering work of Nobel Prize winner, Linus Pauling, who demonstrated that naturally occurring vitamins, minerals and micronutrient levels can have a profound impact on health and body functions.

Bohr effect – Danish physiologist Christian Bohr described haemoglobin's oxygen binding affinity during respiration in 1904, where increased carbon dioxide concentration results in haemoglobin proteins releasing oxygen and decreased carbon dioxide levels cause the proteins to absorb more oxygen.

Borrelia burgdorferi – the main bacterium that causes the symptoms of Lyme disease.

Bradykinesia – slowness of movement, a common symptom of Parkinson's disease.

Bupropion *(Aplenzin, Budeprion SR, Buproban, Forfivo XL, Wellbutrin, Wellbutrin SR, Wellbutrin XL, Zyban, Zyban Advantage Pack, Budeprion XL)* – used as a quit-smoking aid and psychiatric drug for depression.

Buteyko Institute Method (BIM) – a breathing training program for people with asthma, sleep disordered breathing and other breathing-related conditions. It is based on standard medical principles of respiration, the normalisation of breathing and the Bohr effect.

CA 125 (Carbohydrate Antigen 125) – a protein tumour marker present in greater concentration in ovarian cancer cells.

Candida 'die off' is a 'Herxheimer' response – when yeast in the gut dies off too quickly and resulting toxins overwhelm the body, causing symptoms. Austrian dermatologist brothers Jarisch and Karl Herxheimer discovered the phenomenon in 1895.

CAT scan, or CT scan (Computed Axial Tomography) – a diagnostic medical imaging procedure that examines cross sections of the body allowing a three dimensional view.

CCSVI (chronic cerebrospinal venous insufficiency) – compromised blood flow in veins draining the central nervous system, which may be part of the cause of multiple sclerosis.

CDC – Centers for Disease Control and Prevention in the US, which monitors the status of many diseases, including infectious diseases. *www.cdc.gov*

C-section (Caesarean section) – surgery where an incision is made into the uterus to deliver a baby.

Carpal tunnel syndrome – compression of the median nerve travelling through the wrist, causing intermittent numbness of the thumb, index and middle fingers.

CFS (Chronic Fatigue Syndrome) – see ME

Chelation – use of oral or intravenous agents to remove heavy metals from the body.

Chelating agent – a substance that enables unwanted minerals to bond with metal ions, resulting in a water-soluble complex which allows the metal to enter the bloodstream and be harmlessly excreted.

Chemo – popular term used for chemotherapy, the use of chemical substances used to treat serious illness such as cancer.

Cimzia (certolizumab pegol) – an anti-tumour necrosis factor medication.

Clostridium difficile (C. diff) – bacterium found in the gut after antibiotic use that causes symptoms ranging from diarrhoea to life-threatening inflammation of the colon.

Co Enzyme Q10 (CoQ10) – a nutrient discovered by Professor Fredrick L Crane in 1957. Peter Mitchell received a Nobel prize for his work on CoQ10 in 1978, which demonstrated a deficiency of CoQ10 in heart disease.

Cold nodules – non-malignant growths on the thyroid gland.

CPK (creatine phosphokinase) – an enzyme found in the heart, brain and skeletal muscle.

Craniosacral therapy (CST) – a body therapy based on regulating the flow of cerebrospinal fluid by manipulating the joints of the cranium and developed by osteopath John Upledger in the 1970s. Based on the work of William Garner Sutherland in the 1930s.

CRP (C-reactive protein) – a blood test that measures general levels of inflammation.

CT or CAT scan (Computed Axial Tomography) – a diagnostic medical imaging procedure that examines cross sections of the body allowing a three dimensional view.

Detox (detoxification) – the elimination of toxic material from the body.

Diclofenac (has 130+ trade names, including *Voltaren*) – a non steroidal anti-inflammatory drug (NSAID) used to reduce inflammation and pain.

DO – Doctor of Osteopathy.

ELISA (enzyme-linked immunosorbent assay) – antibody test that measures the body's response to a specific bacterial infection, like *Borrelia burgdorferi* in Lyme disease, or food and environmental allergens.

EEG (electroencephalogram) – measures the electrical activity of the brain along the scalp for up to 40 minutes to help diagnose epilepsy.

Electromyography – electrical activity of muscles tested on an electromyograph.

ENAR (Electro Neuro Adaptive Regulator) – a hand-held biofeedback medical device – see SCENAR.

Enbrel (etanercept) – a biopharmaceutical that treats autoimmune diseases like rheumatoid arthritis.

ENT – ear, nose and throat specialist.

Enthesitis – inflammation of the entheses, where tendons and ligaments attach to the bone. Recurring stress or inflammatory autoimmune disease can cause enthesitis.

Epsom Salts (magnesium sulphate, MgS04) – an organic salt used in bath salts. The salts are used for aches and pains, to remove splinters, and internally as a saline laxative.

Epstein-Barr Virus (EBV) – a human herpes virus which causes glandular fever.

ER – Emergency Room in a hospital.

Erythema nodosum – an inflammatory condition where fat cells under the skin cause tender red nodules or lumps, often on both shins.

ESR (erythrocyte sedimentation rate) – the rate that red blood cells sediment, or settle, over one hour. It is a non-specific measure of inflammation.

Exelon (rivastigmine) – a cholinergic drug that helps improve brain cell function, used for mild dementia and Alzheimer's disease.

Feingold diet – eliminates artificial colours, flavours, preservatives and foods that contain salicylates. Used as a diagnostic tool to determine if certain foods or additives trigger symptoms, and continued as a treatment. Developed by paediatrician Ben Feingold in 1965 when a patient recovered from hives after going on a low salicylate diet.

FMT (faecal microbiota transplantation) – transplantation of faecal matter from a healthy donor to one who suffers from inflammatory bowel disease.

FDA (US Food and Drug Administration) – an agency of the United States Department of Health and Human Services, responsible for protecting and promoting public health.

Flagyl (metronidazole) – an antibiotic used for anaerobic bacteria and parasites.

Flare – a severe worsening of symptoms, caused by inflammation in conditions like ulcerative colitis and multiple sclerosis.

Genotype – the genetic make up of a cell or organism.

Gleason Grade – pathology grading for prostate cancers.

Globus (globus hystericus) – feeling of a lump or foreign body in the throat thought to be psychological in origin.

Glycoside – a type of anti-diabetic medication.

GP – general practitioner who is a medical doctor (MD).

Grand mal seizure – a loss of consciousness with violent muscle contractions, caused by abnormal electrical activity in the brain.

Granuloma annulare – a rare, chronic autoimmune skin condition where reddish bumps on the skin appear in a circle or ring.

Gut microbiome – individual make up of bacterial organisms found in the gut.

Haematoma – a collection of blood outside the blood vessels, often under the skin.

Hair Mineral Analysis – test of a hair sample to identify mineral deficiencies and toxicities. Its most widely accepted use is in forensic and environmental toxicology. It is also used to detect recreational drugs to check compliance in drug treatment programmes.

Haldol (haloperidol) – an antipsychotic medication used to treat schizophrenia, acute psychosis, mania and other nervous system disorders.

HCV – hepatitis C virus.

Humira (adalimumab) – *Humira* is an acronym for 'human monoclonal antibody in rheumatoid arthritis' and is a tumour necrosis factor (TNF) inhibiting drug.

Jarisch-Herxheimer reaction – a response to endotoxins released by the death of harmful organisms within the body causing a range of symtoms.

Ibuprofen (100+ brand names including *Nurofen, Advil*) – non-steroidal anti-inflammatory (NSAID) drug used for musculoskeletal and other pain.

Idiopathic – a condition that has no known cause.

IgG (Immunoglobulin G) Food Sensitivity Panel – a blood test that identifies sensitivity reactions to foods.

Imuran (azathioprine) – an immunosuppressant drug used for autoimmune diseases and during organ transplantation.

Intal (cromoglicic acid) – an inhalant drug that prevents the release of inflammatory chemicals like histamine to reduce the allergic response to asthma.

Interferon – one of a group of drugs that act as antiviral agents. They modulate functions of the immune system to treat autoimmune conditions like multiple sclerosis.

Ipilimumab (*Yervoy*) – used for the treatment of cancer, including melanoma.

IV – intravenous drip.

Kefir – a fermented milk drink to improve gut bacteria, made with kefir grains.

Keppra (levetiracetam) – an anticonvulsant drug used to treat epilepsy.

Ketogenic diet – a scientifically tested high-fat, low-carbohydrate, adequate-protein diet that has been used in medicine since the 1920s to treat epilepsy in children.

Ketosis – a state of elevated levels of ketones in the body that can be used as an alternative form of energy.

Klonopin (clonazepam) – a benzodiazepine drug which has sedative, hypnotic, anticonvulsant, muscle relaxant, and anti-anxiety actions.

Kryptopyroluria – when bound to kryptopyrrole, zinc and pyridoxine (vitamin B6) are excreted into the urine as pyrroles, making them both unavailable as co-factors in enzyme reactions and metabolism. This then causes a wide range of deficiency symptoms.

Laparoscopy – a surgical procedure where a fibre-optic instrument is inserted through the abdominal wall to view abdominal organs and sometimes conduct small-scale surgery.

Lou Gehrig's Disease – another name for Motor Neurone Disease or ALS (Amyotrophic Lateral Sclerosis).

Low Dose Naltrexone (LDN) – the off-label use of FDA-approved *Naltrexone* in low doses stimulates the immune system by producing endorphins and used to treat autoimmune, central nervous system disorders, and a wide range of other diseases.

Lupus (SLE) – an autoimmune disease which attacks healthy tissue, causing inflammation, swelling, and damage to joints, skin and organs. Symptoms can be vague, making diagnosis difficult. Two thirds of patients with Lupus suffer from sun sensitivity.

Lyme disease – a diagnosis caused by the bacteria *Borrelia burgdorferi,* transmitted by a tick bite, which can infect multiple organs and produce a wide range of symptoms.

Lyrica (pregabalin) – an anticonvulsant drug used to treat epilepsy, post-herpetic neuralgia, diabetic peripheral neuropathy and fibromyalgia.

Makaton – a language programme designed to provide a means of communication for people who cannot speak well.

MCT – Medium Chain Triglyceride derived from coconut oil.

MD (*medicinae doctor*) – medical doctor.

ME – Myalgic Encephalomyelitis/Chronic Fatigue Syndrome (CFS) is a severe, complex illness with numerous symptoms related to the dysfunction of the brain, gastrointestinal, immune, endocrine and cardiac systems. ME was classified as a neurological disorder in the World Health Organisation's International Classification of Diseases in 1969.

Mesalamine (*Apriso, Asacol, Delzicol, Lialda, Pentasa*) – an aspirin-based anti-inflammatory drug.

Metformin (*Fortamet, Glucophage, Glucophage XR, Glumetza, Riomet*) – an anti-diabetic drug for people with normal kidney function.

Methotrexate – a chemotherapy drug, also used for autoimmune diseases. It has a range of serious side effects.

Milk thistle (*Silybum marianum*) – a herbal medicine used for liver, kidney and gall bladder problems. The active ingredient *silymarin* protects the liver, due to its antioxidant and anti-inflammatory properties. It is reported to help the liver repair itself by growing new cells.

Minocin, Minomycin (minocycline) – a broad-spectrum tetracycline antibiotic.

Motor Neurone Disease (MND) – also known as Lou Gehrig's Disease or ALS (Amyotrophic Lateral Sclerosis).

MMR – measles, mumps and rubella vaccine.

Modafinil (*Provigil*) – a wakefulness promoting drug for daytime sleepiness.

MRI (magnetic resonance imaging) – used in radiology for a more detailed image than standard X-rays, used in hospitals for diagnosis, without exposure to radiation.

MRSA (Methicillin Resistant *Staphylococcus Aureus*) – a superbug that is unresponsive to most antibiotics.

MSG (monosodium glutamate) – a flavour enhancer found in many processed foods. Common reaction symptoms are headache, flushing, sweating, numbness and burning.

Multiple myeloma – a rare cancer of the bone marrow, similar to lymphoma and leukaemia.

MS – multiple sclerosis.

Pericarditis – pain caused by inflammation of the pericardium, the lining that surrounds the heart.

Myelogram – a test to help find the cause of pain not found by an MRI or CT scan, involving injecting a contrast medium into the cervical or lumbar spine, followed by several X-rays. It is used to locate spinal cord injury, cysts or tumours.

NAET – Nambudripad's Allergy Elimination Technique, a natural method of treating sensitivities and allergies.

Namenda (memantine HCl) – a medication for Alzheimer's disease symptoms.

Niacin – vitamin B3.

Necrosis – death of body tissue.

Neoplasm – an abnormal growth of tissue in the body, usually cancerous.

Novocaine (procaine hydrochloride) – an injectable local anaesthetic.

Off-label – the use of an approved pharmaceutical drug for an unapproved indication.

Orthomolecular nutrition – a term first used by double-Nobel laureate Linus Pauling in a paper he wrote in the journal *Science* in 1968. Orthomolecular medicine corrects nutritional imbalances based on individual biochemistry, using substances natural to the body such as vitamins, minerals, amino acids, trace elements and fatty acids.

OxyContin (oxycodone) – a narcotic analgesic used to treat moderate to severe pain.

Paxil (paroxetine) – a SSRI anti-depressant used for depression and anxiety disorders.

Pentasa (mesalazine) – anti-inflammatory drug used to treat inflammatory bowel disease.

PET (Positron Emission Tomography) – an imaging technique in nuclear medicine that is widely used in oncology, to produce a three-dimensional image of the body.

pH (power of hydrogen) – the acid/alkaline balance of aqueous solutions. Below 7.0 is acidic, above 7.0 is alkaline.

PhD – Doctor of Philosophy.

Plasmacytoma – cancer usually found in soft tissue.

PSA (Prostate Specific Antigen) – a screening blood test to detect prostate cancer.

Pulmonary embolism – a potentially life-threatening event caused by a blood clot obstructing the main artery of a lung.

Prednisone – a synthetic corticosteroid drug, used to treat inflammatory diseases.

Prozac (fluoxetine) – a SSRI antidepressant drug.

Quetiapine (*Seroquel, Seroquel XR*) – an antipsychotic medication used to treat schizophrenia, bipolar disorder, autism and depression.

Raynaud's disease – a circulatory disorder that causes discolouration of the fingers and toes, in a characteristic 'glove and stocking' effect, usually triggered by stress or cold.

RDI – Relationship Development Intervention® is a parent-led approach that focuses on teaching children how to develop social skills.

Rebif® (interferon beta 1a) – a medication for the treatment of patients with relapsing forms of multiple sclerosis.

REM sleep behaviour disorder (RBD) – paralysis that normally occurs during REM sleep is incomplete or absent, characterised by the acting out of dreams, including talking, yelling, punching, kicking, sitting and jumping from bed.

Remicade (infliximab) – artificial antibody given intravenously for autoimmune diseases.

Requip (Levodopa, L-dopa) – the most commonly prescribed drug for controlling the symptoms of Parkinson's disease, particularly tremors and rigidity.

Rheumatoid factor (RF) – autoantibody found in rheumatoid arthritis.

Ritalin (methylphenidate) – a central nervous system stimulant which affects the chemicals in the brain that contribute to hyperactivity and impulse control.

Sauerkraut (sour cabbage) – finely cut cabbage fermented with salt, to form lactic acid bacteria beneficial to gut bacteria.

Scleroderma (hard skin) – a life threatening autoimmune connective tissue disorder with no known cause or cure.

SCENAR (Self Controlled Energy Neuro Adaptive Regulator) – a battery-powered device used for the medical treatment of a range of diseases, most notably for pain relief. It was developed as a part of the 1970s Soviet space program, to create a portable, effective, non-invasive device to maintain the health of astronauts while in space.

Serenace (haloperidol) – an antipsychotic medication used to treat schizophrenia, acute psychosis, mania and other nervous system disorders.

Sinemet (carbidopa-levodopa) – a combination drug for Parkinson's disease.

Sonogram – ultrasound-based diagnostic imaging technique.

Specific Carbohydrate Diet (SCD) – a low carbohydrate diet created by Doctor Sidney Valentine Haas (1870-1964) to heal the gut in digestive disorders.

Spinal tap (lumbar puncture) – a diagnostic procedure performed on the lower spine to collect a sample of cerebrospinal fluid for analysis.

Statins – a class of drugs used to lower cholesterol levels.

Stevia – a natural sugar substitute made from the leaves of the *Stevia rebaudiana* plant.

Sulfasalazine (*Azulfidine, Salazopyrin, Sulazine*) – a sulfa drug developed in the 1950s for rheumatoid arthritis, when it was believed the cause was bacterial in origin.

Superbug – a bacterium unresponsive to most antibiotics, known as 'multi-drug resistant'.

Systemic Lupus Erythematosus (SLE) – commonly called 'Lupus', SLE is an autoimmune disease that attacks healthy tissue, causing inflammation, swelling and damage to joints and organs. Symptoms can be vague, making diagnosis difficult. Two thirds of patients with Lupus suffer from sun sensitivity.

Tamoxifen (*Nolvadex, Istubal, Valodex, Genox*) – a medication used to treat oestrogen receptor-positive breast cancer.

Tracheostomy – a surgical incision made in the neck through the windpipe.

TSH (Thyroid Stimulating Hormone) – checked by a blood test to assess thyroid function.

TMJ Dysfunction (Temporomandibular Joint Dysfunction) – an umbrella term used to describe pain and other symptoms felt in the jaw when chewing.

Trileptal (oxcarbazepine) – an anticonvulsant drug used primarily for the treatment of epilepsy, anxiety, mood disorders and tics.

Tylenol, Panadol (acetaminophen) – a common medication used to reduce fever and pain.

Valium (diazepam) – a drug that has a relaxant effect, used for a wide range of anxiety disorders, muscle spasms and alcohol withdrawal.

Vancomycin (derived from the term 'vanquish') – used for the treatment of MRSA (methicillin resistant *staphylococcus aureus*) and life-threatening infections that are unresponsive to less toxic antibiotics.

Ventolin (salbutamol) – a prescription medication used via a puffer to dilate the bronchi in the lungs to improve the lung capacity.

Vicodin (hydrocodone/paracetamol) – a combination opioid-narcotic analgesic medication.

VSL#3® – a high-potency probiotic medical food for the dietary management of patients with severe gut disorders.

Western Blot – a test used to detect specific proteins in a sample of tissue. Compared to ELISA, Western blotting has higher specificity for the diagnosis of Lyme disease.

Whipple procedure – removal of the head of the pancreas, the duodenum, a portion of the common bile duct, gallbladder and part of the stomach.

Yervoy (Ipilimumab) – used for the treatment of cancer, including melanoma.

Zonegran (Zonisamide) – a sulphonamide drug used as an adjunctive therapy for a range of seizure types in adults.

RESOURCES

Asthma

The Buteyko Institute Method (BIM)

http://www.buteyko.info

Official website of the Buteyko Institute of Breathing & Health.

Allergies

Autoimmune Therapies

http://autoimmunetherapies.com

Resource on immunotherapy based on the use of helminths, or helminthic therapy – the result of a theory published in The Lancet in 1986, *The Hygiene Hypothesis.*

Foods Matter

http://www.foodsmatter.com

Vast resource of dietary information for food allergies and allergy-related conditions, autism, coeliac disease, chronic fatigue, eczema, complementary therapies and recipes.

NAET® Nambudripad's Allergy Elimination Techniques

http://www.naet.com

Natural allergy treatment using testing and treatment procedures from acupuncture/acupressure, allopathy, chiropractic, nutrition and kinesiology.

Alzheimer's Disease

Fife, B & Blaylock, R 2011, *Stop Alzheimer's Now! How to Prevent & Reverse Dementia, Parkinson's, ALS, Multiple Sclerosis & Other Neurodegenerative Disorders,* Piccadilly Books Ltd, Colorado.

Describes the use of coconut oil for neurological diseases.

Newport, MT 2011, *Alzheimer's – What if There Was a Cure?* Basic Health Publications Inc, California.

Neonatologist Doctor Mary Newport describes her husband's Alzheimer's disease and what happened when he started taking coconut oil. Includes scientific data and research.

Newport, MT 2013, *Alzheimer's – What if There Was a Cure?* 2nd edn, Basic Health Publications Inc, California.

Continues the story of her husband Steve's progress and provides the most recent research on the possible connection between Alzheimer's disease, the herpes simplex virus and nitrosamine substances, as well as how infection, inflammation and genetic makeup may affect an individual's response to fatty acid therapy.

Autism

The Global Autism Collaboration (GAC)

http://www.globalautismcollaboration.com

Lists over 100 non-profit organisations throughout the world, which aim to share information to improve the standard of care for children and adults on the autism spectrum.

Campbell-McBride, N 2010, *Gut and Psychology Syndrome – Natural Treatment for Autism, Dyspraxia, ADD, Dyslexia, ADHD, Depression, Schizophrenia,* Revised & enlarged edn, Medinform Publishing.

An easy to read and understand book on the specific carbohydrate diet (SCD), based on the work of Doctor Sidney Haas (1870-1964), who pioneered and successfully used a low-carbohydrate diet to treat coeliac disease for over 50 years.

Haas, S & Haas, M 2011, *The Management of Celiac Disease,* Literary Licensing, LLC, Montana.

Written in the 1950s, Doctor Sidney Haas successfully treated Celiac Disease with the SCD, or Specific Carbohydrate Diet. Mainstream medicine rejected the SCD in favour of the easier to follow gluten-free diet. Doctor Haas points out autistic type behaviour in his severe patients and covers the history of the research done on Celiac disease.

McCandless, J 2009, *Children With Starving Brains: A Medical Treatment Guide for Autism Spectrum Disorder,* 4th updated edn, Bramble Books, Florida.

A step-by-step treatment guide for parents and doctors. Doctor McCandless is a psychiatrist whose grandchild was diagnosed with autism at two years of age. She now treats autistic children using a broad spectrum approach and describes important diagnostic tools needed to select appropriate treatment programs. Explains major therapies and identifies safe and effective options for parents and physicians.

Cancer

Cancer Treatment Centers of America

http://www.cancercenter.com

Integrative health treatment for cancer.

The Gerson Institute

http://gersontherapy.eu/therapy/gerson_therapy

Gerson, C & Walker, M 2013, *The Gerson Therapy – The Proven Nutritional Program for Cancer and Other Illnesses,* Re-issue edn, Twin Streams, Kensington Pub Corp.

Alternative medicine therapist Charlotte Gerson and medical journalist Morton Walker outline how juicing reverses the effects of many degenerative illnesses.

Gerson, M 2002, *A Cancer Therapy: Results of Fifty Cases and the Cure of Advanced Cancer by Diet Therapy,* 6th edn, Gerson Institute.

First published in 1958, based on thirty years of clinical experimentation, Doctor Gerson explains how the Gerson therapy reactivates the body's healing mechanisms in chronic degenerative diseases, explaining his scientific research and the exact practice of the therapy. Includes fifty documented cured cancer cases.

Dying to Have Known 2006, documentary, Kroshel Films, USA. Produced & directed by Steve Kroshel.

Documents a 52-day journey around the world to Alaska, Japan, Holland, Spain and Mexico, questioning the effectiveness of Gerson Therapy. Includes interviews with patients, scientists, surgeons and nutritionists who testify to the therapy's efficacy in curing cancer and other degenerative diseases.

Burzynski Patient Group

http://www.burzynskipatientgroup.org

A website run by patients who have been successfully treated with antineoplastons. The group's mission is to raise public awareness of Doctor Stanislaw Burzynski's treatment for cancer using antineoplastons and gene-targeted therapy. Includes patient testimonials and current information on the future of the Burzynski Research Institute.

Burzynski – The Movie 2010, documentary, Merola Productions, USA. Produced & directed by Eric Merola.

Tells the story of PhD biochemist Doctor Stanislaw Burzynski winning a complex legal battle against the US Food & Drug Administration in Texas, USA. In the 1970s, he discovered antineoplastons, which, if approved by the FDA, will mark the first time in history a single scientist will hold the exclusive patent and distribution rights on a life-saving medical breakthrough. Awarded the Humanitarian Vision Award at the Newport Beach Film Festival in 2010.

Burzynski – Cancer is Serious Business, Part 2 2013, documentary, Merola Productions, USA, UK, Japan. Produced & directed by Eric Merola.

Explores the current status of clinical testing of antineoplastons sanctioned by the United States Food & Drug Administration. Interviews with board-certified oncologists, surgeons and neurosurgeons who witnessed patients leave their care and return in good health after being treated with antineoplastons. Winner of the Sedona International Film Festival Audience Choice Best Documentary, 2014.

Turner, K 2014, *Radical Remission, Surviving Cancer Against All Odds,* HarperOne, New York, NY.

Doctor Turner travelled to ten different countries to interview fifty holistic healers and over one hundred cancer survivors. After studying one thousand more such cases, she presents nine common elements that have helped even terminal cancer patients recover.

Doctors Nicholas Gonzalez and Linda Isaacs

http://www.dr-gonzalez.com

Fully describes treatment for pancreatic and other cancers, treatment programmes, case reports and research.

Epilepsy

The Charlie Foundation for Ketogenic Therapies

www.charliefoundation.org

The Charlie Foundation has expanded its mission to champion ketogenic diet therapy not only for epilepsy, but for variations of cancer, autism, ALS, Parkinson's Disease, type-2 diabetes and traumatic brain injury.

Matthew's Friends

http://www.matthewsfriends.org

This UK-based website has been written largely by parents, with the aim of aiding and supporting parents in managing the ketogenic diet. Emma Williams, Founder of Matthew's Friends and mum to Matthew, has been awarded an MBE[1] in Her Majesty Queen Elizabeth II's Birthday Honours for her services to children with epilepsy.

First Do No Harm 1997, DVD recording, Walt Disney Video, USA. Directed by Jim Abrahams.

An ABC (USA) telemovie starring Meryl Streep, depicting one family's inspirational true story about finding the ketogenic diet and curing their child's epilepsy.

General

Bland, J 2014, *The Disease Delusion*, HarperWave, New York, NY.

Heralds the new era of 'functional medicine', which identifies health issues using cutting edge testing. Outlines prevention and treatment of chronic disease. Easy to follow guide on scientifically based, individualised treatments.

1 MBE – Member of the Most Excellent Order of the British Empire.

DoctorYourself.com

A non-commercial internet resource with an extensive alphabetical index of illnesses and health topics, sourcing scientifically based nutritional information.

Fat, Sick and Nearly Dead 2010, documentary, Reboot Media, USA. Produced by Stacey Offman, directed by Joe Cross & Kurt Engfehr.

A multi award-winning documentary by Australian entrepreneur Joe Cross, about his 60-day fruit and vegetable juice fast while on a road trip, to treat his autoimmune disease and stop his medications. On the road, Joe meets a truck driver who suffers from the same rare condition. *Fat, Sick & Nearly Dead 2* was released in September, 2014.

Helminthic Therapy Success Stories

http://www.foodsmatter.com/natural_medicine_comp_therapies/helminthic_therapy/articles/ht_success_stories.pdf

A list of over 60 conditions that have been successfully treated using helminthic therapy, with testimonials.

Extraordinary Medicine: The Truth About Homeopathy

http://www.extraordinarymedicine.org

Describes the science and research on homeopathy.

Low Dose Naltrexone (LDN)

http://www.lowdosenaltrexone.org

An overview of LDN, includes research, the range of conditions it treats and patient testimonials.

Patients Like Me

http://www.patientslikeme.com

A site for patients to connect with others to compare treatments, symptoms and experiences, and to give and find support.

Riding for the Disabled (RDA)

www.frdi.net

A worldwide movement represented internationally by the Federation of Horses in Education and Therapy International (HETI). It is a charitable organisation that forms worldwide links between countries, offering therapeutic horse riding and driving opportunities for anyone with a disability.

SCENAR Therapy

Many websites offer information on SCENAR therapy, which is available worldwide through individual therapists. Some countries have SCENAR associations. The originators of SCENAR therapy, Alexander Karasev and Alexander Revenko, offer key information on their websites:

http://www.scenar-revenko.ru/en/ http://www.rexresearch.com/scenar/kasarev.htm

To find a SCENAR therapist, search on the internet: SCENAR therapy + your country. For example: 'SCENAR therapy London, England'.

Inflammatory Bowel Disease (IBD)

Clostridium difficile, Crohn's disease, ulcerative colitis

Breaking the Vicious Cycle

http://www.breakingtheviciouscycle.info/p/about-the-diet/

In-depth website about the role of the Specific Carbohydrate Diet (SCD) in gut diseases. Shows recent scientific research on the SCD.

Gottschall, E 1994, *Breaking the Vicious Cycle: Intestinal Health Through Diet,* The Kirkton Press.

Elaine and Herb Gotschall's four-year-old daughter was diagnosed with ulcerative colitis, which was unresponsive to standard medical therapy. The last resort treatment recommended was to remove her colon to save her life. Doctor Sidney Haas, then 92, put Judy on a diet, from which she began to improve after just ten days. This book is Elaine's effort to get Doctor Haas's message out to those who need it.

Haas, S & Haas, M 2011, *The Management of Celiac Disease,* Literary Licensing, LLC, Montana.

Written in the 1950s, Doctor Sidney Haas successfully treated Celiac disease with the Specific Carbohydrate Diet. Mainstream medicine rejected this in favour of the easier to follow gluten-free diet. Doctor Haas points out autistic type behaviour in his severe patients.

The Faecal Transplant Foundation

http://thefecaltransplantfoundation.org

Foundation comprised of professionals and survivors of IBD. Provides current information to raise awareness of faecal transplants (FMT) and lobbies for research funding.

Power of Poop

http://thepowerofpoop.com

A patient guide to safe, accessible faecal microbiota transplants (FMT) with success stories and a database of clinics that offer FMT.

Curtis, S 2013, *The Fecal Transplant Guidebook: Treatment for Crohn's Disease, Ulcerative Colitis, C. difficile, Irritable Bowel Disease, Constipation, Diarrhea, and More*, Eagle Bay Publishing.

Helminthic Therapy Forum

https://groups.yahoo.com/neo/groups/helminthictherapy/info

A support group on helminthic therapy for autoimmune disease and allergies.

Legal and Ethical

Jaffe, RA 2008, *Galileo's Lawyer*, Thumbs Up Press, Houston, Texas.

Jaffe, a lawyer, describes courtroom battles in alternative healthcare.

Prescriber Checkup: The Doctors and Drugs in Medicare Part D

http://projects.propublica.org/checkup/

Lists the financial connections between pharmaceutical companies and doctors.

All Trials

http://www.alltrials.net

A movement to compel the results of all clinical trials to be published, instead of the 50 per cent that are currently published. An initiative of *Bad Science, British Medical Journal, Centre for Evidence Based Medicine, Cochrane Collaboration, James Lind Initiative, PLoS and Sense About Science*.

Liver Disease

Berkson, B 1998, *Alpha Lipoic Acid Breakthrough,* Three Rivers Press, New York, NY. Describes the role of Alpha Lipoic Acid in liver and other diseases.

Lyme Disease

International Lyme and Associated Diseases Society (ILADS)

http://www.ilads.org

A nonprofit, medical society dedicated to the diagnosis and treatment of Lyme and associated diseases through research, education and policy.

Under Our Skin 2008, documentary, Open Eye Pictures, USA. Produced & directed by Andy Abrahams Wilson.

An Oscar-shortlisted film about the Lyme disease epidemic.

A sequel, *Under Our Skin: Emergence,* was released in 2014.

Mental, Emotional & Spiritual

The Gawler Foundation

http://gawler.org

A non-profit, non-denominational organisation that offers conferences, wellbeing retreats and workshops on mind, health and immunity for health professionals and people with chronic illnesses. It uses current mind-body medicine research and is associated with The Australasian Integrative Medical Association.

Healing Strong

http://www.healingstrong.com

A volunteer support network of cancer thrivers who have joined together and are dedicated to supporting individuals in their healing journeys.

Pfeiffer, C 1988, *Nutrition and Mental Illness: An Orthomolecular Approach to Balancing Body Chemistry*, Healing Arts Press, Vermont.

Documents Doctor Pfeiffer's approach in treating psychological problems by tracing them to biochemical imbalances. In 1973, he opened the Brain Bio Center in Princeton, New Jersey. With a team of scientists, he succeeded in treating a wide range of mental conditions by adjusting diet and providing specific nutritional supplements.

The Connection 2014, documentary, Elemental Media, Australia. Directed by Shannon Harvey.

A film about how research is proving a direct connection between the mind and health. Features scientists, researchers, writers and doctors, as well as stories of people recovering from severe back pain, heart disease, infertility, cancer and multiple sclerosis.

http://www.theconnection.tv/screenings/

Motor Neurone Disease

Coconut Research Center

http://www.coconutresearchcenter.org/books.htm

Research, success stories and books, available in 11 languages.

Low Dose Naltrexone (LDN)

http://www.lowdosenaltrexone.org

Overview of LDN, includes research, the range of conditions it treats and patient testimonials.

Healing ALS – Motor Neurone Disease – Lou Gehrig's Disease, documentary, Indiegogo, USA. Produced by Patricia Tamowski and directed by Alan Scott Douglas.

A full-length documentary in the making on people who have healed from ALS – the link below shows interviews with 11 patients who have survived ALS and the doctors who treated them.

https://www.indiegogo.com/projects/healing-als-mnd-lou-gehrig-s-disease

Multiple Sclerosis (MS)

Jelinek, G 2010, *Overcoming Multiple Sclerosis, An Evidence Based Guide to Recovery,* Allen & Unwin, Sydney. An MS sufferer himself, Professor Jelinek delved into medical literature and found that it was full of answers.

Helminthic Therapy Success Stories

http://www.foodsmatter.com/natural_medicine_comp_therapies/helminthic_therapy/articles/ht_success_stories.pdf

A list of over 60 conditions including MS that have been successfully treated using helminthic therapy.

Low Dose Naltrexone (LDN)

http://www.lowdosenaltrexone.org

Overview of LDN. Includes research, the range of conditions it treats and patient testimonials.

Nutrition

Erasmus, U 1998, *Fats That Heal, Fats That Kill: The Complete Guide to Fats, Oils, Cholesterol and Human Health,* Revised & enlarged edn, Alive Books, Summertown.

Foods Matter

http://www.foodsmatter.com

Vast resource of dietary information about food allergies and allergy-related conditions, autism, coeliac disease, chronic fatigue and eczema.

Orthomolecular Health

http://www.orthomolecularhealth.com

Dedicated to the advancement of orthomolecular medicine internationally. Educates the public and health professionals on the nutrition-based approach to healing with the use of vitamins and nutrients through diet and supplements to promote mental and physical health.

Saul, A, Cathcart, R, Cott, A & Foster, H 2014, *The Orthomolecular Treatment of Chronic Disease: 65 Experts on Therapeutic and Preventive Nutrition,* Basic Health Publications, Incorporated, California.

Cites the use of nutritional supplements throughout the 20th century, curing multiple sclerosis, arthritis, cardiovascular disease, mental illness, influenza, pneumonia, hepatitis and cancer. Presents orthomolecular pioneers, maverick doctors, nutrition scientists and selected research. Describes which illnesses best respond to nutrition therapy and includes clinical and experimental evidence from expert researchers and clinicians.

Rheumatoid Arthritis

Scammell, H 1998, *The New Arthritis Breakthrough: The Only Medical Therapy Clinically Proven to Produce Long-term Improvement and Remission of RA, Lupus, Juvenile RS, Fibromyalgia, Scleroderma, Spondyloarthropathy, & Other Inflammatory Forms of Arthritis*, 2nd edn, M Evans & Company, Maryland.

Describes the work of eminent physician Doctor Thomas McPherson-Brown, who pioneered antibiotic treatment for rheumatoid arthritis and treated over 10,000 patients. His work was scientifically verified in 1995, six years after his death in 1989.

The Road Back Foundation

www.roadback.org

Informs the public about research, treatment and practitioners around the world who use the Antibiotic Protocol (AP) for musculoskeletal diseases.

Parkinson's Disease

Fife, B & Blaylock, R 2011, *Stop Alzheimer's Now! How to Prevent & Reverse Dementia, Parkinson's, ALS, Multiple Sclerosis & Other Neurodegenerative Disorders*, Piccadilly Books Ltd, Colorado, USA.

Describes the use of coconut oil for neurological diseases.

Michael J Fox Foundation

https://www.michaeljfox.org

Dedicated to finding a cure for Parkinson's disease through funded research.

Parkinson's Recovery

www.parkinsonsrecovery.com

Provides information about options that help people with Parkinson's disease reverse their symptoms.

Acknowledgements

So many people have made this project possible.

For their contribution in the initial stages, Joanne Barry and Tina Mulholland. Jo Wing has been generous with her expertise and time in assisting with each stage of the book. For their belief in the purpose of this book and making referrals, Jim Abrahams, Mary Jo Bean, Melissa Cabral, Nick Gonzalez, Gabrielle Hogg, Fae Hueston, Paul and Colleen Keetley, Victoria Kleeberg, Tracy Mac, Sue Mison, Crystal Nason, Mary Newport, Silvana Procopio, John Scott, Julia Schopick and Mary Jo Siegel. To my editor, Louise de Villiers, and Michael Cowdroy for the book design, who have been invaluable and a pleasure to work with. To my husband Jon Gamble, for his support and critiques throughout. To my daughter Rose, who at ten years old, provided the idea for the cover. To every person I interviewed, for their willingness to share their personal experiences. To my patients, who have taught me so much.

"I'd rather be a live anecdote than a dead statistic."

– Ian Gawler, cancer survivor

About the Author

Nyema Hermiston, RN, ND, Adv Dip Hom

Working first as a Registered Nurse in New Zealand, England and Australia, Nyema then trained as a naturopath and has been in practice as a natural therapist in Sydney and the Southern Highlands of New South Wales since the early 1990s.

She has a keen interest in public health and has written articles on health in *Southern Highlands News* and contributed to national journals in Australia since 1998, including *Wellbeing Magazine*. She has co-authored and edited practitioner texts and treatment manuals, including *Mastering Homeopathy – Accurate Daily Prescribing for a Successful Practice, Mastering Homeopathy 2 – The Treatment of Irritable Bowel Syndrome* and *Treat Your Child Yourself – A Parent's Guide to Drug-Free Solutions for Common Complaints.*

Good News For People With Bad News is Nyema's first book on public healthcare.